Breast Image Reconstruction and Cancer Detection Using Microwave Imaging

Online at: https://doi.org/10.1088/978-0-7503-2592-9

Breast Image Reconstruction and Cancer Detection Using Microwave Imaging

Hardik N Patel
Assistant Professor, ICT, Pandit Deendayal Energy University, India

Deepak K Ghodgaonkar
Professor at Dhirubhai Ambani Institute of Information and Communication Technology, India

Jasjit S Suri
AtheroPoint LLC, Roseville, CA, USA

IOP Publishing, Bristol, UK

ISBN 978-0-7503-2592-9 (ebook)
ISBN 978-0-7503-2590-5 (print)
ISBN 978-0-7503-2593-6 (myPrint)
ISBN 978-0-7503-2591-2 (mobi)

DOI 10.1088/978-0-7503-2592-9

Version: 20221201

IOP ebooks

British Library Cataloguing-in-Publication Data: A catalogue record for this book is available from the British Library.

Published by IOP Publishing, wholly owned by The Institute of Physics, London

IOP Publishing, No.2 The Distillery, Glassfields, Avon Street, Bristol, BS2 0GR, UK

US Office: IOP Publishing, Inc., 190 North Independence Mall West, Suite 601, Philadelphia, PA 19106, USA

I would like to dedicate this work to my guru, my parents, my wife and my kid 'Tanay'.

Contents

Preface **xiii**

Acknowledgements **xiv**

Author biographies **xv**

1 Introduction to breast cancer **1-1**

1.1 Introduction to cancer 1-1
1.2 Worldwide cancer statistics 1-2
1.3 Breast cancer statistics 1-3
1.3.1 Breast cancer prediction 1-7
1.4 Breast anatomy and breast cancer 1-10
1.5 Summary 1-14
References 1-14

2 Introduction to breast cancer detection techniques **2-1**

2.1 Imaging modalities for breast cancer screening 2-1
2.2 Mammography 2-2
2.2.1 History of mammography 2-3
2.2.2 Basic understanding of mammography 2-4
2.2.3 Advantages and disadvantages of mammography 2-6
2.3 Ultrasound imaging 2-6
2.3.1 History of ultrasound 2-7
2.3.2 Physics of ultrasound 2-8
2.3.3 Current status of ultrasound imaging 2-8
2.3.4 Advantages and disadvantages of ultrasound 2-8
2.4 Magnetic resonanace imaging 2-9
2.4.1 Short history of MRI 2-9
2.4.2 Working principle of MRI 2-10
2.4.3 Advantages and disadvantages of MRI 2-11
2.5 Positron emission tomography 2-11
2.5.1 Short history of PET 2-12
2.5.2 Advantages and disadvantages of PET 2-12
2.6 Diffuse optical tomography 2-12
2.6.1 Short history of optical tomography 2-12
2.6.2 Advantages and disadvantages of diffuse optical tomography 2-13

2.7 Electrical impedance tomography 2-13
2.7.1 Advantages and disadvantages of EIT 2-13
2.8 Computed tomography (CT) 2-13
2.8.1 Short history of CT 2-13
2.8.2 Advantages and disadvantages of CT 2-14
2.9 Microwave imaging 2-14
2.9.1 Passive microwave imaging 2-14
2.9.2 Active microwave imaging 2-14
2.10 Comparison of mammography, MRI and ultrasound 2-15
2.11 Overview of image reconstruction methods 2-15
2.11.1 Algebraic reconstruction 2-15
2.11.2 Analytic reconstruction 2-17
2.11.3 Statistical reconstruction 2-17
2.11.4 Learned iterative reconstruction 2-18
2.12 Summary 2-18
References 2-18

3 Introduction to microwave imaging 3-1

3.1 Introduction 3-1
3.2 Introduction to passive microwave imaging 3-2
3.2.1 Emission principles 3-2
3.2.2 Radiative transfer 3-3
3.2.3 Bio-heat transfer 3-4
3.2.4 Temperature resolution 3-4
3.3 Microwave radiometry for cancer detection 3-5
3.3.1 Multiprobe radiometric imaging 3-7
3.3.2 Multi-frequency microwave radiometry 3-11
3.4 Active microwave imaging 3-12
3.5 Summary 3-15
References 3-15

4 Finite difference time domain method for microwave breast imaging 4-1

4.1 Overview of computational electromagnetic methods 4-1
4.1.1 Low frequency methods 4-1
4.1.2 High frequency methods 4-3
4.2 Motivation 4-3

4.3 Overview of FDTD 4-4
4.4 Derivation of basic FDTD update equations 4-5
4.5 Polarization current density equation derivation for numerical breast phantom region 4-14
4.6 Electric field update equation derivation for numerical breast phantom region 4-17
4.7 Derivation of electric field update equations for PML region 4-19
4.8 Magnetic field update equations 4-22
4.9 Steps for FDTD implementation 4-24
4.10 Simulation parameters 4-24
4.11 Results 4-24
4.12 Summary 4-26
References 4-29

5 3D level set based optimization 5-1

5.1 Multiple frequency inverse scattering problem formulation 5-1
5.2 Introduction 5-1
5.3 Problem formulation 5-2
5.4 Review of previous work 5-4
5.5 Theoretical foundations 5-9
5.5.1 Evolution approach 5-11
5.5.2 Optimization approach 5-12
5.6 Single 3D level set function based optimization 5-13
5.7 Two 3D level set function based optimization 5-15
5.7.1 3D level set based regularized optimization 5-18
5.7.2 Steps for 3D level set based optimization implementation 5-20
5.8 Simulation parameters 5-20
5.9 Results 5-21
5.10 Summary 5-27
References 5-29

6 Method of moments 6-1

6.1 Theoretical background 6-1
6.2 Problem formulation 6-6
6.3 Computation reduction using group theory 6-8
6.3.1 Human breast models 6-8
6.3.2 Symmetry exploitation using group theory 6-10

6.4 Inverse scattering problem formulation 6-12
6.5 Simulation parameters and noise consideration 6-13
6.6 Results 6-13
6.7 Summary 6-14
References 6-16

7 Finite difference time domain for microwave imaging 7-1

7.1 Introduction to finite difference time domain 7-1
7.1.1 Grid size and stability 7-1
7.1.2 Input wave for Yee grid computations 7-2
7.1.3 Two-dimensional FDTD analysis of microwave breast imaging 7-3
7.1.4 Healthy breast tissue dielectric properties 7-4
7.1.5 Design of antenna array 7-6
7.2 Microwave image formation using confocal technique 7-8
7.3 Space–time beamforming 7-11
7.4 Removal of skin–breast artifact 7-11
7.5 FDTD based time reversal for microwave breast cancer detection 7-14
7.5.1 Matched filter FDTD based time reversal 7-15
7.6 Summary 7-17
References 7-17

8 Review of machine learning based image reconstruction for different imaging modalities 8-1

8.1 Introduction 8-1
8.1.1 Image reconstruction (inverse) problem formulation 8-2
8.2 Traditional image reconstruction techniques 8-2
8.3 Machine learning techniques for image reconstruction 8-4
8.3.1 Machine learning based solution of inverse problems 8-5
8.3.2 Machine learning in computed tomography 8-7
8.3.3 Physics of low dose x-ray CT 8-16
8.4 Performance analysis of proposed approaches 8-16
8.5 Summary 8-19
References 8-19

9 Review of machine learning based image reconstruction for microwave breast imaging 9-1

9.1 Motivation 9-1

9.2 Machine learning in microwave imaging 9-2
9.2.1 Current challenges in microwave breast diagnosis systems 9-5
9.2.2 Challenges in the development of robust machine learning classification models 9-5
9.3 Flow of the machine learning based microwave breast imaging for cancer diagnosis 9-6
9.3.1 Data collection through microwave scanning 9-7
9.3.2 Data processing 9-8
9.3.3 Diagnosis 9-9
9.4 Variational Bayesian inversion for microwave breast imaging 9-12
9.5 Deep neural networks for microwave breast imaging 9-16
9.6 Summary 9-18
References 9-18

10 Microwave image reconstruction methods 10-1

10.1 Levenberg–Marquardt method 10-1
10.1.1 Forward problem 10-2
10.1.2 Inverse problem solution by using Levenberg–Marquardt 10-3
10.1.3 Choice of the regularization parameter 10-5
10.2 Gauss–Newton method 10-8
10.2.1 Forward problem formulation 10-12
10.2.2 The inverse problem formulation 10-12
10.2.3 Gauss–Newton optimization in general 10-13
10.2.4 Gauss–Newton method for the least squares 10-15
10.2.5 The BFGS quasi-Newton method 10-17
10.3 Born iterative method 10-17
10.4 Stochastic optimization methods for microwave imaging 10-19
10.4.1 Genetic algorithm 10-19
10.5 Summary 10-20
References 10-20

11 The role of AI in diagnosis, treatment and monitoring of breast cancer during COVID-19 and ahead 11-1

11.1 Introduction 11-2
11.2 AI architectures 11-3
11.3 The role of artificial intelligence in diagnosis of breast cancer 11-6

11.4 The role of AI in treatment of breast cancer 11-7
11.5 The role of AI in monitoring of breast cancer 11-11
11.6 AI based integrated system for breast cancer management 11-12
11.7 Summary 11-14
References 11-14

Appendix A: Numerical breast phantom, antenna placement and immersion (surrounding) medium A-1

Appendix B: Important derivations B-1

Preface

Breast cancer incidence and mortality are both increasing at a global level. Breast cancer diagnosis depends on the noninvasive imaging techniques which reconstruct the internal structure of the breast. This book covers diverse topics related to breast cancer diagnosis techniques, microwave breast imaging and the role of machine learning and artificial intelligence in the diagnosis, treatment and monitoring of breast cancer. This book will be useful to research and the academic community for the diverse topics covered in it.

Chapter 1 is an introduction to different types of breast cancer and its statics with respect to different criteria.

Chapter 2 is an introduction to mammography, ultrasound imaging, magnetic resonance imaging (MRI), positron emission tomography, diffuse-optical tomography, electrical impedance tomography, computed tomography and microwave imaging. Comparison of mammography, MRI and ultrasound, and an overview of image reconstruction methods are also covered in this chapter.

Chapter 3 is about introduction to passive and active microwave imaging. Chapter 4 is about finite difference time domain (FDTD) for microwave breast imaging. FDTD equations are derived for a numerical breast model with perfectly matched layer. Chapter 5 is about multi-frequency inverse scattering problem formulation and 3D level set based optimization.

Chapter 6 is about problem formulation using method of moments for breast cancer detection. Chapter 7 is about finite difference time domain for microwave imaging. It includes a literature review related to FDTD for microwave breast imaging. Chapter 8 is a review of different machine learning methods based image reconstruction for different imaging modalities. Chapter 9 is a review of different machine learning based image reconstruction methods for microwave breast imaging. Chapter 10 is about different optimization methods for microwave image reconstruction. Chapter 11 is about the role of AI in diagnosis, treatment and monitoring of breast cancer during COVID19 and ahead. This chapter includes integration of AI based diagnosis, treatment and monitoring of breast cancer, irrespective of the imaging modalities.

Diverse contents around breast image reconstruction for cancer detection are covered in this book. This book will be a good platform for researchers, beginners and students in this field.

Acknowledgements

I would like to thank my guru and God for providing me with this opportunity. This work is possible due to the grace of my guru Avadhut Baal swami maharaj and God. I would express sincere gratitude to my supervisor Professor Deepak K Ghodgaonkar for his support and contribution throughout this book writing journey. His philosophy of a balanced life is an inspiration for me. He always motivates me whenever I feel down. He always encourages me to experiment with new things. I would like to thank him for providing his precious time for discussions and problem solving.

I would like to thank Dr Jasjit Suri for his support and motivation throughout this book writing journey. I would like to thank Dr Raymond C Rumpf (PhD, FSPIE, SMIEEE) for his prompt support and permissions. I would like to thank the authors of all the references and figures for their support and permissions.

I would like to thank my father Nayankumar and mother Jashodaben for their support and patience during this journey. I am very thankful to my sister Brinda for encouraging me throughout the book writing. I would like to thank my little kid Tanay who taught me about unconditional inner happiness. His smile and joy gave me so much confidence. I would like to thank my wife Poonam for her support during this journey. I would like to thank all other family members who have supported me directly or indirectly in this journey.

I would like to thank my school teachers and University professors for their direct or indirect contribution in this book writing journey. I would like to thank the team members of IOP for their continuous support and cooperation during this journey.

Author biographies

Hardik N Patel

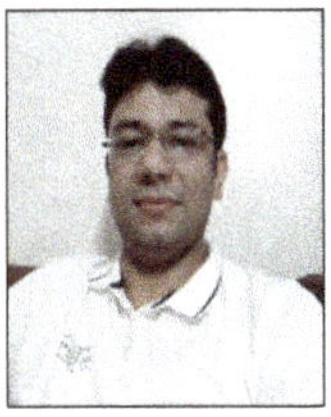

Hardik N Patel completed his BE (Electronics and Communication) from Sardar Patel University in 2007. He has obtained all India 779 rank in GATE 2008. He completed his MTech (Communication Systems) from SVNIT in 2010. He has worked as an associate system engineer at IBM India Pvt Ltd from 2010 to 2011. He completed his PhD from DA-IICT in 2019. He has worked as an assistant professor at centre of excellence (Victoria University Melbourne, ECA and Ganpat University) in 2019. He is working as an assistant professor at Pandit Deendayal Energy University from 2020. He is a member of IEEE, IEEE-MTT, IEEE-ComSoc, IEEE young professional. He is also working as a secretary of IEEE-ComSoc, Gujarat section. His areas of interests are AI in healthcare, decision making using AI and Data Science.

Deepak K Ghodgaonkar

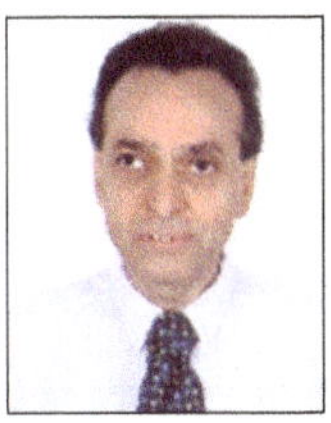

Deepak K Ghodgaonkar received his Bachelor of Engineering in Electronics Engineering from the University of Indore in 1976, Master of Technology in Electrical Engineering, Communication Engineering from IIT Bombay in 1978 and Doctorate in Electrical Engineering from the University of Utah, USA in 1987. He worked as Scientific Officer in Special Microwave Products Unit, Tata Institute of Fundamental Research, Bombay, from 1978 to 1980. Dr Deepak has more than **30** years of teaching and research experience. He has published over **80** papers in peer-reviewed journals and conferences. He got **11** honors and awards in his career. His research interests are radio frequency and microwave engineering, microwave sensors, microwave instrumentation, microwave characterization of composite materials, biomedical applications of microwaves, electromagnetic imaging of complex dielectric bodies and wireless data communications.

Jasjit S Suri

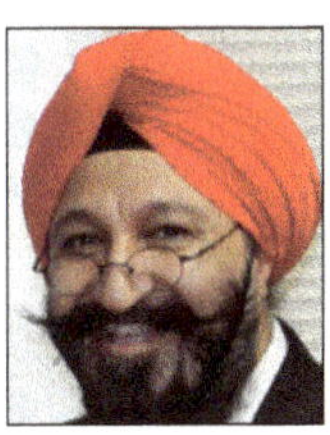

Jasjit S Suri, an innovator, a visionary, a scientist, and an internationally known world leader, a well-known speaker, and has spent over **30** years in the field of biomedical engineering/sciences, software and hardware engineering and its management. Dr Suri has over **700+** peer-reviewed articles which includes books, book chapters and patents with an H-index **56**. He received his Masters from University of Illinois, Chicago, USA, Doctorate from University of Washington, Seattle, USA and

Executive Management from Weatherhead School of Management, Case Western Reserve University (CWRU), Cleveland, USA. Dr Suri was crowned with President's gold medal in 1980, one of the youngest Fellow of American Institute of Medical and Biological Engineering (AIMBE) for his outstanding contributions at Washington DC in 2004 and also a recipient of Marquis Life Time Achievement Award for his outstanding contributions in 2018.

IOP Publishing

Hardik N Patel, Deepak K Ghodgaonkar and Jasjit S Suri

Chapter 1

Introduction to breast cancer

Breast cancer incidence and mortality are increasing globally, so this chapter focuses on the different breast cancer affecting factors with statistics of incidence and mortality. Comparison of different types of cancer statistics is made with that of breast cancer in females. It clearly indicates that breast cancer has the highest global incidence and mortality in females. The impacts of different factors like human development index (HDI), income, and geography on breast cancer incidence and mortality are represented to understand it in better way. Developed countries are much more affected by breast cancer in spite of their high income and health facilities. Predictions are made about breast cancer incidence and mortality for the year 2040. Predictions are quite alarming because they show an increase in breast cancer incidence and mortality in 2040. Breast anatomy is covered here to understand different types of breast cancers. Ductal carcinoma *in situ* (DCIS), lobular carcinoma *in situ* (LCIS), invasive ductal carcinoma (IDC), invasive lobular carcinoma, inflammatory breast cancer etc are covered with pictorial overviews in this chapter.

1.1 Introduction to cancer

Cancer is a mysterious disease of the 21st century because all the causes of the disease are still not found. 'Uncontrollable cell growth in any body part' is the simplest definition of tumor. This tumor can be classified as benign or malignant, and malignant tumor is often known as cancer. Tumor can be found in any of the body part so there are chances of having cancer in any of the body parts. It is a merciless disease because the whole family of its victim suffers. Breast cancer incidence and mortality are both very high in developing as well as developed countries. The best way to prevent this disease is to detect it at an early stage. The Global Cancer Observatory (GCO) is an interactive web-based platform presenting

doi:10.1088/978-0-7503-2592-9ch1

global cancer statistics to inform cancer control and research [1]. It is an initiative of World Health Organization (WHO) for fighting against this merciless disease. Breast cancer is one of the leading causes of mortality in many countries. From a tumor detection point of view, it is extremely important to know the tumor cell properties given below [2].

1. Dielectric properties of tumor tissues are different from healthy tissues in microwave frequency range [3–7].
2. Cell reproduction rate is higher.
3. Glucose and blood consumption are high due to abnormal reproduction rate.
4. Temperature is high due to abnormal reproduction rate.
5. Shape and size are abnormal.
6. Electrical properties are also different.
7. They neither become mature nor commit suicide.
8. They do not follow commands of surrounding healthy cells.

The above properties are common in any type of cancer. This uncontrollable growth leads to tumor which may be benign or malignant. Most of the cancers are diagnosed during their advanced stage which makes survival of the patient difficult. Worldwide cancer statistics are represented in the next section.

1.2 Worldwide cancer statistics

Worldwide breast cancer incidence and maortality statistics can provide a better idea about the status of this cancer type. GCO provides data on 36 types of cancers from 185 countries to estimate the incidence, mortality, and prevalence of this disease. Country-wise data clearly indicate the mortality due to particular cancer types in each of the 185 countries. Worldwide cancer incidence and mortality rate statistics are provided by GCO. Worldwide cancer statistics are shown in figure 1.1 for both genders. Breast cancer incidence is highest among all the cancer types. Mortality rate is second highest in breast cancer. Lung cancer mortality rate is highest among all the cancer types followed by that of breast cancer. The analysis of figure 1.1 is for both genders. It is important to analyze breast cancer incidence and mortality for females before concluding anything about breast cancer. Figure 1.1 shows the highest incidence or new cases for breast cancer. Prostate, lung, colorectum, cervix uteri, stomach, liver, corpus uteri, thyroid and ovary follow the breast cancer incidence. Liver cancer incidence and mortality are almost the same as for breast cancer, which indicates its severity. Worldwide cancer incidence statistics in females for the year 2018 are shown in figure 1.2 [1]. The cancer statistics of figure 1.2 clearly show that the breast, colorectum, lung and cervix uteri cancer incidences are about 24%, 10%, 8% and 7%, respectively. Breast cancer is the dominating cancer type in females worldwide because its new incidence is quite high as compared to other cancer types. Breast cancer has highest incidence as compared to all other types of cancers globally in females.

Worldwide cancer mortality rate statistics are shown in figure 1.3. Mortality rate due to breast, lung, colorectum and cervix uteri cancer are 15%, 14%, 10% and 7%,

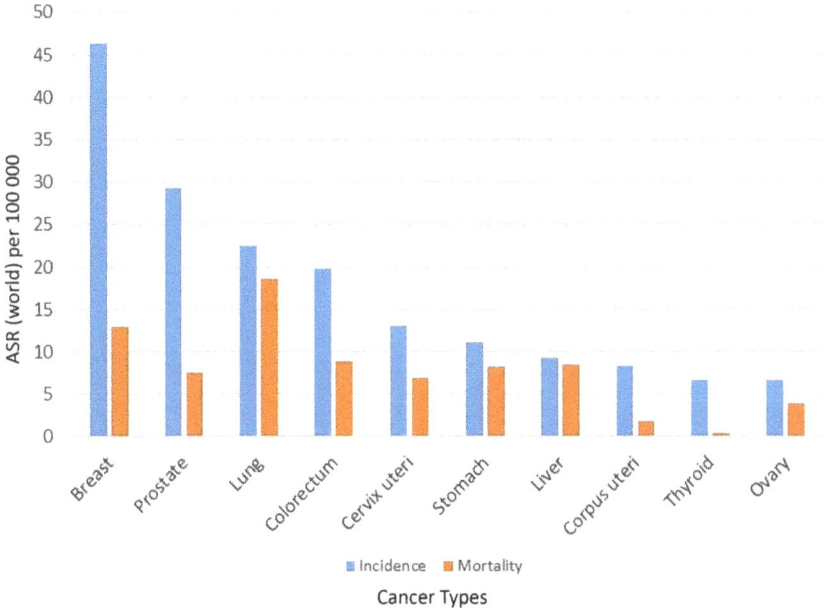

Figure 1.1. Worldwide cancer incidence in males and females. Data source: https://gco.iarc.fr/.

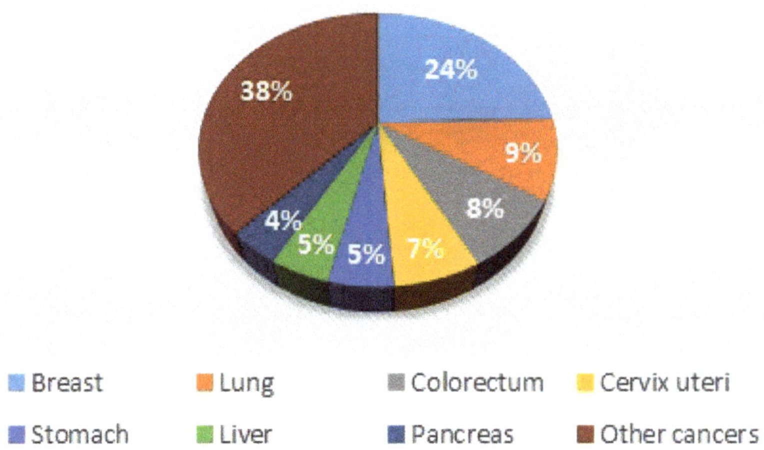

Figure 1.2. Worldwide cancer incidence in females. Data source: https://gco.iarc.fr/.

respectively. Breast cancer mortality rate is highest in females throughout the globe. It clearly indicates that breast cancer is spreading very fast.

1.3 Breast cancer statistics

It is better to understand this statistics according to human development index (HDI), income, country, continent and the world. It shows a better picture of breast

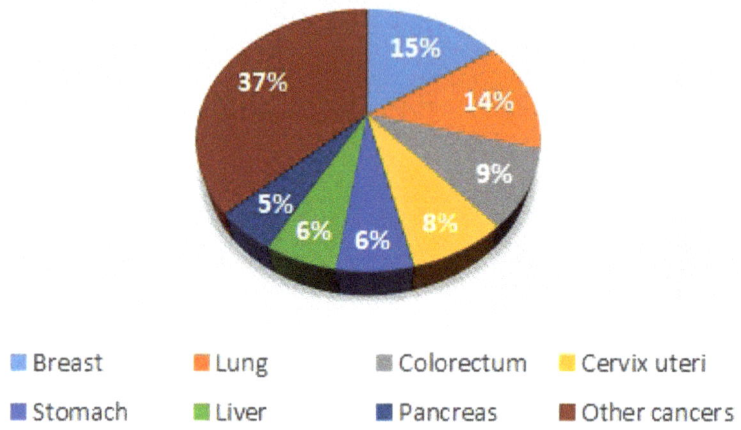

Figure 1.3. Worldwide mortality due to cancer in females. Data source: https://gco.iarc.fr/.

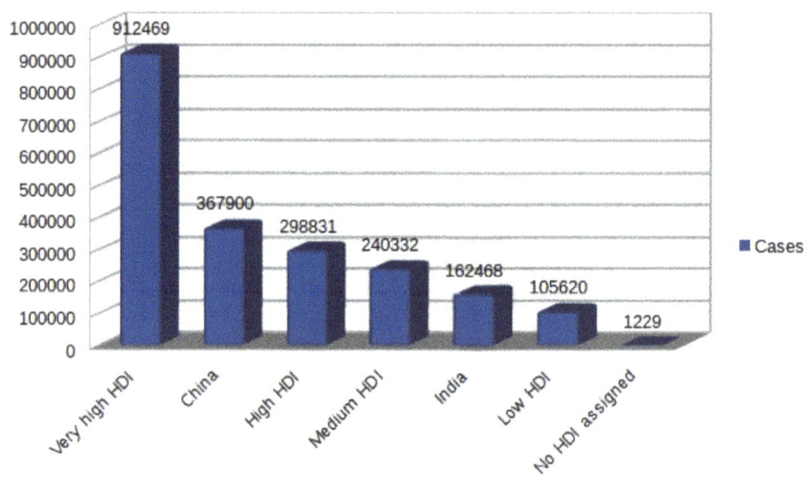

Figure 1.4. Human development index-wise breast cancer incidence cases in 2018. Data source: https://gco.iarc.fr/.

cancer incidence and mortality. Figure 1.4 shows the relationship between HDI and breast cancer incidence. The regions with very high HDI have almost 912 469 breast cancer cases or incidences in 2018. The higher development index has highest breast cancer cases in 2018. China had 367 900 breast cancer cases in 2018 which is the second highest. The mortality rate due to breast cancer also plays a major role in the prediction of this disease. The relationship between breast cancer mortality rate and HDI is shown in figure 1.5 for the year 2018. According to figure 1.5, the regions with very high HDI have 205 616 deaths due to breast cancer in the year 2018. China is second in breast cancer deaths in 2018.Breast cancer deaths are high in medium HDI regions and India as compared to high HDI regions. Income-wise breast cancer cases in the year 2018 are shown in figure 1.6. Breast cancer cases are shown in figure 1.6 for different income brackets. There were 823 638 breast cancer cases from

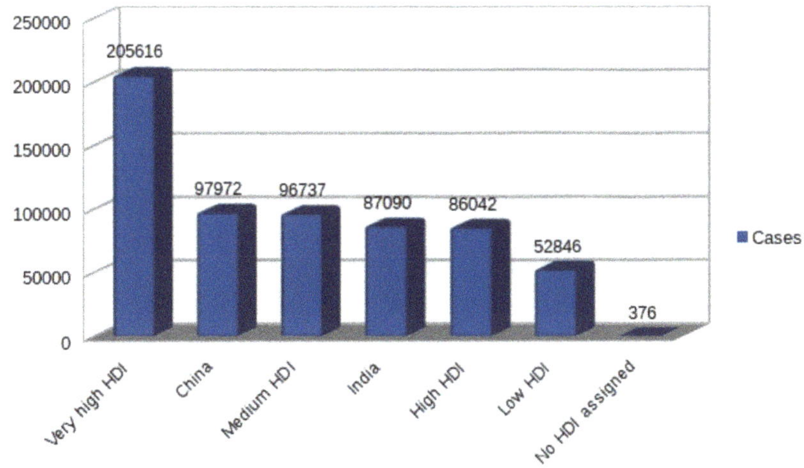

Figure 1.5. Human development index-wise breast cancer death cases in 2018. Data source: https://gco.iarc.fr/.

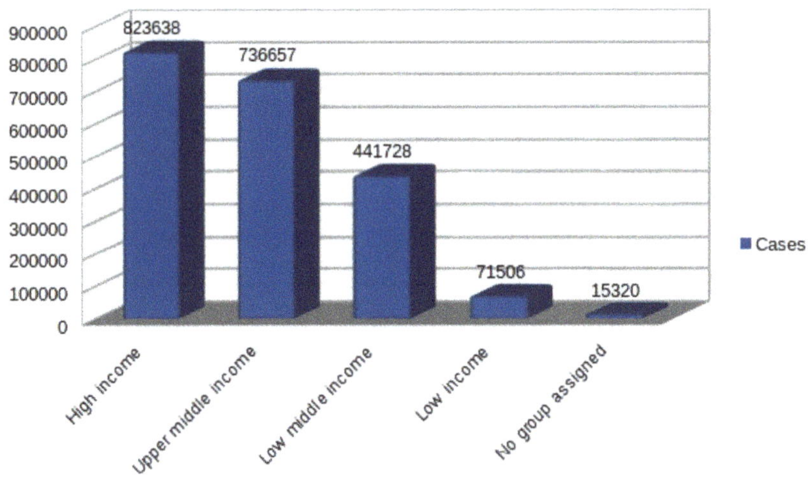

Figure 1.6. Income-wise breast cancer incidence cases in 2018. Data source: https://gco.iarc.fr/.

the high income group in 2018. There were only 71 506 breast cancer cases from the low income group. Figure 1.6 shows that the number of breast cancer cases is directly proportional to the income. Breast cancer deaths are shown in figure 1.7 for different income brackets. The low middle income bracket has the highest number of breast cancer deaths in the year 2018. The high income bracket has the third highest breast cancer deaths in the year 2018. So higher income has highest breast cancer incidences and low deaths in the year 2018. Country-wise breast cancer cases in the year 2018 are shown in figure 1.8. China has the highest number of breast cancer cases in the year 2018. USA and India have second and third highest breast cancer cases, respectively, in the year 2018. The country-wise breast cancer deaths are shown in figure 1.9. It shows an alarming situation for countries like China and

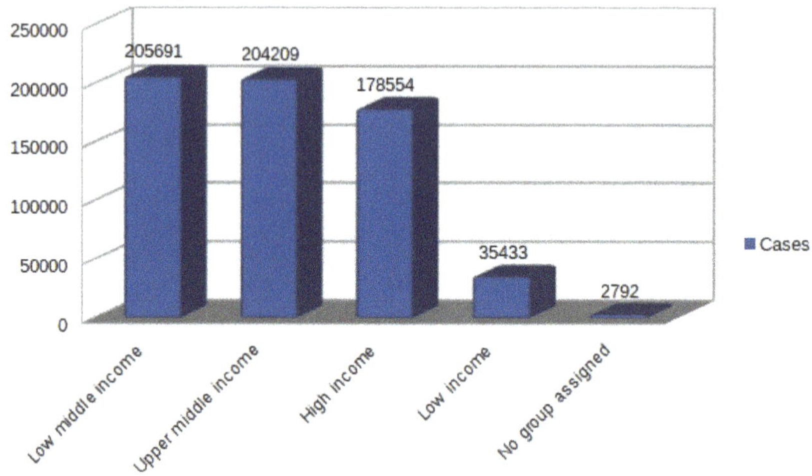

Figure 1.7. Income-wise breast cancer death cases in 2018. Data source: https://gco.iarc.fr/.

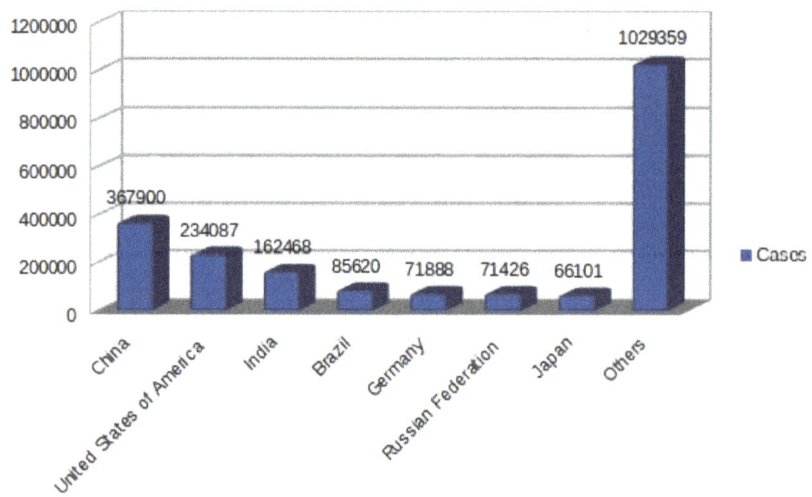

Figure 1.8. Country-wise breast cancer incidence cases in 2018. Data source: https://gco.iarc.fr/.

India because of higher breast cancer deaths as compared to other countries. Continent-wise analysis is shown in figure 1.10 for breast cancer cases. Asia, Europe and north America have higher breast cancer cases among all the continents in 2018. Analysis of continent-wise breast cancer deaths is shown in figure 1.11. Asia, Europe and Africa have higher breast cancer deaths among all the continents in 2018. Worldwide breast cancer cases and deaths are shown in figures 1.12 and 1.13, respectively. It is clear from figure 1.12 that eastern Asia has the highest number of breast cancer cases. North America is second and it is followed by south central Asia, western Europe, south America, central-eastern Europe and south eastern Asia. Mortality due to breast cancer is not following the same trend as

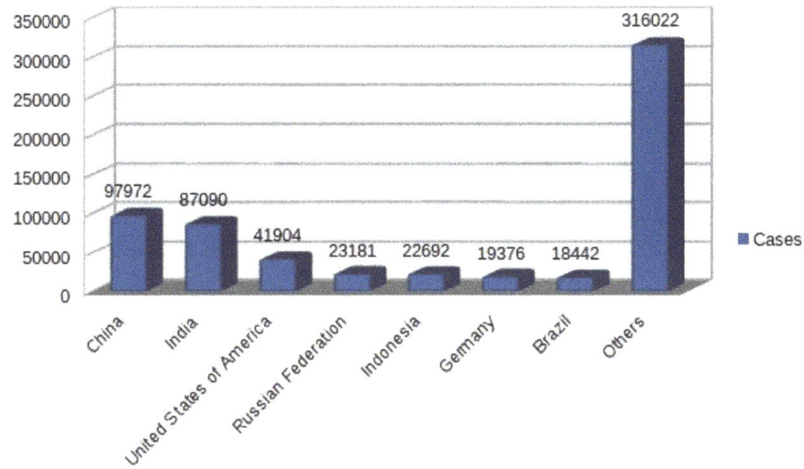

Figure 1.9. Country-wise breast cancer death cases in 2018. Data source: https://gco.iarc.fr/.

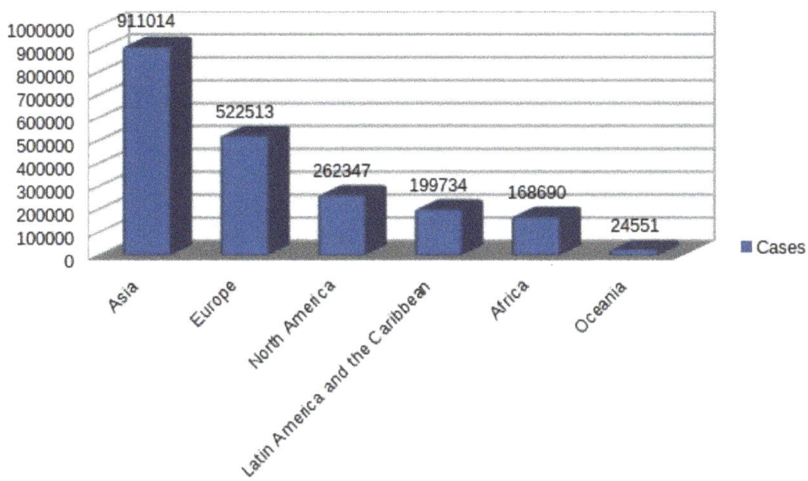

Figure 1.10. Continent-wise breast cancer incidence cases in 2018. Data source: https://gco.iarc.fr/.

incidences. It is clear from figure 1.13 that south central Asia has the highest mortality rate due to breast cancer. Eastern Asia is second followed by south eastern Asia, central-eastern Europe, north America, western Europe and south America. Mortality trend shows that there is a relationship between healthcare facilities, breast cancer awareness and mortality rate. The next section is about breast cancer prediction in 2040.

1.3.1 Breast cancer prediction

Breast cancer prediction is extremely important to enhance healthcare facilities and awareness about breast cancer disease. Worldwide breast cancer incidence prediction is shown in figure 1.14 for the year 2040. Breast cancer incidences are predicted

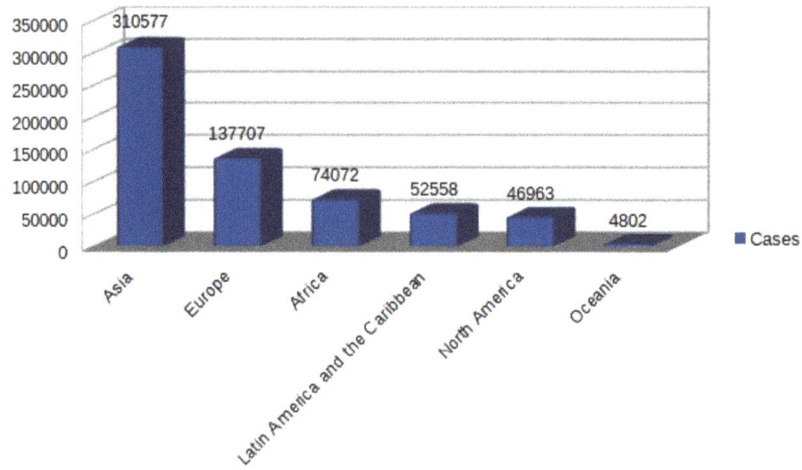

Figure 1.11. Continent-wise breast cancer death cases in 2018. Data source: https://gco.iarc.fr/.

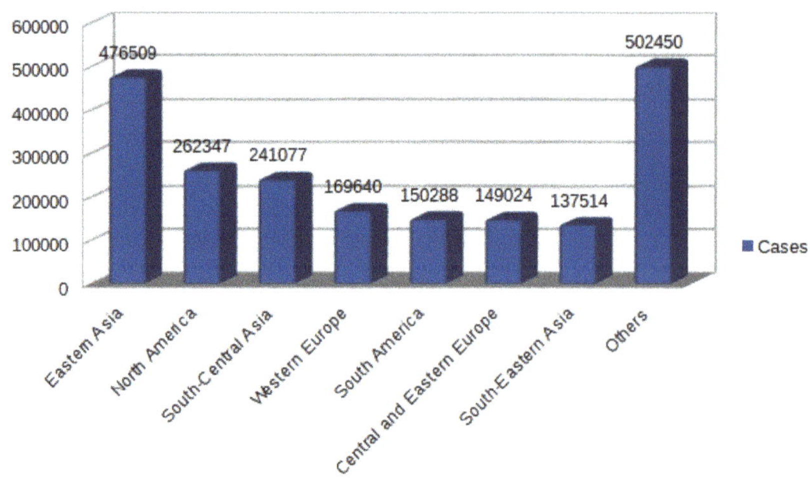

Figure 1.12. Worldwide breast cancer incidence cases in 2018. Data source: https://gco.iarc.fr/.

to increase by almost 1 million globally by 2040. Worldwide breast cancer mortality prediction is shown in figure 1.15 for the year 2040. Mortality is predicted to be almost double in the year 2040. Country-wise breast cancer incidences are shown in figure 1.16. Asia and africa could have the highest increase in breast cancer incidences in the year 2040. It is an alarming situation for the developing countries. Country-wise breast cancer mortalities are shown in figure 1.17. Asia and Africa have the highest increase in mortality rate in 2040. It clearly indicates a relationship between healthcare infrastructure, breast cancer awareness, breast cancer incidences and mortality. The above analysis is useful for making policy and strategies to combat breast cancer disease. An overview of breast anatomy and different types of breast cancer is given in the next section.

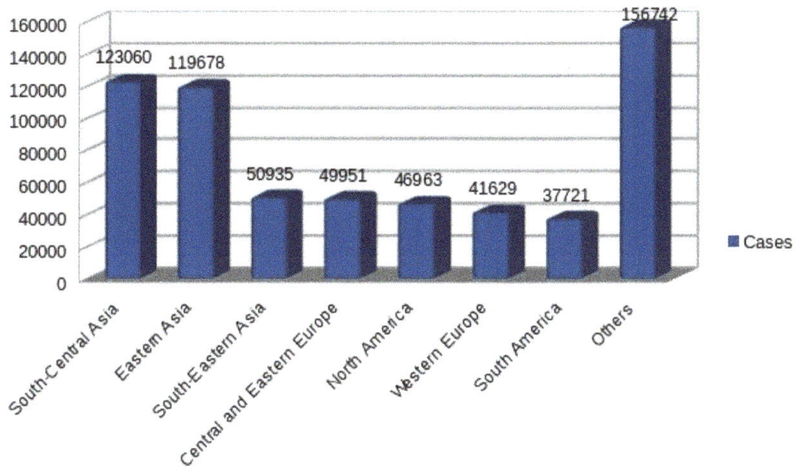

Figure 1.13. Worldwide breast cancer death cases in 2018. Data source: https://gco.iarc.fr/.

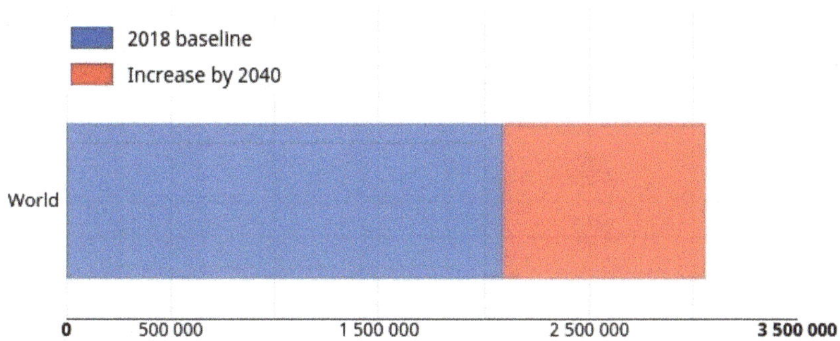

Figure 1.14. Worldwide breast cancer incidence prediction in 2040. Source: https://gco.iarc.fr/tomorrow/en.

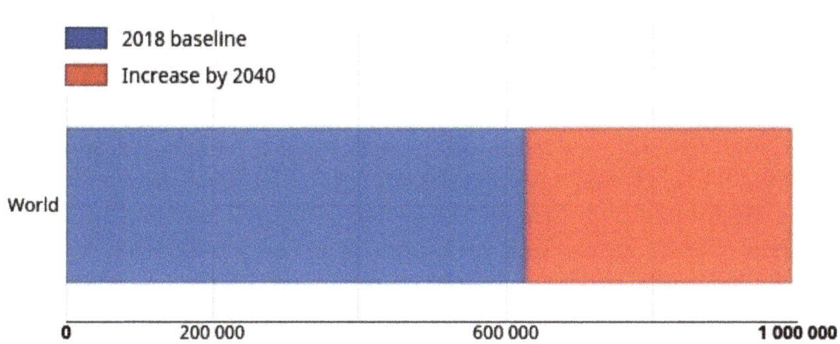

Figure 1.15. Worldwide breast cancer mortality prediction in 2040. Source: https://gco.iarc.fr/tomorrow/en.

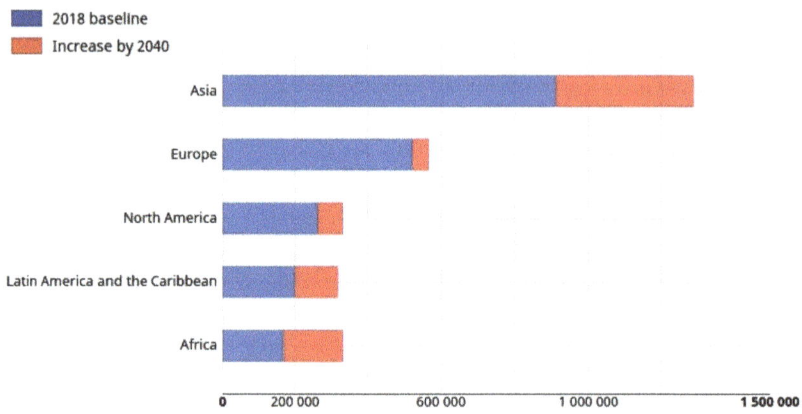

Figure 1.16. Country-wise breast cancer incidence prediction in 2040. Source: https://gco.iarc.fr/tomorrow/en.

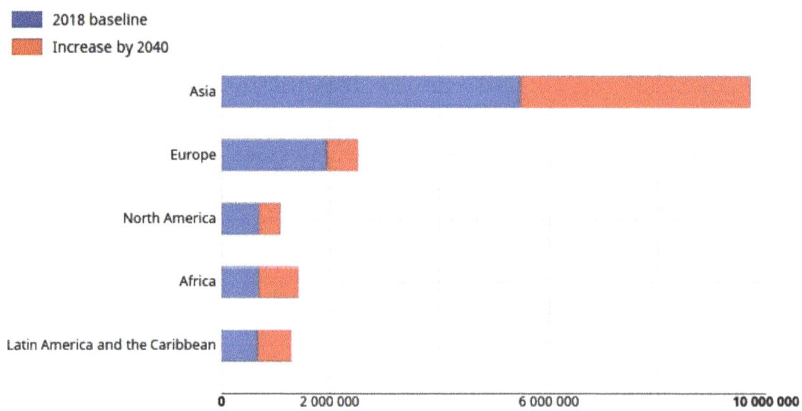

Figure 1.17. Country-wise breast cancer mortality prediction in 2040. Source: https://gco.iarc.fr/tomorrow/en.

1.4 Breast anatomy and breast cancer

Breast cancer incidence and mortality are both increasing globally according to GCO data. Early breast cancer detection can reduce mortality rate considerably. It is quite important to understand anatomy of breasts for breast cancer detection system development. Internal structure of the human female breast is shown in figure 1.18 [8, 9]. Each breast has approximately 14–20 lobes as shown in figure 1.18. These lobes are formed by a structure known as lobules. There are bulbs at the end of each lobule which can produce milk and ducts carry milk from lobules to the nipple. The whole milk producing network is surrounded by fatty tissues. Lymph nodes have the ability to filter harmful bacteria. Therefore, lymph nodes are key locations because cancer can spread to other body parts through them. Breasts have

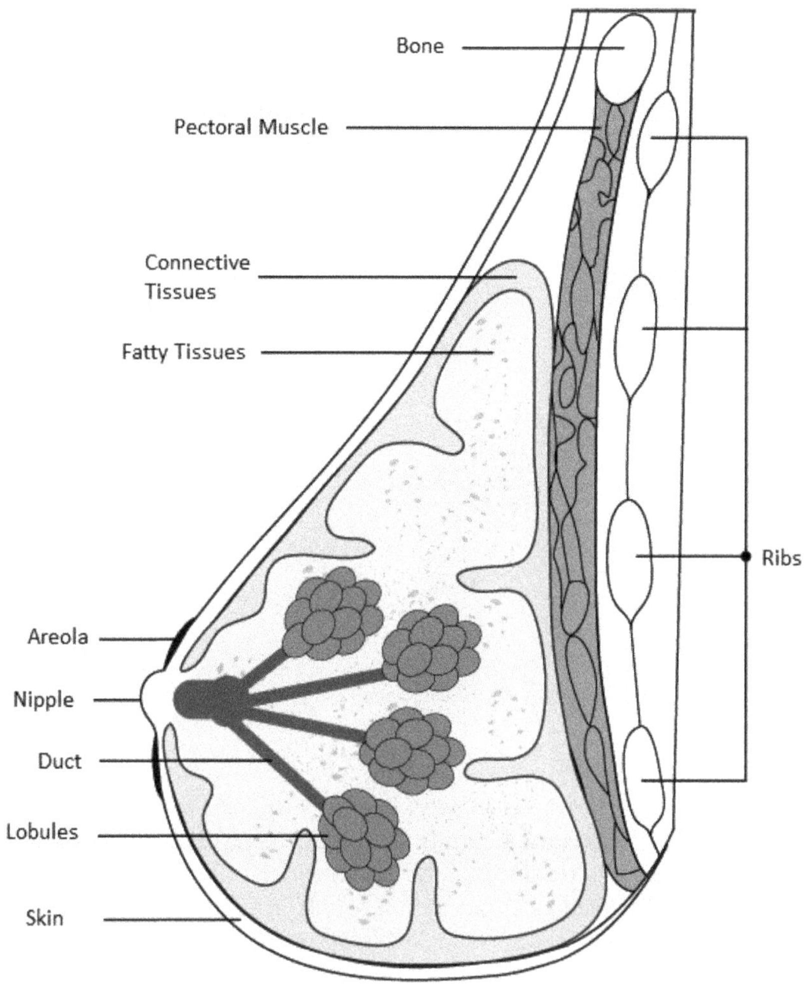

Figure 1.18. Human female breast internal structure. Source: http://www.cancer.ca/en/cancer-information/cancer-type/breast/breast-cancer/the-breasts/?region=on.

two main types of tissues, fatty (adipose) and fibro-glandular, as shown in figure 1.19. Fibro-glandular tissues are surrounded by fatty tissues. These two types of breast tissues are modeled using numerical phantom models. There are four classes of breasts according to the Breast Imaging Reporting and Data System (BI-RADS). There are four classes of breasts according to mammography based tissue densities [19, 20].

Class I breasts have only 25% glandular tissues which make them almost entirely fatty. Class II breasts have 25% to 50% scattered glandular tissues. Class III breasts are heterogeneously dense due to 51% to 75% glandular tissues. Class IV breasts are known as extremely dense due to more than 75% of glandular tissues. Women with class III and class IV breasts have high breast cancer risk [18–21]. The color of breast

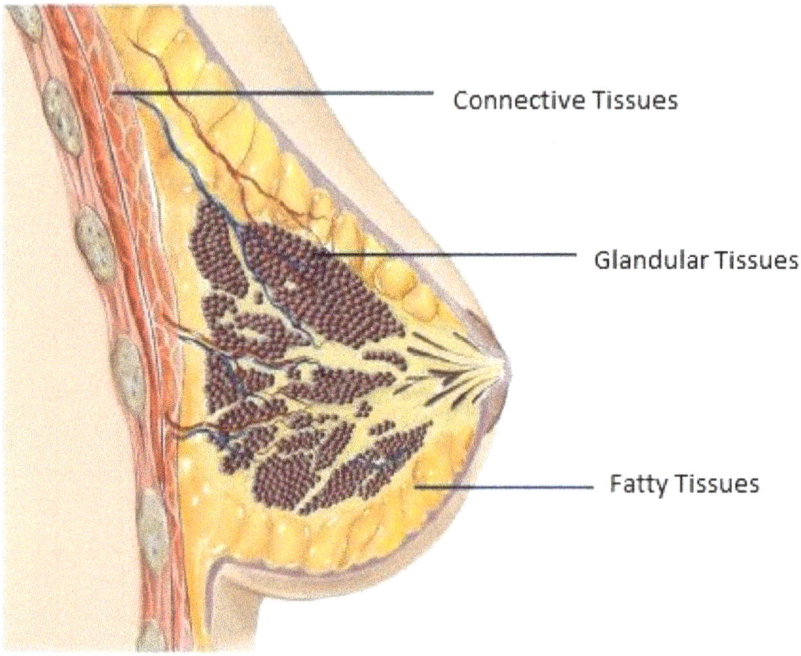

Figure 1.19. Breast anatomy showing main tissues. Source: https://aboutbrachytherapy.com/de/krebsarten/brustkrebs/.

tumor is white in mammography images. It is very difficult to detect tumor in class III and class IV breasts because of white glandular tissues. If tumor is hidden inside glandular tissues then it results in false negative detection. If higher density of glandular tissues is detected as tumor then it results in false positive detection. False positive and false negative rates are higher in class III and class IV breasts [21].

In general, breast cancer is broadly divided into non-invasive and invasive categories. Non-invasive types of cancers stay within some part of the breast; they do not grow beyond the breast. On the other hand, invasive types of cancers do spread to normal healthy tissues. Unfortunately, most breast cancers are invasive, so the patient's survival depends on early detection of breast cancer.

Ductal carcinoma *in situ* (DCIS), lobular carcinoma *in situ* (LCIS), invasive ductal carcinoma, (IDC), invasive lobular carcinoma, inflammatory breast cancer, molecular subtypes of breast cancer, Paget's disease of the nipple, phyllodes tumors of the breast, metastatic breast cancer are different types of breast cancer. The DCIS type of breast cancer stays inside milk ducts, so it is a non-invasive type of breast cancer. LCIS type indicates risk of developing invasive breast cancer. IDC type of breast cancer starts in milk ducts and it spreads to normal healthy breast tissues.

DCIS is commonly found inside the milk ducts of the breast. Most of the time DCIS is limited to milk ducts due to its non-invasive nature. Normal milk ducts do not have abnormal growth of cells while ducts with DCIS have abnormal growth of cells. If carcinoma spreads beyond ducts then it is known as invasive ductal

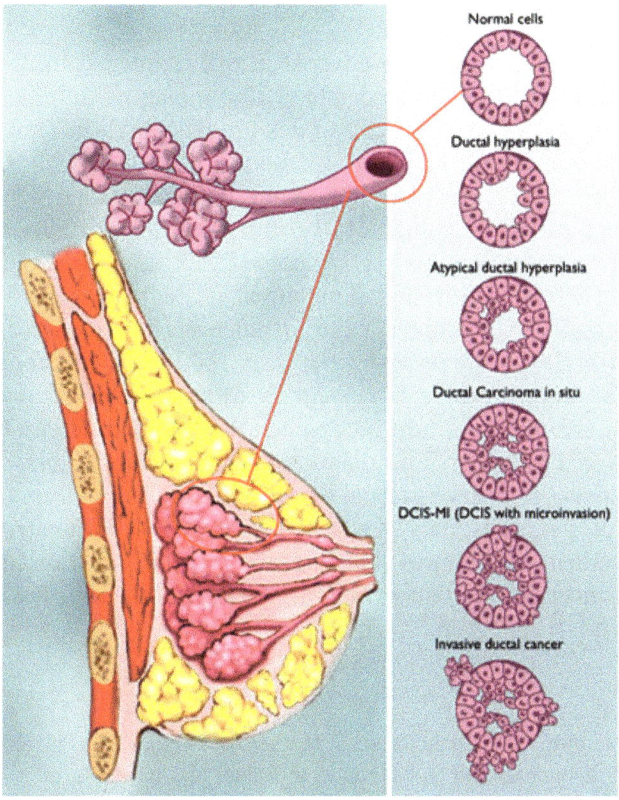

Figure 1.20. Invasive ductal carcinoma (IDC). Source: http://www.breastcancer.org/pictures/types/dcis/dcis_range.

carcinoma (IDC). IDC is clearly shown in figure 1.20 for better understanding. Ductal hyperplasia, atypical ductal hyperplasia and ductal carcinoma *in situ* have abnormal cell growth within milk ducts. DCIS with microinvasion and IDC have abnormal cell growth inside as well as outside of milk ducts. Mortality rate is higher due to IDC because of its invasive nature. LCIS is commonly found in lobules of breasts. LCIS can easily spread outside of lobules and breasts due to its invasive nature. Normal lobules do not have abnormal growth of cells while lobules with LCIS have abnormal growth of cells.

A patient with LCIS has high risk of inavsive cancer development. LCIS has higher mortality rate as compared to DCIS. Redness, swelling and enlargement, pain or itchiness, breast skin thickening and texture change, and swelling of lymph nodes are the early signs of this type of cancer. This type of cancer can be diagnosed easily by regular breast examination in initial stage.

This chapter has covered cancer definition, statistics of different types of cancer, statistics of breast cancer, breast anatomy and an overview of different types of cancer.

1.5 Summary

Cancer properties and statistics are covered in this chapter. Cancer incidences and mortality rate are important to understand the impact of different cancer types. Breast cancer incidences and mortality rates are both high in females worldwide. Breast cancer incidence and mortality statistics are mapped with different factors like HDI, income and geography. It is interesting to see the high breast cancer incidences in high income and high HDI regions but the mortality rate is lower as compared to low income and low HDI regions. The awareness about breast cancer, good healthcare infrastructure and population are main reasons behind this low mortality rate despite of high breast cancer incidences. Breast cancer incidences and mortality rates both will increase by the year 2040. Low income and low HDI countries should focus more on breast cancer awareness campaigns and improvement of healthcare infrastructure. Breast anatomy and different types of breast cancers are covered to understand diagnosis techniques in details. There are fatty and glandular tissues in the breasts and breasts are classified in four categories based on the density of these two types of tissues. Invasive and non-invasive both types of cancers are described with figures. This chapter gives introduction to breast cancer, incidence and mortality statistics and different factors affecting incidence and mortality rates.

References

[1] Ferlay J, Colombet M, Soerjomataram I, Mathers C, Parkin D M, Piñeros M, Znaor A and Bray F 2019 Estimating the global cancer incidence and mortality in 2018: GLOBOCAN sources and methods *Int. J. Cancer* **144** 1941–53

[2] Hanahan D and Weinberg R A 2011 *Hallmarks of Cancer: The Next Generation* vol 144 (Amsterdam: Elsevier) pp 646–74

[3] Campbell A M and Land D V 1992 Dielectric properties of female human breast tissue measured *in vitro* at 3.2 GHz *Phys. Med. Biol.* **37** 193–210

[4] Lazebnik M, McCartney L, Popovic D, Watkins C B, Lindstrom M J, Harter J and Sewall S *et al* 2007 A large-scale study of the ultrawideband microwave dielectric properties of normal breast tissue obtained from reduction surgeries *Phys. Med. Biol.* **52** 2637–56

[5] Lazebnik M, McCartney L, Popovic D, Watkins C B, Lindstrom M J, Harter J and Sewall S *et al* 2007 A large-scale study of the ultrawideband microwave dielectric properties of normal, benign and malignant breast tissues obtained from cancer surgeries *Phys. Med. Biol.* **52** 6093–115

[6] Fear E C, Meaney P M and Stuchly M A 2003 Microwaves for breast cancer detection *IEEE Potentials* **22** 12–8

[7] Fear E C, Hagness S C, Meaney P M, Okoniewski M and Stuchly M A 2002 Enhancing breast tumor detection with near field imaging *IEEE Microw. Mag.* **3** 48–56

[8] The Breasts http://www.cancer.ca/en/cancer-information/cancertype/breast/breast-cancer/the-breasts/?region=on

[9] Jesinger R A 2014 Breast anatomy for the interventionalist *Techniques in Vascular and Interventional Radiology* **17** 3–9

[10] Introduction to Breast Cancer https://aboutbrachytherapy.com/de/krebsarten/brustkrebs/, Accessed March 2015.

[11] Available at http://www.cancervic.org.au/preventing-cancer/attend-screening/breasts-health/ductal-carcinoma-in-situ, Accessed on 10 June 2019
[12] Ductal Carcinoma In Situ (DCIS) http://www.breastcancer.org/pictures/types/dcis/dcis_-range, Accessed on 10 June 2019.
[13] Available at http://www.aboutcancer.com/lcis.gif, Accessed on 11 June 2019.
[14] About the Inflammatory Breast Cancer Program http://www.dana-farber.org/inflammatory-breast-cancer-program/diagnosis-and-treatment/, Accessed on 12 June 2019
[15] Zhou C, Chan H P, Petrick N, Helvie M A, Goodsitt M M, Sahiner B and Hadjiiski L M 2001 Computerized image analysis: estimation of breast density on mammograms *Med. Phys.* **28** 1056–69
[16] Lemieux J 2016 Both Doctors and Patients Confused by Dense Breasts http://www.acsh.org/news/2016/09/07/both-doctors-and-patients-confused-dense-breasts-9960
[17] Vacek P M and Geller B M 2004 A prospective study of breast cancer risk using routine mammographic breast density measurements *Epidemiol. Prev. Biomarkers* **13** 715–22
[18] Boyd N F, Lockwood G A, Byng J W, Tritchler D L and Yaffe M J 1998 Mammographic densities and breast cancer risk *Epidemiol. Prev. Biomarkers* **7** 1133–44
[19] Vachon C M, VanGils C H, Sellers T A, Ghosh K, Pruthi S, Brandt K R and Pankratz V S 2007 Mammographic density, breast cancer risk and risk prediction *Breast Cancer Res.* **9** 217–25
[20] Freer P E 2015 Mammographic breast density: impact on breast cancer risk and implications for screening *Radiographics* **35** 302–15
[21] Nelson H D, O'meara E S, Kerlikowske K, Balch S and Miglioretti D 2016 Factors associated with rates of false-positive and false-negative results from digital mammography screening: an analysis of registry data false-positive and false-negative digital mammography screening results *Ann. Intern. Med.* **164** 226–35

IOP Publishing

Breast Image Reconstruction and Cancer Detection
Using Microwave Imaging

Hardik N Patel, Deepak K Ghodgaonkar and Jasjit S Suri

Chapter 2

Introduction to breast cancer detection techniques

In this chapter, breast cancer detection techniques are introduced with their brief history, operation, current status, comparison and advantages–disadvantages. At present, mammography is used as the gold standard technique for breast cancer screening. Magnetic resonance imaging (MRI) and computed tomography (CT) are also used along with mammography for breast cancer screening. Ultrasound imaging, positron emission tomography (PET), diffuse optical tomography, electrical impedance tomography and microwave imaging have the potential to be either alternative or complementary breast imaging techniques. However, most of the above techniques are at the research stage. Almost all breast cancer detection techniques are covered in this chapter. Algebraic, analytic, statistical and learned iterative image reconstruction methods are introduced at the end with simple mathematical formulas. Mammography provides good cancer diagnosis for fatty breasts but at the same time it cannot do well for dense breasts. MRI is also used for breast cancer diagnosis but it is costly. Computed tomography is good but it also uses ionizing x-rays. Ultrasound, PET, diffuse optical tomography and microwave imaging techniques are very promising for breast cancer diagnosis at the research level.

2.1 Imaging modalities for breast cancer screening

Breast cancer incidence and mortality is increasing worldwide. Early detection is the key for the survival of breast cancer patients. There are many non-invasive techniques for breast cancer detection. A list of different imaging modalities or techniques for breast cancer screening is given below.

1. Mammography;
2. Ultrasound imaging;

doi:10.1088/978-0-7503-2592-9ch2

3. Magnetic resonance imaging (MRI);
4. Positron emission tomography (PET);
5. Diffuse optical tomography;
6. Electrical impedance tomography;
7. Computed tomography;
8. Microwave imaging.

2.2 Mammography

At present, mammography is the gold standard technique for breast cancer detection. Extensive research work is ongoing in all breast cancer detection techniques. Each of the techniques have its advantages and disadvantages which motivated researchers to develop hybrid imaging modalities. Mammography is still used extensively in breast cancer screening. A typical mammography setup is shown in figure 2.1.

Mammography screening uses x-rays for breast imaging and cancer diagnosis. Frequent mammography screenings may lead to cancer due to ionizing x-ray radiation. X-ray dose is also a crucial factor because of different breast sizes. Mammography has poor contrast which results in high false positive and false negative rates. High radiation dose of x-ray or frequent mammography screening increases risk of cancer because x-rays are an ionizing radiation. False negative and false positive rates are about 15% and 13%, respectively, in mammography which leads to additional imaging and biopsies [1, 2]. Breasts are compressed between two plates to enhance contrast in mammography, which makes it uncomfortable and painful for patients. In mammography, the patient's breast is placed and compressed between two flat plates. The x-ray machine generates small bursts of x-rays which are passed through the breast and detected on the other side. An image is formed based on detected signals for diagnosis. There are three types of mammography.

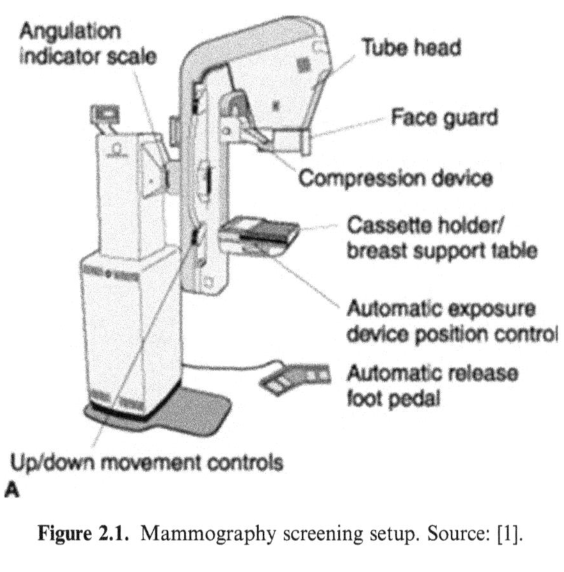

Figure 2.1. Mammography screening setup. Source: [1].

1. Film based mammography;
2. Digital mammography;
3. Tomosynthesis (3D mammography).

In film based mammography, low density tissues like fatty tissues appear as darker shades of gray, whereas dense tissues like glandular tissues and tumor are white on grayscale. In digital mammography, working principal remains the same but film is replaced by a solid-state detector. The solid-state detector receives x-rays after they pass through the breast. Then these received signals are sent to the computer for image formation. In tomosynthesis, x-rays pass at different angles to generate different cross-sections of the breast. Now, images are represented in 3D by using a standard developed for computed tomography. Women with class III and class IV breasts have high breast cancer risk [3–6].

2.2.1 History of mammography

Mammography is quite old and the gold standard technique for breast cancer detection. The evolution of mammography is shown below using a timeline diagram (figure 2.2). As depicted in the timeline, x-rays were discovered by Wilhelm Roentgen in 1895. The next major event was the first attempt of Albert Solomon to detect breast cancer using x-rays in 1913. This can be considered as the foundation of mammography.

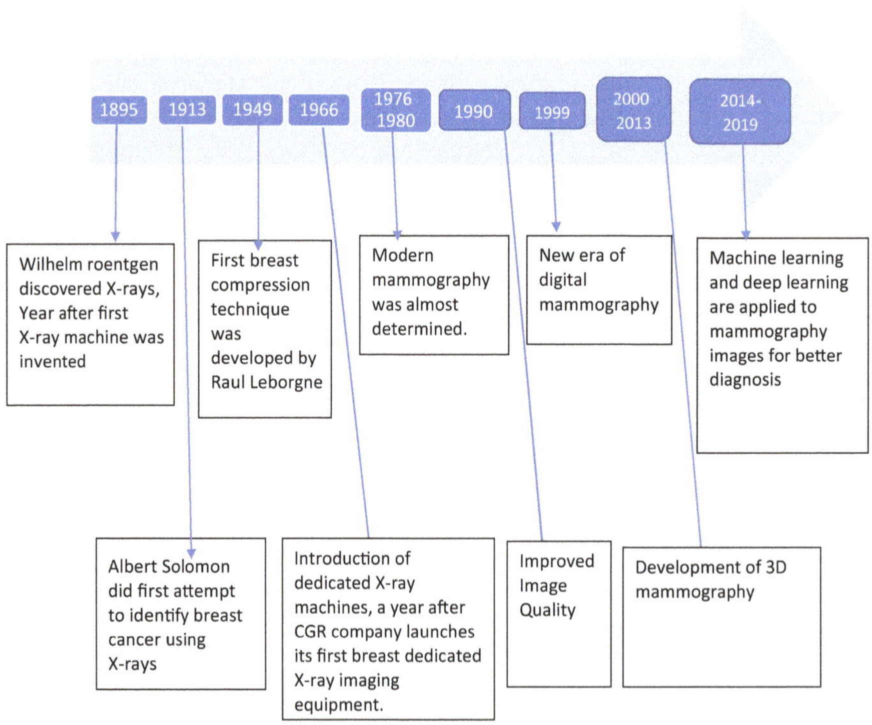

Figure 2.2. History of mammography.

Raul Leborgne invented the breast compression technique for cancer detection using x-rays in 1949. This compression technique increased contrast and resolution of x-ray based images. A dedicated x-ray based breast imaging machine was designed in 1966. Modern mammography was established completely during 1976–80. Mammography image quality was improved by different techniques in 1990. Digital mammography research was started in 1999. 3D and digital mammography research dominated during 2000–13. Machine learning and deep learning based algorithms have been used to improve mammography based diagnosis during the last five years.

2.2.2 Basic understanding of mammography

Mammography technology understanding is very important. Important parts of a mammography machine are shown in figure 2.3.

X-ray tube anodes are made up of tungsten in most cases. Mammography x-ray tube anodes are generally made up of molybdenum. Some manufacturers use rhodium with molybdenum. The spectrum provided by these materials is suitable for breast imaging. Filters are used to reduce unnecessary exposure of x-rays to patients. Focal spots are used to reduce blurring and at the same time provide good visibility of details to detect small tumors. Breast compression is extremely important because it can provide the advantages listed below. A grid is used to absorb scattered radiation and it also improves contrast sensitivity. Film and digital receptors are used in mammography (table 2.1). The colour of a breast tumor is white in mammographic images. It is very difficult to detect tumor in class III and class IV breasts because of white glandular tissues. If the tumor is hidden inside

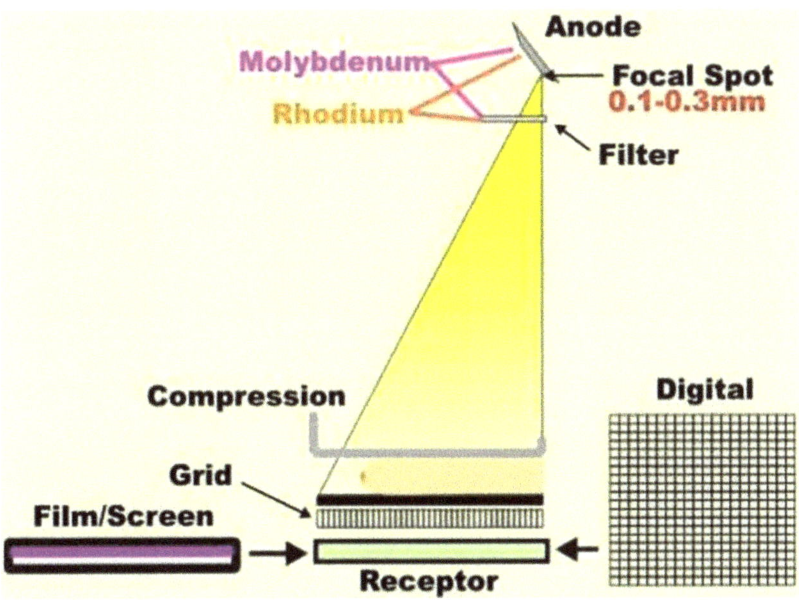

Figure 2.3. Important parts of mammography setup. Reprinted with permission from Sprawls: http://www.sprawls.org/resources/MAMMO/module.htm.

Table 2.1. Comparison of different mammography techniques [9].

Imaging modality	Description	Limitations	Summary of performance
Mammography	It is performed on a woman with no clinical symptoms or complaints to detect early stage breast cancer	It depends on type of mammography.	Variable
Film mammography	1. X-rays are passed through the breast to create a grayscale image on film. 2. Sufficient breast compression is required. 3. More than two views are required for women with large breasts. 4. Average radiation dose is 4.7 mGy.	1. Sensitivity is limited in dense breasts. 2. Subject to artifacts. 3. Inability to manipulate image after exposure.	**All women** Sensitivity: 0.41 ± 0.03 Specificity: 0.98 ± 0.001 PPV: 0.13 ± 0.01 **Women < 50** Sensitivity: 0.35 ± 0.06 Specificity: 0.98 ± 0.001 PPV: 0.07 ± 0.01
Digital mammography	1. X-ray photons are converted to electronic signals and these signals are processed to form an image. 2. It is more effective than film. 3. Average radiation dose is 3.7 mGy.	1. Spatial resolution is less as compared to film. 2. More expensive.	**All women** Sensitivity: 0.41 ± 0.03 Specificity 0.98 ± 0.001 PPV 0.12 ± 0.01 **Women < 50** Sensitivity: 0.49 ± 0.06 Specificity 0.97 ± 0.001 PPV 0.08 ± 0.01
Tomosynthesis	1. Breasts are scanned at multiple angles. 2. Series of images are reconstructed. 3. Average radiation dose is 1 or 2 times that of digital mammography.	Patient is exposed to high radiation dose as compared to other modalities.	PPV for recall $6.4\% \pm 2.1\%$.

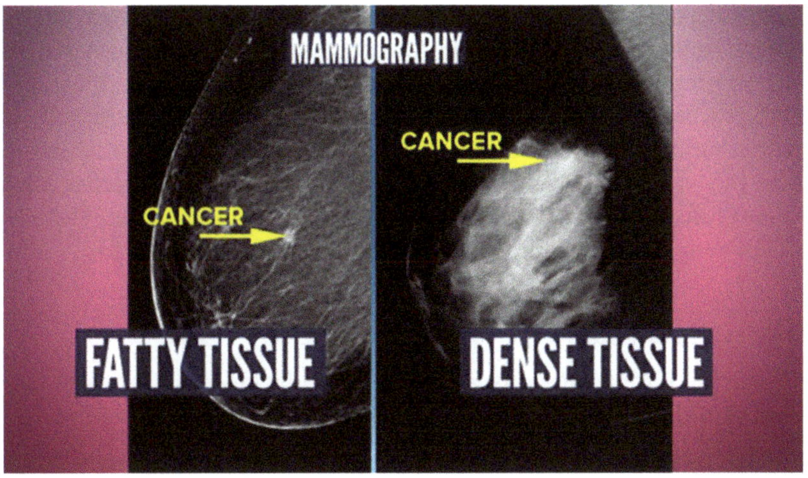

Figure 2.4. Tumor in fatty and dense breast tissues. Source: http://www.today.com/health/do-you-have-dense-breasts-you-may-need-more-mammogram-t104102.

glandular tissues then it results in false negative detection. If higher density of glandular tissues is detected as a tumor then it results in false positive detection. False positive and false negative rates are higher in class III and class IV breasts [7]. Tumor detection is very difficult in dense tissues, as shown by figure 2.4. Advantages and disadvantages of mammography are given below.

2.2.3 Advantages and disadvantages of mammography

Advantages

- High sensitivity.
- Good resolution.
- Short image formation time.

Disadvantages

- Sensitivity is less for dense breasts.
- Low contrast.
- Painful for patients because breasts are pressed to improve image quality.
- It uses ionizing radiation.
- Molecular level imaging is not possible.

2.3 Ultrasound imaging

Sound or sonic waves are used in ultrasound imaging. Sound waves are transmitted to the breast through probe; based on internal structure of the breast, sound waves are echoed back at the probe. Received signals are sent to a computer for image formation. Ultrasound imaging for breast cancer detection is an emerging research area. Ultrasound basically refers to acoustic waves with frequency higher than 20 kHz. An ultrasound scanner works in the 2–18 MHz frequency range. The resolution of the image depends on the frequency or range of frequencies chosen for imaging. Higher frequencies have better image resolution than lower frequencies. Acoustic waves are transmitted into body tissues through a transducer, and these waves are reflected back when they hit interface areas with different densities. Reflected waves are received by transducer and the depth of the interface area is calculated by using the travel time of the reflected sound waves. Higher frequencies have higher attenuation losses so lower frequencies have better penetration depth inside tissues. There is a clear trade off between resolution and depth of penetration.

2.3.1 History of ultrasound

A brief history of ultrasound is given in table 2.2. It includes all the major inventions in the field of ultrasound.

Table 2.2. History of ultrasound.

Year	Events
1794	Lazzaro Spallanzani laid the foundation of ultrasound physics by revealing his research related to echolocation among bats.
1877	Piezoelectricity was discovered by Pierre and Jacques Curie. Ultrasound transducers use the piezoelectric principle during transmission and reception of sound waves.
1915	A device was designed to detect objects at the bottom of the sea by Paul Langevin.
1920–1940	Sonography was used to treat European soccer team members.
1942	Karl Dussik was the first to use sonography for medical diagnosis. Ultrasound was used to detect brain tumor.
1948	George Ludwig made ultrasound equipment to detect gallstones.
1949–1951	Douglas Howry and Joseph Holmes developed B-Mode ultrasound equipment. John Reid and John Wild invented a handheld B-Mode device to detect breast tumors.
1953	Inge Edler and Engineer C Hellmuth Hertz performed the first successful echo cardiogram.
1958	Ian Donald incorporated ultrasound into the field of medicine.
1966	Pulsed Doppler ultrasound technology was developed by Don Baker, Dennis Watkins and John Reid.
1970	Continuous wave Doppler, spectral wave Doppler and Color Doppler ultrasound equipment were developed.
1980	Kazunori Baba developed 3D ultrasound technology and captured 3D images of a fetus in 1986.
1989	Daniel Lichtenstein started incorporating lung and general sonography in intensive care units.
1990	Improved image quality and 3D imaging capabilities were added to ultrasound imaging. Ultrasound guided biopsies started in this year.
2000–present	Ultrasound technology is evolving and more compact devices are developed. Artificial intelligence will be part of ultrasound diagnosis sooner or later.

2.3.2 Physics of ultrasound

The physics of ultrasound is important for understanding of imaging process. Acoustic wave characterization is given below.

$$c = \sqrt{\frac{1}{k\rho}} \tag{2.1}$$

In equation (2.1) c is speed of sound in medium, k is compressibility, ρ is density. Acoustic pressure is related to impedance as shown in equation (2.2).

$$p = Zv \tag{2.2}$$

Characteristic impedance of a medium is given in equation (2.3).

$$Z = \rho c = \sqrt{\frac{\rho}{k}} \tag{2.3}$$

Acoustic energy density is given by equation (2.4).

$$w = \frac{1}{2}(\rho v^2 + kp^2) \tag{2.4}$$

A three-dimensional wave equation is given in equation (2.5)

$$(\nabla)^2 p(x, y, z, t) = \frac{1}{c^2} p_{tt}(x, y, z, t) \tag{2.5}$$

where $\nabla^2\ p = p_{xx} + p_{yy} + p_{zz}$ and c is the speed of sound. If a plane wave in the z direction is assumed then the above relationship is represented by equation (2.6).

$$(\nabla)^2 p_{zz}(z, t) = \frac{1}{c^2} p_{tt}(z, t) \tag{2.6}$$

As shown in equation (2.7), a general solution of the above equation is a combination of forward and backward traveling waves.

$$p(z, t) = \phi_{\mathrm{f}}(t - c^{-1}z) + \phi_{\mathrm{b}}(t - c^{-1}z) \tag{2.7}$$

Equation (2.7) is used in the ultrasound imaging of the object. This technique has long been used to diagnose disease and abnormalities in different body parts. It is a very well established technique for some of the applications.

2.3.3 Current status of ultrasound imaging

Table 2.3

2.3.4 Advantages and disadvantages of ultrasound

Advantages

- Non-ionizing radiation.
- Examination of dense breasts and implants is possible.
- Good resolution.

Table 2.3. Current status of ultrasound breast imaging [8, 9].

Imaging Modality	Description	Limitations	Summary of Performance
Ultrasound	1. Sound or acoustic waves are used to create images of breast. Accuracy of diagnosis depends on the expertise of the operator. Recently, FDA approved whole breast ultrasound of patients with dense breasts. 2. It is not part of routine screening at this stage. 3. Some medical practitioners recommend breast ultrasound for patients with dense breasts 4. Radiation is not involved.	1. It is not an appropriate initial screening modality for breast cancer detection. It is accepted as an addition with mammography screening for women with dense breasts. 2. High false positive and false negative rates 3. There is no standard for performance in the case of breast cancer detection 4. Image quality as well as diagnosis depends on operator and observer. 5. Limited ability to detect DCIS type of breast cancer.	—

Disadvantages

- Technician skill based system performance.
- Difficult to distinguish solid masses.
- Lesions lying deep inside the breast are difficult to detect.

Ultrasound breast images are different than mammography breast images. Ultrasound has the ability to detect breast cancer. Ultrasound breast images are shown in figure 2.5.

2.4 Magnetic resonanace imaging

Magnetic resonance imaging (MRI) uses magnetic field and radio waves to generate images of internal structure of the human body.

2.4.1 Short history of MRI

The foundation of MRI was laid by Nikola Tesla when he discovered the rotating magnetic field. Isidor I Rabi, Felix Bloch and Edward Mills Purcell demonstrated the quantum phenomenon known as nuclear magnetic resonance (NMR). The structure of molecules can be seen in detail by using this technique. Until 1970, MRI was mainly used in chemical and physical analysis. Raymond Damadian started using it to detect disease in living organisms. In 1971, he found that cancerous tissues have more water than normal healthy tissues. He started designing the full-body

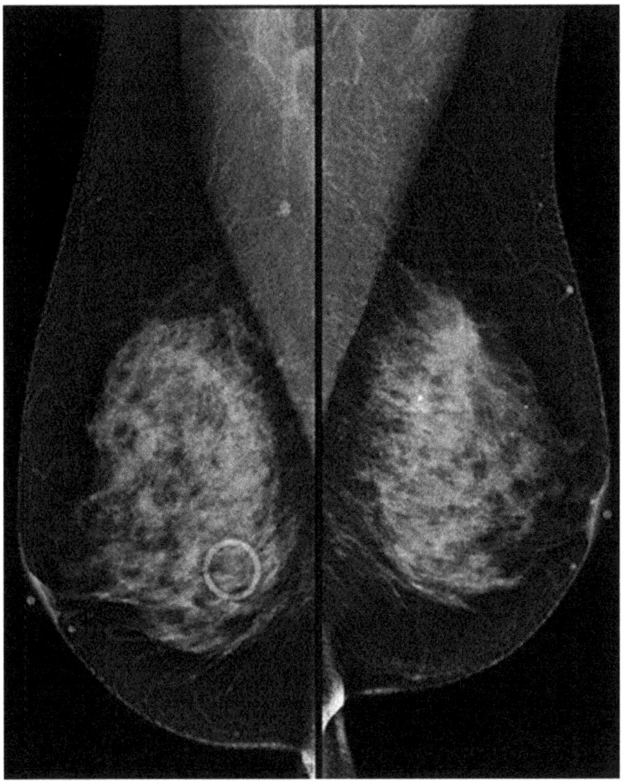

Figure 2.5. Ultrasound images of breast. Reprinted with permission from [9], copyright American Roentgen Ray Society (2015).

MRI scanner. The first true MR image was published by Paul Lauterbur in 1973. The ability of a gradient magnetic field to form two-dimensional images was found by Lauterbur. The first image of a live body was published in 1977. Different technological modifications have been made to date in MRI.

2.4.2 Working principle of MRI

The human body contains around 70% water. Hydrogen nuclei (protons) of water molecules become aligned in a magnetic field. An MRI scanner applies a very strong magnetic field which aligns the protons. The scanner also produces a radio frequency current that produces a varying magnetic field. The aligned protons absorb the energy from the magnetic field and change their spins. When the field is turned off, the protons gradually return to their normal spin, a process called precession. The return process produces a radio signal that can be measured by receivers in the scanner and converted into an image. Advantages and disadvantages of MRI are given below.

2.4.3 Advantages and disadvantages of MRI

Advantages

- Non-ionizing technique.
- Capability of detecting small tumors.
- Multi focal cancers can be detected.

Disadvantages

- It is extremely expensive.
- It is immobile.
- Contrast agent injection is needed.
- Time consuming.

2.5 Positron emission tomography

Positron emission tomography (PET) uses radioactive biomarkers to diagnose cancer. In PET, glucose with radioactive biomarker is injected in the body to trace changes at metabolism level. A PET scanner setup is shown in figure 2.6.

PET is a three-dimensional nuclear medicine based imaging technique. It detects the γ rays emitted through the nucleus of a radioactive biomarker injected in the human body. As discussed above, malignant tumours are detected based on their glucose consumption as compared to surrounding healthy cells. Contrast in the reconstructed images is very good due to the working principal of PET. Basically, It provides the metabolism information and chemical functions inside tissues and organs.

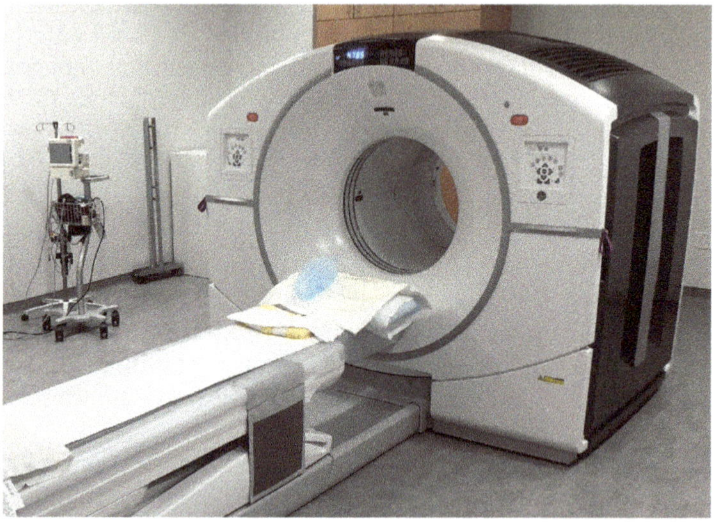

Figure 2.6. PET machine or setup. Source: https://zhuanlan.zhihu.com/p/53827823.

2.5.1 Short history of PET

David E Khul, Luke Chapman and Roy Edwards introduced the concept of emission and transmission tomography in the late 1950s. James Robertson and his team built the first single plane PET scan in 1961. The first PET instrument was designed in 1968–69. The work was reported in 1972. The radioactive compound was tested on two normal human volunteers by Abass Alavi in 1976. Now, PET is used for breast cancer detection using radioactive biomarkers. Advantages and disadvantages of PET imaging are given below.

2.5.2 Advantages and disadvantages of PET

Advantages

- Good contrast.
- Tissue level chemical and metabolism information.
- Real time.

Disadvantages

- Poor resolution.
- High cost.
- Radioactive biomarkers are used.
- Patients are exposed to radiation.

2.6 Diffuse optical tomography

Diffuse optical tomography is a special case of computed tomography in which photons of the near infrared regime have significant scattering during their propagation through the body. Near infrared light penetrates several centimeters into tissues but it suffers from a large amount of scattering. Scattering effect results in blurring of reconstructed images where optical inhomogeneities are present in the tissues. Diffuse tomography setup is shown in the literature [10, 11].

There are source and detector plates in the breast box. Source fiber carries optical light waves generated by the source and detector fiber carries the scattered waves collected by detector plate. Images are created by processing scattered light wave data.

2.6.1 Short history of optical tomography

The first paper on optical coherence tomography was published by Huang *et al* in 1991 [30]. The first time human retina study was done using OCT was in 1993, and it was first used commercially for retinal imaging in 1997. A high-speed and better-resolution OCT machine was launched in 2003. The first time OCT was used commercially for vascular imaging in 2010. FDA clearance was given to OCT for one application in 2012. Different versions of OCT machines were launched after 2012. Diffuse optical tomography was also included in the research. Advantages and disadvantages of diffuse optical tomography are given below.

2.6.2 Advantages and disadvantages of diffuse optical tomography

Advantages

- Low cost technique.
- Safe for patients.
- Good for imaging of moving objects.

Disadvantages

- Expert user is required.
- Cell level imaging is difficult.

2.7 Electrical impedance tomography

Human body tissues allow electric current or signals so they have electrical impedance. It has been established that malignant cancerous tissues have lower impedance as compared to normal tissues. In this technique, 2D or 3D images are reconstructed from impedance values which are captured by electrodes surrounding breasts.

2.7.1 Advantages and disadvantages of EIT

Advantages

- It is cheap.
- Non-invasive technique.
- No radiation.
- Differential EIT can be used to cancel errors.
- High temporal resolution.

Disadvantages

- Poor availability.
- It is not widely accepted.
- Small errors in voltage measurements can result in misleading diagnosis.
- Less spatial resolution than computed tomography and MRI.

2.8 Computed tomography (CT)

Computed tomography uses x-rays for the image reconstruction of internal body structure. Images are taken from different views to reconstruct the image with better quality. A short history of CT is given below.

2.8.1 Short history of CT

Tomography was invented by radiologist Alessandro Vallebona in the early 1900s. Conventional tomography was not able to do soft tissue imaging. The first CT scanner was invented by Godfrey Hounsfield using x-rays in 1967. The first brain CT was performed in the UK in 1971. The first CT scanner was installed in the USA in 1973. Three million CT scans had been performed by 1980, and 68 million were performed annually by 2005. 64 slice CT scanners were installed by 2007. In 2008, a new generation of CT scanner was developed which can take images of beating hearts or coronary arteries in less than one second. Low-dose CT scanners were developed after 2010 to reduce effects of harmful x-ray radiation.

2.8.2 Advantages and disadvantages of CT

Advantages

- Rapid acquisition of images.
- Non-invasive technique.
- Clear and specific information.
- Large portion of body is visible.

Disadvantages

- Ionizing radiation is used.
- Radiation dose determination.
- molecular imaging is not possible.

2.9 Microwave imaging

Microwave imaging is a non-invasive technique which uses non-ionizing radiation. The frequency band of 300 MHz to 300 GHz is known as the microwave band. Electromagnetic signals with microwave band frequencies are used in microwave based tomography. Microwave imaging started with frequency domain analysis. Initially, research was done for weapon detection, material characterization, remote sensing, etc, and microwave imaging of the human body started around the 1950s. Microwave imaging applications are attracting industry due to increase in computation power. At present, there are many commercial opportunities in microwave imaging. Two basic microwave imaging techniques are given below.

1. Passive microwave imaging.
2. Active microwave imaging.

2.9.1 Passive microwave imaging

Every hot thing radiates electromagnetic energy in this Universe. The human body also radiates electromagnetic energy. In passive microwave imaging, the electromagnetic energy of a human body part is captured for cancer diagnosis. A radiometer is used to capture the microwave signals generated by human body parts. This technique is still used in healthcare, weather and space applications

2.9.2 Active microwave imaging

Microwave signals are transmitted through antennas on the object or body part to be imaged. These signals are scattered after their interaction with the object or body part. A scattered field is measured using antennas around the object. Active microwave imaging is an emerging research field. There are many applications of active microwave imaging in healthcare, security and space.

2.10 Comparison of mammography, MRI and ultrasound

Mammography, MRI and ultrasound are used for breast cancer screening. Performance comparison of these three techniques for breast cancer detection is given in table 2.4.

2.11 Overview of image reconstruction methods

There are different image reconstruction methods for breast cancer imaging modalities. Different types of image reconstruction algorithms are given below.

1. Algebraic reconstruction.
2. Analytic reconstruction.
3. Statistical reconstruction.
4. Learned iterative reconstruction.

2.11.1 Algebraic reconstruction

In 1970, algebraic reconstruction technique (ART) was first introduced by Gordon and Herman for three-dimensional image reconstruction from its projections [20, 21]. Estimator function in a higher dimensional space is deconvoluted with lower dimensional space measured projections. X-ray film represents the two-dimensional projection of three-dimensional distribution of x-ray densities within the body. A finite number of photographs taken at different angles are used to reconstruct the three-dimensional densities within the body. In order to understand ART, consider the equation given below. Let's consider f_i^q as the qth estimate for f_i.

Table 2.4. Comparison of mammography, MRI and ultrasound for breast cancer detection.

	Sardanelli *et al* [14]	Kuhl *et al* [15]	Lehman *et al* [16]	Leach *et al* [17]	Warner *et al* [18]	Morris *et al* [19]	Vreemann *et al* [20]
Study period	2000–2007	2002–2005	2005	1997–2004	1997–2003	2000–2001	2003–2014
Number of participants	501	687	195	648	256	367	2463
Number of cancers	52	27	6	35	22	14	170
Sensitivity (%)							
MRI	91	93	100	77	77	100	81.4
Mammography	50	33	33	40	36	0	51.7
Ultrasound	52	37	17	NA	33	NA	NA
PPV (%)							
MRI	65	48	43	7	49	17	28
Mammography	71	39	50	10	83	NA	40
Ultrasound	62	33	25	NA	23	NA	NA

$$P_j^q = c_j \sum_{r_i \in g_j} f_i^q \tag{2.8}$$

where $j = 1, \ldots, m$.

In the above equation, P_j^q is the value of the projection of the qth estimate. Let $\bar{f}$ be the mean density of the object in finite region R then the ART algorithm is

$$f_i^0 \equiv \bar{f} \tag{2.9}$$

where $i = 1, \ldots, n$.

$$f_i^{q+1} = \max\left[0, f_i^q + \left(\frac{\frac{P_j}{c_j} - \frac{P_j^q}{c_j}}{N_j}\right)\right] \tag{2.10}$$

where $\left(\frac{\frac{P_j}{c_j} - \frac{P_j^q}{c_j}}{N_j}\right)$ is correction factor.

In words, the iterative process starts with all reconstruction elements set to $f_i^0 = \bar{f}$. At each iteration the calculation is carried out to get a difference between actual measurement data for projection elements and the sum of the reconstructed projection elements. The correction factor is divided by the number of reconstructions N_j here. If the correction factor in the above equation is negative then it is set to zero. The same calculation is repeated in each of the iterations till convergence. There are different convergence criteria for the ART algorithm. The difference between measured and reconstructed projections of equation (2.11) can be used as convergence criteria.

$$D^q = \sqrt{\frac{1}{m}\sum_{j=1}^{m} \frac{\left(\frac{P_j}{c_j} - \frac{P_j^q}{c_j}\right)^2}{N_j}} \tag{2.11}$$

Convergence is reached if D^q tends to zero as q increases. Variance of reconstructed object at qth projection and mean density of object given by equation (2.12) can also be used as convergence criteria.

$$V^q = \sum_{i=1}^{n} (f_i^q - \bar{f})^2 \tag{2.12}$$

convergence is reached when V^q tends to be a minimum as q increases. Entropy convergence criteria is shown by equation (2.13).

$$S^q = \frac{-1}{\ln(n)} \sum_{i=1}^{n} \frac{f_i^q}{\bar{f}} \ln\left(\frac{f_i^q}{\bar{f}}\right) \tag{2.13}$$

convergence is reached when S^q tends to be a minimum as q increases. There are several variants of ART due to divergence and other issues. Generalized, multiplicative, unconstrained, constrained, ART2, ART3, ART with binary constraint and ART with damping factor are different variants of ART given in [22, 23].

2.11.2 Analytic reconstruction

There are two analytic reconstruction techniques mainly used in tomography.

1. Back projections.
2. Filtered back projections.

The radon transform is used in the back projection method. Radon transform of a function $f(x, y)$ is given by equation (2.14)

$$r(s, \phi) = \int_{x=-\infty}^{\infty} \int_{y=-\infty}^{\infty} f(x, y) \cdot \delta(x \cos\phi + y \sin\phi - s)\, \mathrm{d}x\, \mathrm{d}y \tag{2.14}$$

The role of delta function is quite clear in this equation. The integral is zero everywhere except on the line $L(s, \phi)$. The back projected image is the inverse radon transform given by equation (2.15).

$$b(x, y) = \int_0^{\pi} r(s, \phi)\Big|_{S=x\cos\phi+y\sin\phi}\, \mathrm{d}\phi \tag{2.15}$$

Important information is there in the half so integration over 180° is required. The reconstructed image is blurred in this case. In the filtered back projection, filters are applied to projection data before the back projection process [24]. The quality of the reconstructed image is drastically improved due to application of filters before back projection.

2.11.3 Statistical reconstruction

There are different statistical methods for image reconstruction. The five basic steps of any statistical reconstruction method are given below.

1. Choose a suitable model to express unknown parameters to be determined through image reconstruction.
2. A model used to express unknown parameters should consider noise because actual measurements are always noisy.
3. Gaussian or Poisson models are generally used to model noisy measurement data.
4. Cost function to be minimized is calculated using proper technique.
5. An algorithm with proper stopping criteria is used to minimize cost function iteratively. The image is properly reconstructed at the end of this step.

Genetic algorithms, differential evolution methods, memetic algorithms, particle swarm optimization, Simulated annealing, maximum likelihood estimation, and hybrid techniques are some examples of statistical methods for image reconstruction [25–27].

2.11.4 Learned iterative reconstruction

Learned iterative reconstruction involves machine learning, deep learning and artificial intelligence. This area is new and very rapidly changing. A review of different learned iterative algorithms or methods is given in [28].

2.12 Summary

Imaging modalities like mammography, ultrasound imaging, MRI, PET, diffuse optical tomography, electrical impedance tomography, computed tomography, and microwave imaging are briefly explained with working principle, history, and typical setup. Mammography uses ionizing x-rays to reconstruct images of internal structure of different body parts. Operation, limitations and performance are compared for mammography, film mammography, digital mammography and tomosynthesis. Ultrasound imaging uses acoustic waves to reconstruct images of internal structure of different body parts. Physics and current status of ultrasound imaging are described with advantages and disadvantages of this technique. MRI uses magnetic resonance to reconstruct images of internal structure of body parts. History and working principle of MRI are described with advantages and disadvantages. PET uses a radioactive biomarker to track glucose consumption in the cells. The history of PET and advantages and disadvantages are discussed here. Diffuse optical tomography, electrical impedance tomography and computed tomography are described with history, advantages and disadvantages. Passive and active microwave imaging techniques are described with block diagram. Mammography, MRI and ultrasound are compared with number of participants, number of cancers, sensitivity and positive predictive value (PPV). Algebraic, analytic, statistical and learned iterative reconstructions are explained with a mathematical overview.

References

[1] Fear E C, Hagness S C, Meaney P M, Okoniewski M and Stuchly M A 2002 Enhancing breast tumor detection with near field imaging *IEEE Microw. Mag.* **3** 48–56

[2] Fear E C, Meaney P M and Stuchly M A 2003 Microwaves for breast cancer detection *IEEE Potentials* **22** 12–8

[3] Vacek P M and Geller B M 2004 A prospective study of breast cancer risk using routine mammographic breast density measurements *Cancer Epidemiol. Biomarkers Prev.* **13** 715–22

[4] Boyd N F, Lockwood G A, Byng J W, Tritchler D L and Yaffe M J 1998 Mammographic densities and breast cancer risk *Cancer Epidemiol. Biomarkers Prev.* **7** 1133–44

[5] Vachon C M, VanGils C H, Sellers T A, Ghosh K, Pruthi S, Brandt K R and Pankratz V S 2007 Mammographic density, breast cancer risk and risk prediction *Breast Cancer Res* **9** 217–25

[6] Freer P E 2015 Mammographic breast density: impact on breast cancer risk and implications for screening *Radiographics* **35** 302–15
[7] Nelson H D, O'meara E S, Kerlikowske K, Balch S and Miglioretti D 2016 Actors associated with rates of false-positive and false-negative results from digital mammography screening: an analysis of registry data false-positive and false-negative digital mammography screening results *Ann. Intern. Med.* **164** 226–35
[8] Ko E S and Morris E A 2019 Abbreviated magnetic resonance imaging for breast cancer screening: concept, early results, and considerations *Korean J. Radiol.* **20** 533–41
[9] Brem R F, Lenihan M J, Lieberman J and Torrente J 2015 Screening breast ultrasound: past, present, and future *Am. J. Roentgenol.* **204** 234–40
[10] Choe R *et al* 2009 Differentiation of benign and malignant breast tumors by in-vivo three-dimensional parallel-plate diffuse optical tomography *J. Biomed. Opt.* **14** 024020
[11] Choe R *et al* 2009 Differentiation of benign and malignant breast lesions by in-vivo three-dimensional diffuse optical tomography *Cancer Res.* **69** 805
[12] Wagenaar J 2015 Electrical impedance tomography in 3D: characterization and evaluation *PhD Thesis* Carleton University
[13] Sardanelli F, Podo F, Santoro F, Manoukian S, Bergonzi S and Trecate G *et al* 2011 Multicenter surveillance of women at high genetic breast cancer risk using mammography, ultrasonography, and contrast-enhanced magnetic resonance imaging (the high breast cancer risk Italian 1 study): final results *Invest. Radiol.* **46** 94–105
[14] Kuhl C *et al* 2010 Prospective multicenter cohort study to refine management recommendations for women at elevated familial risk of breast cancer: the EVA trial *J. Clin. Oncol.* **28** 1450–7
[15] Lehman C D, Lee J M, DeMartini W B, Hippe D S, Rendi M H and Kalish G *et al* 2016 Screening MRI in women with a personal history of breast cancer *J. Natl. Cancer Inst.* **7** 108
[16] Leach M O, Boggis C R, Dixon A K, Easton D F, Eeles R A and Evans D G *et al* 2005 Screening with magnetic resonance imaging and mammography of a UK population at high familial risk of breast cancer: a prospective multicentre cohort study (MARIBS) *Lancet* **365** 1769–78
[17] Warner E, Plewes D B, Hill K A, Causer P A, Zubovits J T and Jong R A *et al* 2004 Surveillance of BRCA1 and BRCA2 mutation carriers with magnetic resonance imaging, ultrasound, mammography, and clinical breast examination *JAMA* **292** 1317–25
[18] Morris E A, Liberman L, Ballon D J, Robson M, Abramson A F and Heerdt A *et al* 2003 MRI of occult breast carcinoma in a high-risk population *Am. J. Roentgenol.* **181** 619–26
[19] Vreemann S, Gubern-Mérida A, Schlooz-Vries M S, Bult P, van Gils C H and Hoogerbrugge N *et al* 2018 Influence of risk category and screening round on the performance of an MR imaging and mammography screening program in carriers of the BRCA mutation and other women at increased risk *Radiology* **286** 443–51
[20] Gordon R 1974 A tutorial on ART (algebraic reconstruction techniques) *IEEE Trans. Nucl. Sci.* **21** 78–93
[21] Brooks M 2010 A survey of algebraic algorithms in computerized tomography *PhD Thesis* University of Ontario Institute of Technology
[22] Gordon R 1974 A tutorial on ART (algebraic reconstruction techniques) *IEEE Trans. Nucl. Sci.* **21** 78–93

[23] Tepe J, Schuster T and Littau B 2017 A modified algebraic reconstruction technique taking refraction into account with an application in terahertz tomography *Inverse Probl. Sci. Eng.* **25** 1448–73
[24] Kim C, Lee K Y, Shin C, Kang E Y, Oh Y W, Ha M, Ko C S and Cha J 2018 Comparison of filtered back projection, hybrid iterative reconstruction, model-based iterative reconstruction, and virtual mono energetic reconstruction images at both low-and standard-dose settings in measurement of emphysema volume and airway wall thickness: a CT phantom study *Korean J. Radiol.* **19** 809–17
[25] Fessler J A 2002 Statistical methods for image reconstruction. NSS-MIC short course on statistical image reconstruction methods (annotated slides for attendees)
[26] De Man B and Qi J 2005 Statistical methods for image reconstruction
[27] Pastorino M 2007 Stochastic optimization methods applied to microwave imaging: a review *IEEE Trans. Antennas Propag.* **55** 538–48
[28] Wang G, Ye J C, Mueller K and Fessler J A 2018 Image reconstruction is a new frontier of machine learning *IEEE Trans. Med. Imaging* **37** 1289–96
[29] Sree S V, Ng E Y K, Acharya R U and Faust O 2011 Breast imaging: a survey *J. Clin. Oncol.* **2** 171
[30] Huang D *et al* 1991 Optical coherence tomography *Science* **254** 1178–81

IOP Publishing

Breast Image Reconstruction and Cancer Detection Using Microwave Imaging

Hardik N Patel, Deepak K Ghodgaonkar and Jasjit S Suri

Chapter 3

Introduction to microwave imaging

Microwave imaging is a very important technique for breast cancer diagnosis due to its unique advantages. Passive and active microwave imaging have both been explored in medical imaging of breasts. Passive imaging relies on thermal image reconstruction of breasts. The working principle and mathematics of passive microwave imaging are covered in a simplified manner. Passive microwave breast imaging requires very sensitive radiometers because human breasts radiate very weak electromagnetic radiation. The sensitive radiometers even pick up noise so it is difficult to avoid errors completely. Active microwave imaging is better than passive microwave imaging but it is also complex. It requires lots of signal processing and good calibration to achieve best results. Microwave tomography and UWB RADAR are two main techniques of active microwave imaging. Passive and active microwave imaging can both offer unique advantages and applications in medical imaging of breasts.

3.1 Introduction

Microwaves have frequency range of 300 MHz to 300 GHz. Microwave imaging is a technique to detect and locate hidden or embedded objects in different structures. Quantitative and qualitative are two types of techniques used in microwave imaging. Quantitative imaging reconstructs parameters of imaging objects by solving non-linear inverse problems. Nonlinear inverse problems are generally converted into linear inverse problems by using approximations. Iterative forward solvers are preferred over direct inversion due to large ill- posed matrices. In qualitative microwave imaging, qualitative images of hidden or embedded objects are reconstructed. Imaging problems are simplified by using approximations and then back propagation is used to reconstruct the unknown object profile. Synthetic aperture

doi:10.1088/978-0-7503-2592-9ch3

radar (SAR) and ground penetrating radar (GPR) are popular qualitative microwave imaging algorithms. Two types of microwave imaging are given below.

1. Passive microwave imaging.
2. Active microwave imaging.

3.2 Introduction to passive microwave imaging

All hot matter in the Universe radiates electromagnetic energy. So, electromagnetic signals coming from objects are received by a radiometer and images are reconstructed in terms of temperature. The basic setup of passive microwave imaging is shown in the figure 3.1.

As shown in figure 3.1, a radiometer is used to collect microwave signals coming out of an object (breast). A temperature profile of the object is reconstructed based on microwave energy received by the radiometer. So, cancer or tumour is detected based on the temperature profile of the breast. Passive microwave imaging has a number of applications in remote sensing. Humidity and temperature profiling are two popular applications of passive microwave imaging. Thermography is used to reconstruct an image of the internal structure of human body organs. Skin temperature clinical diagnosis was carried out by using infrared emission of a human body around 1960. The thermal emission is captured from 10 kHz to 100 GHz in passive microwave imaging [1–4]. Subcutaneous temperatures can be measured by using thermography at centimeter and millimeter wavelengths, whereas infrared thermography is limited to measurement of skin temperature only [1]. Subcutaneous thermal abnormalities can be detected and localized by using thermography at centimeter and millimeter wavelengths.

3.2.1 Emission principles

All objects or substances emit electromagnetic radiation due to internal heat. The Rayleigh–Jeans expression of equation (3.1) is useful to approximate the intensity of the electromagnetic radiation at cm and mm wavelengths.

$$I(f,\, T) = e(f)\frac{2kTf^2}{c^2} \tag{3.1}$$

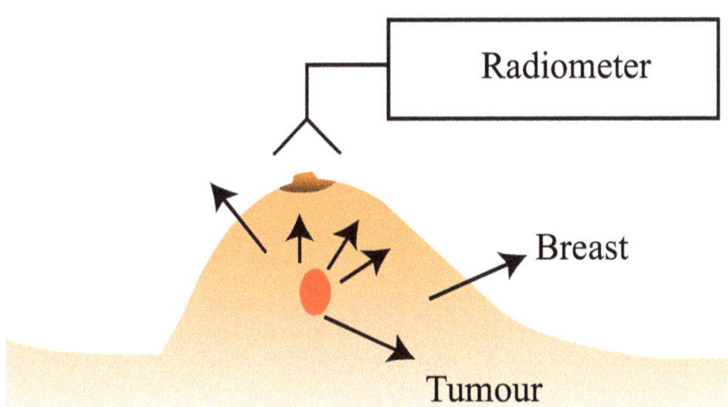

Figure 3.1. Basic setup of passive microwave imaging.

In equation (3.1), k and c are Boltzmann's constant and the speed of light, respectively. The intensity of electromagnetic radiation is proportional to the temperature T so it is possible to get a thermal image of the object. $e(f)$ is a dimensionless quantity known as emissivity, which depends on the permittivities of the emitting and receiving medium, respectively. The Fresnel's equation result is shown in equation (3.2) for a plane-parallel case.

$$e(f) = 1 - |\sqrt{\epsilon_1^*(f)} - \sqrt{\epsilon_2^*(f)}|^2 \cdot |\sqrt{\epsilon_1^*(f)} + \sqrt{\epsilon_2^*(f)}|^{-2} \quad (3.2)$$

The above equation with the measured values of skin and muscle permittivity at cm and mm wavelengths and radiometric measurement of the skin-to-air emission show that the emissivity increases from a relatively low value of 50% at 3 GHz to a thermographically useful value of 96% at 30 GHz [2–7]. Reflections between fat and skin, which are intra-tissue interactions, can lead to major loss contributions and muddling of standing waves of internally produced radiations [8, 9].

3.2.2 Radiative transfer

An internal hot spot of change in temperature ΔT with respect to the surrounding body temperature T results in an increase ΔI of the emitted radiation intensity according to equation (3.1). The associated temperature increase ΔT_E can be measured externally. This temperature increase ΔT_E can be obtained from the equation of radiative transfer [10].

$$\Delta T_E = \Delta T\left[1 - \exp\left(\frac{-d_t}{\delta_t}\right)\right] \cdot \exp\left(\frac{-d_f}{\delta_f}\right) e_{fs} \cdot \exp\left(\frac{-d_s}{\delta_s}\right) e_{sa} \quad (3.3)$$

In equation (3.3), d_t, d_f and d_s are the thickness of the tumor, fat and skin tissues respectively. δ_t, δ_f and δ_s are their $\exp^{-1}$ power penetration depths, e_{fs} and e_{sa} represent power transmission coefficients fat-to-skin and skin-to-air, respectively. The standing waves and their effects between boundaries of various layers are neglected in equation (3.3). $\frac{\delta}{d} \ll 1$ and $e = 1$ for millimeter waves, which simplifies equation (3.3) to equation (3.4) [11].

$$\Delta T_E = \Delta T \exp\left(\frac{-d_f}{\delta_f}\right) \cdot \exp\left(\frac{-d_s}{\delta_s}\right) \quad (3.4)$$

Equation (3.3) has been used to determine incremental tumor temperature ΔT_E which is externally measurable. The incremental tumor temperature is $\Delta T_E = 0.4$ °C at 3 GHz with assumed tumor thickness, internal depth of 2 cm and incremental tumor temperature $\Delta T = 1.5$ °C [12]. Conventional radiometers can measure the above temperature changes very easily. Unfortunately, practical antenna illumination can reduce this externally measurable incremental tumor temperature. It is not possible to detect small internal hot spots through the radiative transfer principal of electromagnetic waves only.

3.2.3 Bio-heat transfer

A more complete model is needed to consider the broad effects of blood flow and thermal tissue conduction. The steady state solution of the bioheat transfer equation can be used to analyze the above effects [13].

$$Q(z) = \zeta_b \cdot c_b \cdot U_b \cdot \nabla T - K \cdot \nabla^2 T \tag{3.5}$$

In equation (3.5), $Q(z)$ is the input at the 'hot spot' as a function of the internal layer depth z, ζ_b is the density of the blood, c_b is the specific heat of the blood, U_h is the average blood velocity vector, K is the coefficient of tissue heat condition, T is the temperature. The first term $\zeta_b \cdot c_b \cdot U_b \cdot \nabla T$ of equation (3.5) represents the contribution of the blood convection to the dissipation of the heat produced by the hot spot. The second term $K \cdot \nabla^2 T$ is due to tissue conduction. Infrared thermography based experimental studies of the above heat transfer to the skin have been performed in [14–16]. The effect of externally applied irradiated microwave power has been reported by using idealized version of equation (3.5) in [17]. It shows strong influence of blood flow and thermal conduction on the internal temperature distributions with tenfold increase of the effective penetration depth [17]. Passive microwave imaging or thermographic imaging can also lead to similar strong effects for internal hot spot detection. Normal and abnormal blood flows and tissue conduction may help to conclude about high tumor detection rates of thermography [6–8, 12, 18, 19].

3.2.4 Temperature resolution

Radiometers that are used in radioastronomy and earth resources receivers can be used to sense or capture radiation emitted by the body [20, 21]. The input to this type of radiometer is rapidly switched between a hot spot of incremental temperature ΔT_E and another normal region. This beam or load switching technique allows the radiometer to measure small incremental power changes as shown by equation (3.6).

$$\Delta P = kB\Delta T_A \tag{3.6}$$

The incremental power changes are proportional to the radiometer bandwidth B and the incremental antenna temperature ΔT_A. The incremental antenna temperature is given by equation (3.7).

$$\Delta T_A = \eta\phi\Delta T_E \tag{3.7}$$

In equation (3.7), η is the antenna efficiency and ϕ is the beam filling factor. ϕ is equal to one for a hot spot with an angular size $\Delta\Omega_B$. The minimum detectable temperature ΔT_{min} or sensitivity of a radiometer is equal to its root mean square (RMS) noise temperature variations [22].

$$\Delta T_{RMS} = \frac{AT_{sys}}{(B\tau)^{1/2}} \tag{3.8}$$

In equation (3.8), A, T_{sys}, B and τ are the receiver mode coefficient, system noise temperature, bandwidth and post detection integration time, respectively.

3.3 Microwave radiometry for cancer detection

Microwave radiometry or microwave thermography is a technique for detection and diagnosis of temperature profile based pathologic state through measurement of natural electromagnetic radiation or emission from the body at microwave frequencies. Early detection and diagnosis of breast cancer is one of the potential microwave radiometry applications. Mammography, ultrasound and optical tomography are used to detect a tumor based on its mass and contrast with respect to surrounding healthy tissues. Non-ionizing radiation and painful diagnosis process are two major drawbacks of mammography. Mammography is not efficient for dense breasts which leads to unnecessary biopsies and other diagnosis procedures. Radiometry offers a passive, non-invasive and non-ionizing procedure to detect thermal activity for tumor detection. It has the ability to provide information beyond physical parameters provided by other techniques like mammography [23]. In the Universe, any object with above absolute temperature radiates electromagnetic energy. A body which transmits, reflects or absorbs all of the incident radiation or energy is often known as a black body. a perfect absorber is also a perfect emitter or radiator according to black body theory. According to Planck's radiation law, any perfectly absorbing body emits radiation at all frequencies [23]. The level of this electromagnetic radiation is a function of both temperature and frequency.

Figure 3.2 shows intensity of radiated electromagnetic signal versus frequency [23]. Transmission loss (attenuation) of tissues with high water content is greater than low water content tissues at a given temperature. Thermography assumes temperature difference between malignant tumor and surrounding healthy tissues in cancer detection. As shown in figure 3.3, the heat production in the human body depends on the doubling time of the tumor volume [23, 24]. High temperature is associated with the tumor growth rate in the body which leads to significant thermal

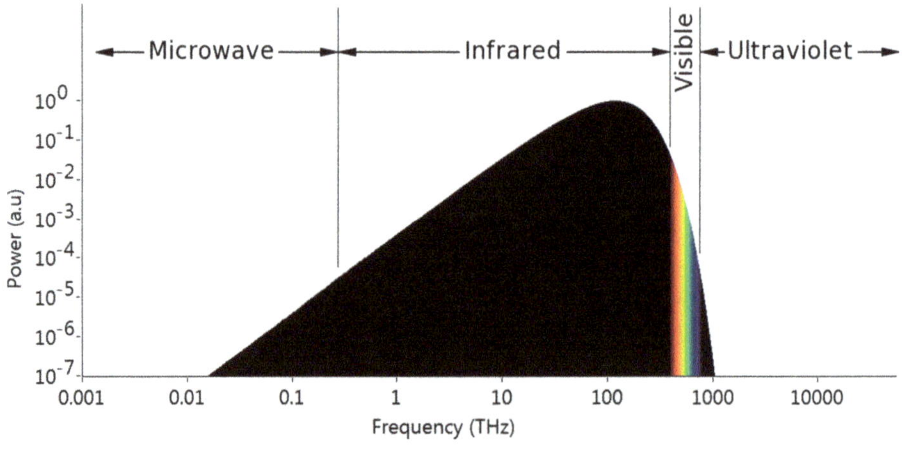

Figure 3.2. Emission intensity versus frequency. Source: [23].

activity in the tumor area. The tumor temperature was found to be 1 °C to 3 °C higher than surrounding healthy tissues in 16 out of 17 patients [23, 25]. The early development was done in infrared frequency range for thermography based diagnosis equipment. Figure 3.2 shows higher levels of emission in the infrared frequency range which is the reason for initial development of thermography equipment [23]. The potential of microwave radiometry to detect malignant tumors in the female breast was reported by [26–31]. Improved transmission characteristics at lower frequencies compensate for the lower level of emission. The research is proposed to calculate or measure dielectric properties of various biological tissues at microwave frequencies in [32–40]. Figure 3.4 shows depth of penetration versus frequency for various types of body tissues with different levels of water [23]. The lower frequencies allow detection at greater depths in the human body. Noise has been generated by all the components of radiometers so the system output has noise received by the antenna as well as noise generated within the system. Gain variations within the system also result in output fluctuations beyond the signal level to be measured. Minimum detectable temperature sensitivity can be calculated by using equation (3.9).

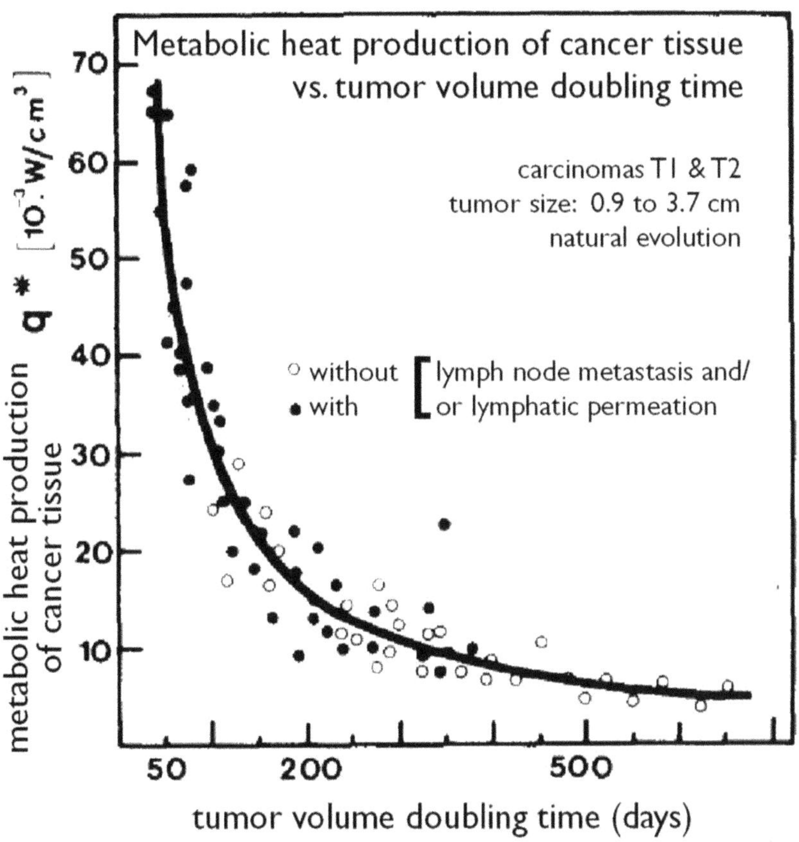

Figure 3.3. Temperature versus doubling time of tumor volume. Reprinted with permission from [45].

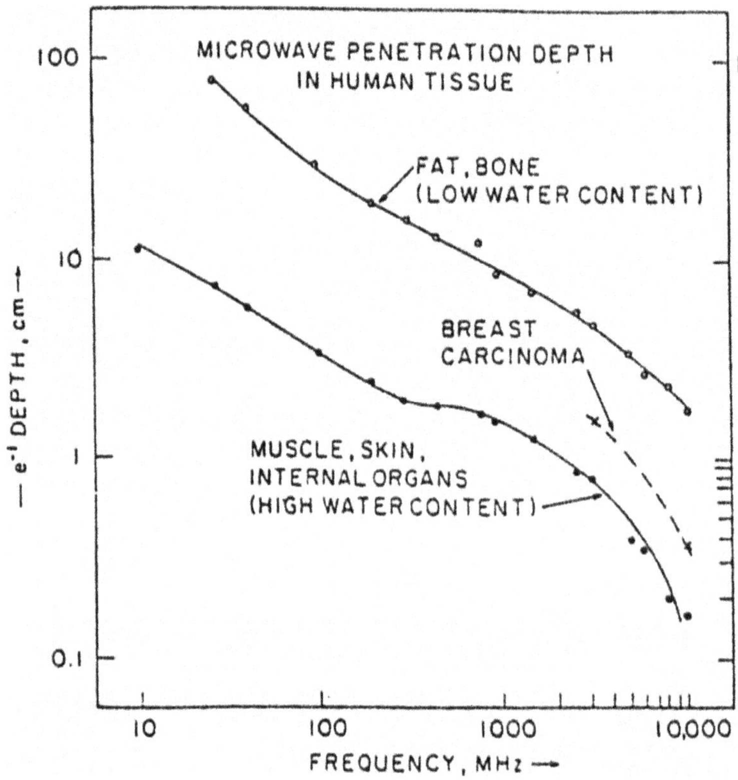

Figure 3.4. Temperature versus doubling time of tumor volume. Source: [23].

$$\Delta T_s = \frac{\Delta G}{G}(T_1 - T_2) \tag{3.9}$$

In equation (3.9), ΔG is change in the gain, G is the receiver gain, T_1 is the reference load temperature in kelvin, T_2 is the antenna temperature in kelvin. Microwave radiometric imaging is presented for the exploration of benign and malignant breast tumors at 3 GHz [41].

3.3.1 Multiprobe radiometric imaging

Small breast tumors cannot be detected or characterized by mammography and these small tumors may be benign most of the time. A multiprobe radiometer based imaging process has been used to improve tumor localization by increasing the number of measurements. Figure 3.5 shows the multiprobe radiometer based imaging process setup [41, 42].

Figure 3.5 shows 12 different locations of the multiprobe on a square area of 6.6 cm × 6.6 cm. Overlapping of elementary areas covered by multiprobes is used for data capturing and processing. Probe positioning logic is shown in figure 3.6 [41]. In figure 3.6, the excess temperature at point A is calculated by equation (3.10).

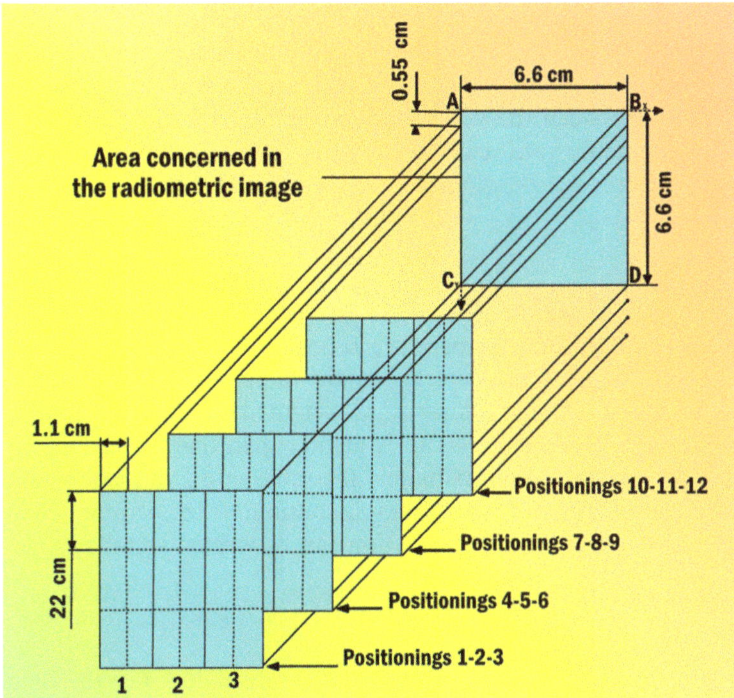

Figure 3.5. Temperature versus doubling time of tumor volume. Copyright (1990) IEEE. Reprinted with permission, from [41].

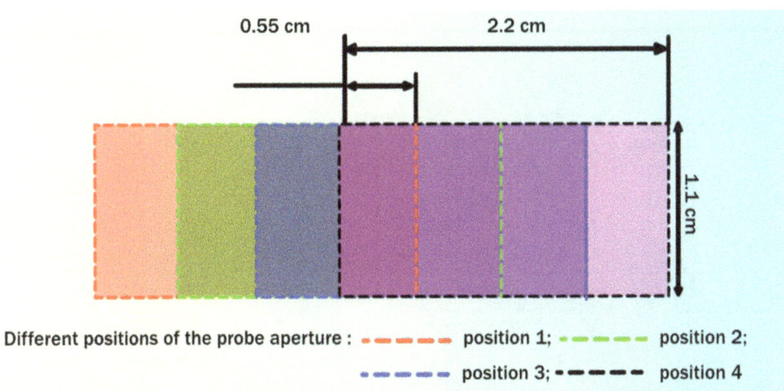

Figure 3.6. Temperature versus doubling time of tumor volume. Copyright (1990) IEEE. Reprinted with permission, from [41].

$$\Delta Tm_{\mathrm{A}} = 0.125\Delta Tm_1 + 0.375\Delta Tm_2 + 0.375\Delta Tm_3 + 0.125\Delta Tm_4 \tag{3.10}$$

In equation (3.10), ΔTm_i is the radiometric temperature measured by the probe i ($i = 1$–4). The image formation using multiprobe radiometry is helpful in detection of small breast tumors. This technique is used to find out the type of breast tumor as well. Pathological and reference breasts are shown in figure 3.7 [41]. It shows the difference of temperature (Δ1) between warmest point image, T_t and the temperature T_r of the symmetrical point image of a reference breast, and the difference of temperature (Δ2) between the warmest point image and the coldest one in set of breast. The radiometric ratio can be found by using quantities Δ1 and Δ2. The temperature measured by a radiometer can be calculated by using equation (3.11).

$$T_{\text{rad}} = \frac{\iiint T(r)P_r(r)\,\mathrm{d}r}{\iiint P_r(r)\,\mathrm{d}r} \tag{3.11}$$

In equation (3.11), $T(r)$ is the temperature at position r, $P_r(r)$ is the antenna receiving pattern, T_{rad} is the temperature detected by the radiometer. Temperature measured by radiometer is the average temperature weighted by field distribution antenna pattern. If the antenna aperture width is greater than one wavelength in the body tissues then $P_r(r)$ decays at approximately the same rate as a plane wave, it decays faster for smaller antennas. There are no discontinuous temperature changes in the body tissues. The bioheat transfer equation can be written as follows.

$$\nabla \cdot (k_t \nabla \cdot T) - w_b c_b (T - T_a) + q = \rho_t c_t \frac{\partial T}{\partial t} \tag{3.12}$$

In equation (3.12), k_t is the tissue thermal conductivity, T is the tissue temperature, T_a is the arterial blood temperature, w_b is the tissue perfusion rate (in units of mass per unit volume per unit time), C_b and c_r are the specific heat of the blood and tissue, ρ_t is the density of the tissue and q is the volumetric rate of heat generation.

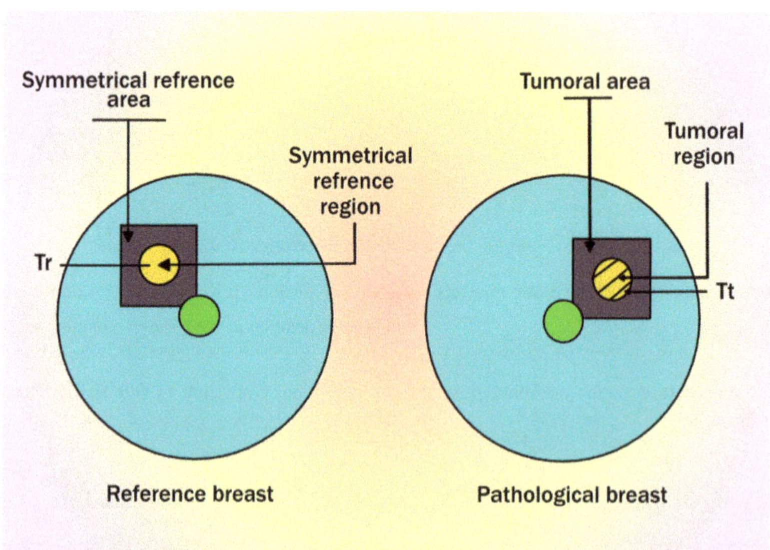

Figure 3.7. Thermological investigation of small breast region. Copyright (1990) IEEE. Reprinted with permission, from [41].

Under steady state condition, constant heat generation in homogeneous medium due to metabolism can be calculated by using equation (3.13).

$$\nabla^2\theta - \beta^2 = 0 \tag{3.13}$$

Geometry of heat transfer problem is applicable in the body tissues as well. However, it gives approximate values of the temperature profiles for human body tissues. The Dicke radiometer signal is described by equation (3.14) [43].

$$S = (1 - |\rho|^2)(T_{\text{app}} - T_{\text{R}}) \tag{3.14}$$

In equation (3.14), ρ is the reflection coefficient between the antenna and the material, T_{R} is the reference temperature, T_{app} is the radiometric temperature. Reference temperature can be adjusted at radiometric temperature to get a zero signal. Spatial resolution has been increased by applying a multiprobe radiometric imaging method as mentioned above. For each patient, two images are formed as shown in figure 3.7. The radiometric coefficient R is calculated by using equation (3.15) [43].

$$R = \frac{T_{\text{T}} - T_{\text{R}}}{\Delta T_{\text{max}}} \times 100 \tag{3.15}$$

In equation (3.15), T_{T} is the radiometric temperature at the suspicious breast region, T_{R} is the radiometric temperature on the symmetrical point on the healthy breast, the maximum radiometric temperature difference between warmer and colder breast regions. Malignant and benign tumors can be distinguished by using the value of radiometric coefficient R. The higher values of R indicate malignant breast tumors, whereas lower values of R are associated with benign breast tumors. The absolute weighting function (AWF) can be calculated by using equation (3.16) to represent the signal emitted by the thermal object [43].

$$C_i(f) = (1 - |\rho|^2)\frac{\sigma_i|E_i(f)|^2}{\sum_{i=0}^{\infty}\sigma_i|E_i(f)|^2} \tag{3.16}$$

In equation (3.16), σ_i is the dielectric conductivity of the elementary volume ΔV_i, E_i is the electric field produced in elementary volume ΔV_i and ρ is the reflection coefficient at the interface. AWF represents the increase in the radiometric degree of an elementary volume for 1 K physical temperature increase. The summation of each elementary cell contribution gives radiometric temperature.

$$T_{\text{app}} = \sum C_i T_i \tag{3.17}$$

The two-dimensional convolution between the excess of physical temperature $\Delta T(x, y)$ and AWF $C_{z_0}(x, y)$ at depth z_0 represents the excess radiometric temperature $\Delta T_{\text{app}}(x, y)$ due to probe displacement. Noise is added to the convolution for a realistic situation.

$$\Delta T_{\text{app}}(x, y) = \Delta T(x, y) * C_{z_0}(x, y) + n(x, y) \tag{3.18}$$

In equation (3.18), C_{z_0} is given by equation (3.19)

$$C_{z_0}(x, y) = \int_{-\text{infty}}^{z_0} C_i(x, y, z)\mathrm{d}z \tag{3.19}$$

It is essential to know AWF for the analysis of radiometric signal. Both structure and permittivity should be known to calculate AWF. A temperature profile of breast tissues is obtained by solving the inverse problem. The resolution is always restricted due to the ill-posed nature of the inverse problem. Equation (3.20) is obtained after applying Fourier transform to equation (3.18).

$$\Delta T_{\text{app}}(u, v) = \Delta T(u, v)C_{z_0}(u, v) + n(u, v) \tag{3.20}$$

Now, a filtering approach is used to improve resolution of the image. Regularization is also widely applied due to the ill-posed nature of the inverse problem. The regularized solution is given by using equation (3.21) [43].

$$\Delta T(u, v) = \frac{C_{z_0}^*}{|C_{z_0}(u, v)|^2 + \lambda(1 + (u^2 + v^2)^2)}\Delta T_{\text{app}}(u, v) \tag{3.21}$$

In the above equation $C_{z_0}^*(u, v)$ is the spectral conjugate of AWF, λ is the regularization parameter. The characterization of breast tumor at an early stage can be achieved by microwave radiometry.

3.3.2 Multi-frequency microwave radiometry

Single frequency microwave radiometry is used to measure average temperature of a certain area of the body. Sometimes information about temperature profile and location of heat source is not available. The area of increased temperature indicates possibility of a tumor inside the body region. It is better to have multi- frequency microwave thermography for accuracy improvement. This method works based on improving thermal radiation intensity and decreasing depth of penetration in body tissues for multiple frequencies. The temperature brightness (T_q) increase is associated with the increased physical temperature (T) of the internal heat source. The following formula expresses the relationship between T_q and T.

$$T_q = T\exp\left(-\frac{d_q}{\delta_q}\right) \tag{3.22}$$

where d_q is a distance and δ_q is a depth of penetration in glandular tissues. Temperature brightness (T_f) increase measured by a radiometer at frequency f relies on the reflection coefficient and tissue interface (Γ_f). T_f is given by equation (3.23).

$$T_f = T_a(1 - |\Gamma_f|^2)K_T = T_q K_f \tag{3.23}$$

In equation (3.23), K_T is a ratio of displayed temperature increase to real temperature increase, K_f is a coefficient for actual antenna tissue matching. The problem is to determine unknown temperature distribution in the particular body area. Here multiple frequency microwave radiometric measurements are done by taking different values of frequencies. Multi-frequency data generates more insights about a tumor present in the body.

3.4 Active microwave imaging

Design complexity of the radiometer is very high in passive microwave imaging. Noise removal is also very challenging because human body tissues radiate a very low power electromagnetic signal. Noise can easily change the thermal profile calculated through microwave radiometry. In order to avoid these drawbacks, active microwave imaging was introduced. In active microwave imaging, low power microwave signals are transmitted towards the object to be imaged. Transmitted signals interact with the body tissues and are scattered in different directions. These scattered signals are captured by the antennas. The setup for active microwave imaging is shown in figure 3.8. Antennas are placed surrounding the body or object to be imaged. Transmitter antennas transmit microwave signals on to the body. These emitted signals from antennas interact with the body or object. Signals get scattered due to the above interactions. Scattered signals are received by the antennas, as shown in the figure. In figure 3.8, transmitter and reciver antennas are different so it is an example of a bi-static imaging system setup. A mono-static microwave imaging setup is shown in figure 3.9. In figure 3.9, all antennas can transmit and receive microwave signals. Forward and inverse scattering are two main types of problems involved in active microwave imaging. In the forward problem, the object or body part dielectric or electric properties and incident signals are known. The scattered electric field at antennas due to body part or object is unknown. In the forward problem scattered electric field at different antenna locations is determined by using known incident electric field and object properties.

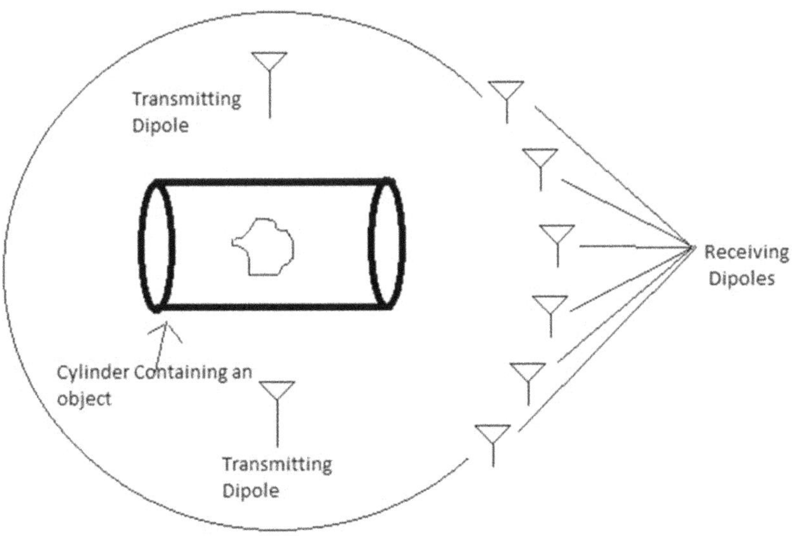

Figure 3.8. General active microwave imaging setup. Source: [44].

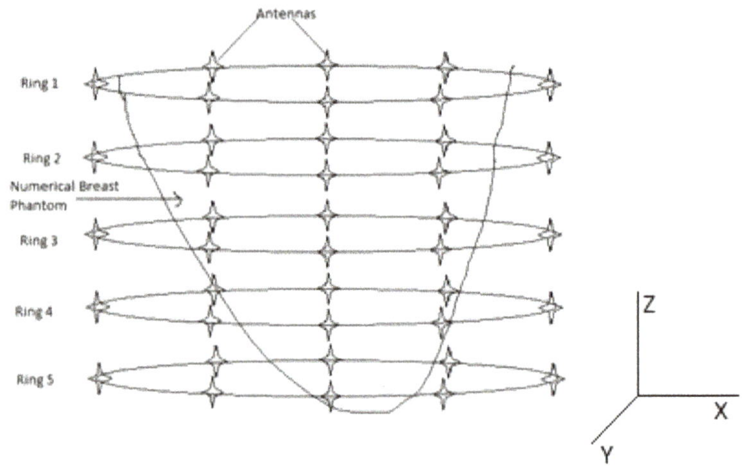

Figure 3.9. Active microwave breast imaging setup. Source: [44].

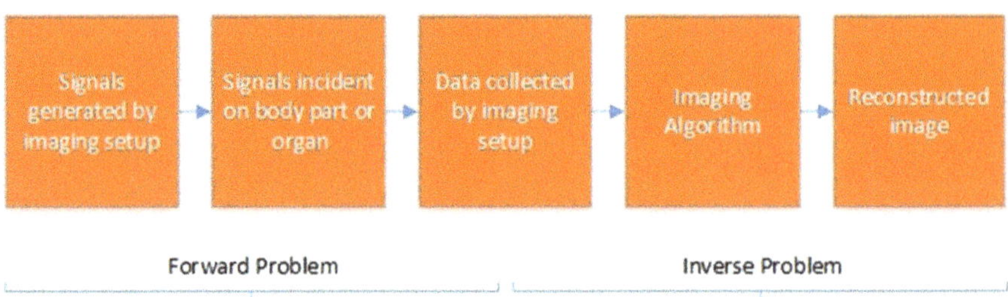

Figure 3.10. Block diagram of forward and inverse problems.

On the other hand, in inverse scattering problems, incident and scattered electric field profiles are known. In inverse scattering problems, the object's electric or dielectric properties are determined by using incident and scattered electric field profiles. Maxwell's equations are shown below in differential form. Forward and inverse problems are solved in medical microwave imaging. Forward and inverse problems of medical microwave imaging are shown in figure 3.10 for basic understanding. Data is collected for diagnosis of the breast using microwave imaging. This data collection process is known as a forward problem. A microwave image of the breast is reconstructed using this collected data, which is often known as an inverse problem. The imaging algorithm of figure 3.10 takes measured data as an input and gives a reconstructed image as an output.

$$\frac{\partial B}{\partial t}(r, t) + \nabla \times E(r, t) = 0 \tag{3.24}$$

In equation (3.24), $\frac{\partial B}{\partial t}(r, t)$ is time changing magnetic flux density, $\nabla \times E(r, t)$ is curl of electric field intensity. Equation (3.24) proves that the spatial variations of electric field generate a time varying magnetic field.

$$\frac{\partial D}{\partial t}(r,\ t) - \nabla \times H(r,\ t) + J(r,\ t) = 0 \tag{3.25}$$

In equation (3.25), $\frac{\partial D}{\partial t}(r,\ t)$ is time varying electric field density, $\nabla \times H(r,\ t)$ is curl of magnetic field intensity, $J(r,\ t)$ is current density. The equation (3.25) proves that the spatial variations of magnetic field generate a time varying electric field.

$$\nabla \cdot B(r,\ t) = 0 \tag{3.26}$$

In equation (3.26), $\nabla \cdot B(r,\ t)$ is divergence of magnetic flux density. Equation (3.26) indicates that the divergence of magnetic flux density is zero. Magnetic field lines originate from the north pole and terminate on the south pole of the magnet so net divergence is zero.

$$\nabla \cdot D(r,\ t) = \rho(r,\ t) \tag{3.27}$$

In equation (3.27), $\nabla \cdot D(r,\ t)$ is divergence of electric flux density, $\rho(r,\ t)$ is the volume charge density. Equation (3.27) proves that the electric flux coming out of any volume is equal to the charge density of that volume. If harmonic time dependence is assumed then the above Maxwell's equations can be written as follows.

$$\nabla \times E(r) = j\omega B(r) \tag{3.28}$$

$$\nabla \times H(r) = -j\omega D(r) + J(r) \tag{3.29}$$

$$\nabla \cdot B(r) = 0 \tag{3.30}$$

$$\nabla \cdot D(r) = \rho(r) \tag{3.31}$$

In the above equations, $\omega = 2\pi f$ is angular frequency and j is $\sqrt{-1}$. By taking divergence of the equation (3.25) and applying the above relations, the following equation is obtained.

$$\frac{\partial \rho}{\partial t}(r,\ t) + \nabla J(r,\ t) = 0 \tag{3.32}$$

Equation (3.32) is related to equation (3.27). The relationship between D and E is specified by equation (3.33).

$$D = \epsilon E \tag{3.33}$$

The relationship between B and H is specified by equation (3.34).

$$B = \mu H \tag{3.34}$$

The above equations specify polarization and magnetization acquired by materials due to incident electromagnetic fields. Human body tissues do not response instantaneously to applied external electromagnetic fields. Permittivity of body tissue is complex due to the above reason. Biological tissues are nonmagnetic so relative permeability is equal to one. Now equation (3.29) can be written as equation (3.35).

$$\nabla \times H(r) + j\omega\left[\epsilon(r, \omega) + j\frac{\sigma(r, \omega)}{\omega}\right]E(r) = J_{\mathrm{a}}(r) \tag{3.35}$$

In the above equation, $J = \sigma E + J_{\mathrm{a}}$, where J_{a} is the applied current density. From equation (3.35), permittivity can be written as shown by equation (3.36).

$$\epsilon_0 \epsilon_{\mathrm{r}}^*(r, \omega) = \epsilon_0\left[\epsilon(r, \omega) + j\frac{\sigma(r, \omega)}{\omega}\right] \tag{3.36}$$

From equation (3.36), the relative permittivity is a complex quantity for biological tissues. The complex permittivity profile of biological tissues is obtained in microwave imaging problems. Resolution, location and accuracy are important metrics for the performance measurement of microwave imaging systems.

3.5 Summary

Passive and active microwave imaging techniques are described in this chapter. Passive microwave imaging emission principles, radiative transfer, bioheat transfer and temperature resolution are discussed. Multiprobe radiometric imaging and multi-frequency microwave radiometry techniques are described for cancer detection. We present an overview of active microwave imaging with block diagram, setup and basic mathematical overview.

References

[1] Enander B and Larson G 1977 Microwave radiometric measurements of the temperature inside a body *Electron. Lett.* **10** 317

[2] Barrett A H and Myers P C 1972 Investigation of microwave radiometry as a medical diagnostic technique

[3] Bigu-del-Blanco J, Romero-Sierra C and Watts D G 1975 Microwave radiometry and its potential applications in biology and medicine: experimental studies *Biotelemetry* **2** 298–316

[4] Edrich J and Hardee P C 1976 Complex permittivity and penetration depth of muscle and fat tissues between 40 and 90 GHz *IEEE Trans. Microw. Theory Techn.* **24** 273–5

[5] Edrich J and Smyth C J 1978 Arthritis inflammation monitored by subcutaneous millimeter wave thermography *J. Rheumatol.* **5** 59–67

[6] Edrich J 1979 Centimeter-and millimeter-wave thermography—A survey on tumor detection *J. Microw. Power* **14** 95–104

[7] Edrich J 1975 Microwave absorption of living human skin between 8 and 96 GHz *Proc. 5th Europ. Microw. Conf., Hamburg* (Tunbridge Wells: Microwave Exhibitions & Publishers Ltd) 361–5

[8] Johnson C C and Guy A W 1972 Nonionizing electromagnetic effects in biological materials and systems *Proc. IEEE* **60** 692–716

[9] Schwan H P 1965 Biophysics of diathermy *Therapeutic Heat and Cold* ed S Licht Sec. 12 (New Haven, CT: Williams & Wilkins) pp 310–20

[10] Chandrasekhar S 1950 *Radiative Transfer* (Oxford: Oxford University Press)

[11] Edrich J 1975 Microwave absorption of living human skin between 8 and 96 GHz *Proc. 5th Europ. Microw. Conf. (Hamburg)* (Tunbridge Wells: Microwave Exhibitions & Publishers Ltd) 361–5

[12] Myers P C and Barrett A H 1977 Microwave thermography: physical principles and diagnostic applications *Proc. Workshop on Physical Basis of Electromagnetic Interactions with Biological Systems (College Park, MD)* 309–25
[13] Wulff W 1974 The energy conservation equation for living tissue *IEEE Trans. Biomed. Eng.* **21** 494
[14] Tabern D L *et al* 1966 Experimental studies on thermal measurements over animal and human tumors *Surgery* **60** 1058
[15] Omai Y, Uchida I and Tomaru T *et al* 1973 Some basic studies on breast thermography using phantoms for detection of tumors *Medical Thermography* (University of Tokyo Press: Tokyo) pp 179–91
[16] Nilson I K 1975 Skin temperature over an artificial heat source implanted in man *Phys. Med. Biol.* **20** 366–14
[17] Foster K R, Kritikos H N and Schwan H P 1978 Effect of surface cooling and blood flow on the microwave heating of tissue *IEEE Trans. Biomed. Eng.* **25** 313–6
[18] Cacak R K, Edrich J, Hendee W R, Shenton D W and Winans D H 1978 Phantom evaluation of millimeter wave thermography *Dig. 20th Ann. Meet. AAPM* 105
[19] Edrich J, Cacak R K and Hendee W R 1979 Centimeter- and millimeter-wave thermography: a survey on tumor detection *J. Microw. Power.* **14** 95–104
[20] Kraus J D 1966 *Radio Atronomy* (New York: McGraw-Hill)
[21] Staelin D H 1969 Passive remote sensing at microwave wavelengths *Proc. IEEE* **57** 427
[22] Kraus J D 1950 *Antennas* (New York: McGraw-Hill)
[23] Carr K L 1989 Microwave radiometry: its importance to the detection of cancer *IEEE Trans. Microw. Theory Tech.* **37** 1862–9
[24] Gautherie M and Albert E 1982 *Clinical Thermohioloa* (New York: Alan R. Liss)
[25] Noell U R, Woodward K, Worde K, Fishbum B R and Miller L 1980 Microwave-induced local hyperthermia in combination with radiotherapy of human malignant tumors *Cancer (Philadelphia)* **45** 638–46
[26] Barrett A H, Myers P C and Sadowsky N L 1977 Detection of breast cancer by microwave radiometry *Radio Sci.* **12** 167
[27] Myers P C, Sadowsky N L and Barrett A H 1979 Microwave thermograph: principles, methods and clinical applications *J. Microw. Power* **14** 105–15
[28] Enander B and Larson G 1974 Microwave radiometric measurements on the temperature inside the body *Electron. Lett.* **10** 317–9
[29] Mamouni A, Bliot F, Leroy Y and Moschetto Y 1977 A modified radiometer for temperature and microwave properties measurements of biological substances *7th European Microwave Conf. (Copenhagen)* 703–7
[30] Carr K L, El-Mahdi A M and Shaeffer J 1981 Dual-mode microwave system to enhance early detection of cancer *IEEE Trans. Microw. Theory, Techn.* **29** 256–60
[31] Porter R A and Miller H H 1978 Microwave radiometric detection and location of breast cancer *ELECTRO (Boston, MA)*
[32] Schwan H P 1968 Radiation biology, medical applications, and radiation hazards *Microw. Power Eng.* **2** 215–34
[33] Schwan H P and Foster K R 1980 RF field interactions with biological systems: Electrical properties and biophysical mechanisms *Proc. IEEE* **68** 104–13
[34] Barber P W, Gandh O P, Hagmann M J and Chattejee I 1979 Electromagnetic absorption in a multi-layered model of man *IEEE Trans. Biomed. Eng.* **BME-26** 400

[35] Schwan H P 1957 Electrical properties of tissues and cells *Adu. Biol. Med. Phys.* **5** 147–209

[36] Barrett A H and Myers P C 1981 Microwave thermography *Progress Report, no. 123* Research Laboratory of Electronics (RLE) at the Massachusetts Institute of Technology (MIT) pp 45–56

[37] Dicke R H 1946 The measurement of thermal radiation at microwave frequencies *Rei. Sci. Inslr.* **17** 268–75

[38] Ludeke K M and Kohler J 1983 Microwave radiometric system for biomedical 'true temperature' and emissivity measurements *J. Microw. Power* **18** 277–83

[39] Carr K L, Bielawa R J, Regan J F, El-Mahdi A M and Shaeffer J 1983 The effect of antenna match on microwave radiometric thermal patterns *in IEEE MTT-S Int. Microwave Sympos. Dig.* 189–91

[40] Shaeffer J, El-Mahdi A M, Bielawa R J, Regan J F and Carr K L 1982 Thermal drift in microwave thermography *in IEEE MTT-S Int. Microwave Sympos. Dig.* 441–3

[41] Bocquet B, Van de Velde J C, Mamouni A, Leroy Y, Giaux G, Delannoy J and Delvalee D 1990 Microwave radiometric imaging at 3 GHz for the exploration of breast tumors *IEEE Trans. Microw. Theory Techn.* **38** 791–3

[42] Cheever E A and Foster K R 1990 Microwave radiometry in living tissue: what does it measure? *IEEE Trans. Biomed. Eng.* **39** 563–8

[43] Mouty S, Bocquet B, Ringot R, Rocourt N and Devos P 2000 Microwave radiometric imaging (MWI) for the characterisation of breast tumours *Europ. Phys. J.: Appl. Phys.* **10** 73–8

[44] Patel H N 2019 Microwave imaging for breast cancer detection using 3D level set based optimization, FDTD method and method of moments *PhD Dissertation* Dhirubhai Ambani Institute of Information and Communication Technology

[45] Vesnin S, Turnbull A K, Dixon J M and Goryanin I 2017 Modern microwave thermometry for breast cancer *J. Mol. Imaging Dynam.* **7** 2

Hardik N Patel, Deepak K Ghodgaonkar and Jasjit S Suri

Chapter 4

Finite difference time domain method for microwave breast imaging

Finite difference time domain (FDTD) was proposed to solve Maxwell's equations on a discrete grid in 1966 by Yee [1]. FDTD offers unique advantages of multi-frequency electromagnetic simulation and the possibility of time domain inversion. Breasts can be discretized in small voxels and FDTD can be applied to find the electromagnetic field absorbed, scattered and transmitted through it. These electric fields can be used to reconstruct breast images for cancer diagnosis. Method of moments and finite element method are used in frequency domain and require large memory and ill-posed matrix inversion. FDTD is advantageous because it can avoid ill-posed matrix inversion. However, FDTD is complex due to perfectly matched layer (PML) and source design. FDTD provides better results up to several gigahertz. All FDTD update equations are derived in this chapter for better understanding of microwave breast imaging.

4.1 Overview of computational electromagnetic methods

Microwave imaging for the human body started around the 1950s. Computational electromagnetic methods (CEM) were developed due to unavailability of an analytical solution of Maxwell's equations. There are two types of computational electromagnetic method for microwave imaging.

1. Low frequency (exact) methods.
2. High frequency (approximate) methods.

4.1.1 Low frequency methods

Low frequency methods solve Maxwell's equations without any approximations. These methods solve small electric size problems due to lack of computational power

doi:10.1088/978-0-7503-2592-9ch4

in the past. Computation time and system memory were two major problems with these type of methods.

4.1.1.1 Finite difference time domain (FDTD)

Finite difference time domain (FDTD) was first proposed by Yee [1]. In FDTD, Maxwell's equation's are solved using a grid-like structure, so this grid is often known as a Yee grid. The structure or object to be imaged is discretized into rectangular or curvilinear elements. Now Maxwell's equations are solved using this discretized structure with a leapfrog in time to calculate electric and magnetic fields. There are several advantages and disadvantages of this method.

Advantages

- Multiple frequency simulation.
- Easy to include different dispersion models.
- Fast as compared to frequency domain methods.

Disadvantages

- Fourier transform is often required at each iteration.
- The grid is truncated at the boundary which increases complexity.
- It is not suitable for higher microwave frequencies.

4.1.1.2 Finite element method (FEM)

Finite element method (FEM) is frequency domain technique to solve boundary value electromagnetic problems. Two- and three-dimensional canonical elements with different shapes can be used to discretize the structure, giving highly accurate results. Advantages and disadvantages of this method are given below.

Advantages

- Accurate discretization.
- Accurate field distribution calculation in cavity and waveguides.

Disadvantages

- Multi-frequency simulation consumes large memory.
- The grid is truncated at the boundary which makes it unsuitable for several problems.
- It is not suitable for higher microwave frequencies.

4.1.1.3 Method of moments (MoM)

Method of moments (MoM) is a frequency domain method [3, 4]. It solves electric field integral equation (EFIE) after discretization of object or structure. Advantages and disadvantages of MoM are given below.

Advantages

- Suitable for radiation and scattering problems.
- Discretization is easy.

Disadvantages

- Large memory space is required for problems with large objects.
- Multiple frequency computation is difficult.
- It is not suitable for higher microwave frequencies.

4.1.2 High frequency methods

Large-size electromagnetic problems existed even before the invention of the computer. Radar cross-section and antenna radiation pattern calculations are considered as large-scale problems. Ray optics and edge diffraction are used to solve high frequency problems with approximations.

4.1.2.1 Geometrical theory of diffraction

Ray optics based electromagnetic wave propagation is used in geometrical theory of diffraction (GTD) [5]. Fermat's principle is used to calculate spreading, amplitude intensity and decay. It is useful to find the electromagnetic field in shadow regions. GTD is fast but it results in poor accuracy for complex geometries.

4.1.2.2 Physical optics (PO) and physical theory of diffraction (PTD)

This is a method for approximation of high frequency surface currents, so that the fields are obtained through boundary integration [6]. PO and MoM are both used to solve the same type of integral equation. MoM directly solves the integral equation, whereas PO solves it through approximations. High frequency reflector antenna analysis and radar cross-section prediction are done by using physical optics. The physical theory of diffraction is used to add nonuniform currents due to diffraction at the edges.

4.1.2.3 Ray optics

Ray optics is used to model multiple back scattering due to complex objects [7, 8]. It determines the path and amplitudes of different rays due to scattering. Wave propagation and scattering in a complex urban environment for cellular services are calculated by using ray optics.

4.2 Motivation

Simultaneous acquisition of multi-frequency vector electromagnetic fields data is possible using 3D FDTD over a large or narrow bandwidth of interest. Multiple frequency total electric field vector data acquisition is achieved in just one FDTD simulation which makes it efficient. In this chapter, 3D FDTD is used to get multiple frequency total field vector data inside a numerical human breast model. Complex permittivity distribution of the human breast model is represented by Debye model. Perfectly matched layer (PML) is required at all boundaries for the absorption of microwave signals. Two different sets of 3D FDTD update equations are required for implementation in numerical breast phantom and PML regions, respectively. In this chapter, the effect of malignant breast tissues on electric field distribution is evaluated.

4.3 Overview of FDTD

Yee showed a novel method to solve Maxwell's equations by using finite difference on a discrete grid. Now it is very well known as the Yee grid for solution of Maxwell's equations [9]. Taflove gave a numerical method to solve the sinusoidal steady state of electromagnetic fields penetration in an arbitrary dielectric or conducting body by introducing lattice truncation conditions and loss factors [10]. Small air-dielectric loss factors are introduced to accelerate the sinusoidal steady state convergence of cavity interior fields. This method was evaluated by using experimental results via application to a dielectric sphere and a cylindrical metal cavity with an aperture. Okonievski *et al* have shown three simple and efficient algorithms to incorporate multi-term Debye or Lorentz dispersion in the FDTD method [11].

Hagness *et al* have shown time-gating and pulsed confocal techniques to enhance tumour detection by suppressing absorption and tissue heterogeneity effects in [12]. A 2D FDTD analysis of the system is done by using published data for the dielectric properties of malignant tumors and normal breast tissues. The FDTD simulation results proved that the small tumors can be detected robustly in the presence of the background clutter. Hagness *et al* have proposed a pulsed microwave confocal system by using 3D FDTD for breast cancer detection in [13].

Bond *et al* have shown microwave imaging via space–time (MIST) beam-forming for detecting early-stage breast cancer in [14]. An ultra wideband (UWB) signal is transmitted sequentially from each antenna of the array. The data-adaptive algorithm is used to remove artifacts in this method. The effectiveness of this algorithm is shown by using a variety of MRI derived numerical breast phantoms. Malignant tumours embedded in the complex fibro-glandular structure are easily detected in [14]. Li *et al* have shown an experimental study of UWB antenna performance for dielectric contrast of malignant to normal breast tissues in [15]. Research work of Li *et al* represents the first experimental demonstration of three dimensions MIST beam-forming for malignant-to-normal dielectric contrasts down to 1.5:1 with a synthetic tumour in multilayer breast phantoms.

Kosmas and Rappaport have proposed a time reversal algorithm to detect breast cancer in [16]. Amplitude and phase information of the tumor response is used to get enough focusing. They have shown that the algorithm is robust to breast inhomogeneities. Guo *et al* have proposed a new FDTD formulation using Cole–Cole model for electromagnetic wave propagation in dispersive biological tissues in [17]. Kosmas and Rappaport have proposed FDTD based time reversal algorithm for three dimensions in [18]. They have shown that the 3D algorithm based reconstructions are better than 2D algorithm based reconstructions. Kosmas and Rappaport have proposed a clutter dominated total signal processing using matched filter approach with FDTD based time reversal algorithm in [19]. A low complexity Cole–Cole model is used with FDTD for human tissues modelling by Kang *et al* [20]. Gedney has proposed a solution to the FDTD lattice truncation problem by using an anisotropic perfectly matched layer (PML) absorbing medium in [21]. Schneider *et al* have proposed FDTD equations which incorporate polarization and different types of dispersions [22]. Taflove and Hagness have proposed FDTD methods and parameters for different cases in [23].

Moll *et al* have proposed a computationally efficient and flexible ray tracing algorithm for microwave based tumor localization in moderate heterogeneous breast tissues in [24]. Easy tumor localization is possible using this proposed method [24]. Moll *et al* have proposed a novel RADAR based beam-forming procedure by using 31 element array configuration and heterogeneous numerical breast phantom for microwave breast cancer detection in [25]. Yin *et al* have proposed a novel adaptive combining through correlation exploration algorithm for breast cancer detection using UWB imaging in [26]. The performance of this algorithm is validated by using accurate 3D FDTD breast models. Song *et al* have proposed a UWB based microwave breast cancer detection system by using MRI derived realistic numerical breast phantom in [27]. Mirza *et al* have implemented 1D, 2D and 3D FDTD numerical methods for breast cancer detection in [28]. They have also discussed the best ways to identify the existence of cancerous tissues in the breast. Wang *et al* have proposed a microwave imaging system with wearable conformal antenna array for breast cancer detection in [29]. A tumor of size 5 mm diameter inside the glandular region can be precisely located and detected by using an FDTD solver of microwave studio in computer simulation technology (CST) [29]. Kwon *et al* have proposed a cost effective breast cancer imaging system with time domain measurements which can reconstruct the breast image in the presence of white noise [30]. The above system can acquire images in a short time so instantaneous microwave imaging is possible.

4.4 Derivation of basic FDTD update equations

Yee proposed a method to solve Maxwell's equations using a discrete grid [1]. This chapter has widely used the concepts of [1, 31, 32]. It is better to understand the basics of the Yee grid before starting derivation of more complex equations. First consider Maxwell's two equations given below.

$$\nabla \times \vec{E} = -\mu \frac{\partial \vec{H}}{\partial t} \tag{4.1}$$

$$\nabla \times \vec{H} = \epsilon \frac{\partial \vec{E}}{\partial t} \tag{4.2}$$

Equations (4.1) and (4.2) are also known as Faraday's and Ampere's laws, respectively. In equation (4.1), $\nabla \times \vec{E}$ is the curl of electric field $\vec{E}$, μ is permeability of the medium, $\frac{\partial \vec{H}}{\partial t}$ is a time varying magnetic field. In equation (4.2), $\nabla \times \vec{H}$ is the curl of magnetic field $\vec{H}$, ϵ is permittivity of the medium, $\frac{\partial \vec{E}}{\partial t}$ is a time varying electric field.

According to equation (4.1), spatial rotation of the electric field generates a time varying magnetic field. According to equation (4.2), spatial rotation of the magnetic

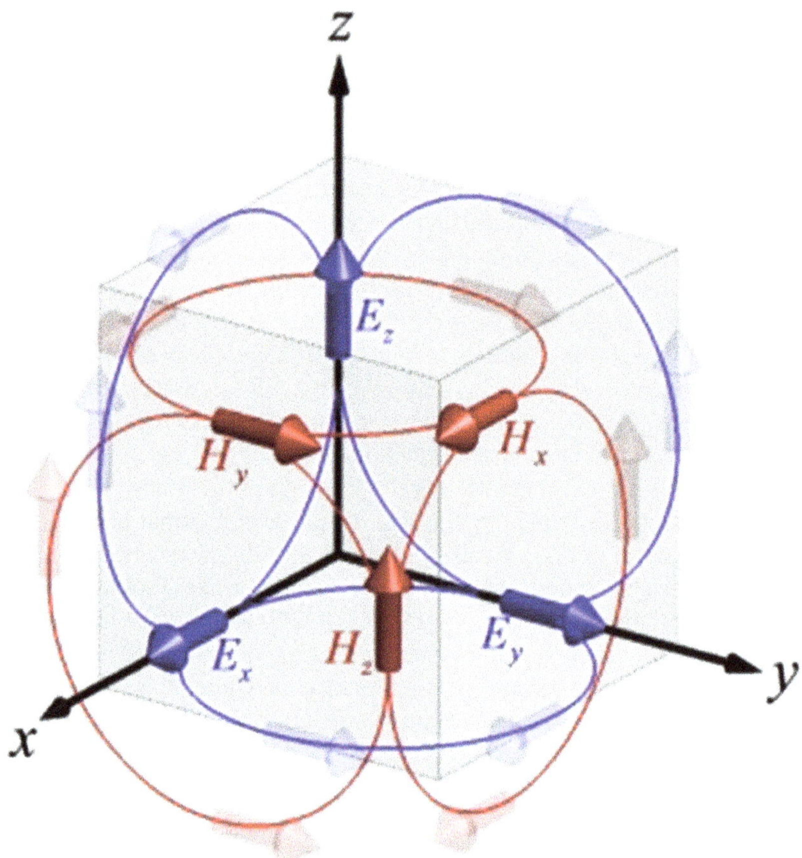

Figure 4.1. Yee grid. Reprinted with permission from Rumpf (2020) https://empossible.net/wp-content/uploads/2020/01/Lecture-Formulation-of-1D-FDTD.pdf.

field generates a time varying electric field. A three-dimensional representation of a Yee grid is shown in figure 4.1.

$$\nabla \times \vec{E} = -\mu_0[\mu_r]\frac{\partial \vec{H}}{\partial t} \tag{4.3}$$

$$\nabla \times \vec{H} = \epsilon_0[\epsilon_r]\frac{\partial \vec{E}}{\partial t} \tag{4.4}$$

It is always good practice to normalize field parameters. Exact impedance is not known ahead of time so free space impedance is used in the normalization process. Consider the equation given below for normalization.

$$\vec{\tilde{H}} = \eta_0\vec{H} \Rightarrow \vec{H} = \frac{\vec{\tilde{H}}}{\eta_0} \tag{4.5}$$

Equations (4.6) and (4.7) are derived by substituting equation (4.5) into equations (4.3) and (4.4). The free space equation of η_0 and some simple steps are used to get the following equations.

$$\nabla \times \vec{E} = -\frac{[\mu_r]}{c_0}\frac{\partial \vec{\tilde{H}}}{\partial t} \tag{4.6}$$

$$\nabla \times \vec{\tilde{H}} = \frac{\epsilon_r}{c_0}\frac{\partial \vec{E}}{\partial t} \tag{4.7}$$

From an implementation point of view, it is very easy to visualize the above equations in terms of matrices. Equations (4.6) and (4.7) are represented in matrix form as shown by equations (4.8) and (4.9).

$$\begin{bmatrix} \hat{i} & \hat{j} & \hat{k} \\ \frac{\partial}{\partial x} & \frac{\partial}{\partial y} & \frac{\partial}{\partial z} \\ E_x & E_y & E_z \end{bmatrix} = -\frac{1}{c_0}\begin{bmatrix} \mu_{xx} & \mu_{xy} & \mu_{xz} \\ \mu_{yx} & \mu_{yy} & \mu_{yz} \\ \mu_{zx} & \mu_{zy} & \mu_{zz} \end{bmatrix}\begin{bmatrix} \frac{\partial \tilde{H}_x}{\partial t} \\ \frac{\partial \tilde{H}_y}{\partial t} \\ \frac{\partial \tilde{H}_z}{\partial t} \end{bmatrix} \tag{4.8}$$

$$\begin{bmatrix} \hat{i} & \hat{j} & \hat{k} \\ \frac{\partial}{\partial x} & \frac{\partial}{\partial y} & \frac{\partial}{\partial z} \\ \tilde{H}_x & \tilde{H}_y & \tilde{H}_z \end{bmatrix} = \frac{1}{c_0}\begin{bmatrix} \epsilon_{xx} & \epsilon_{xy} & \epsilon_{xz} \\ \epsilon_{yx} & \epsilon_{yy} & \epsilon_{yz} \\ \epsilon_{zx} & \epsilon_{zy} & \epsilon_{zz} \end{bmatrix}\begin{bmatrix} \frac{\partial E_x}{\partial t} \\ \frac{\partial E_y}{\partial t} \\ \frac{\partial E_z}{\partial t} \end{bmatrix} \tag{4.9}$$

Some simple matrix calculations and simplification would help to derive the equations given below. Three equations are derived by simplifying equation (4.8) for magnetic field calculations.

$$\frac{\partial E_z}{\partial y} - \frac{\partial E_y}{\partial z} = -\frac{1}{c_0}\left[\mu_{xx}\frac{\partial \tilde{H}_x}{\partial t} + \mu_{xy}\frac{\partial \tilde{H}_y}{\partial t} + \mu_{xz}\frac{\partial \tilde{H}_z}{\partial t}\right] \tag{4.10}$$

$$\frac{\partial E_x}{\partial z} - \frac{\partial E_z}{\partial x} = -\frac{1}{c_0}\left[\mu_{yx}\frac{\partial \tilde{H}_x}{\partial t} + \mu_{yy}\frac{\partial \tilde{H}_y}{\partial t} + \mu_{yz}\frac{\partial \tilde{H}_z}{\partial t}\right] \tag{4.11}$$

$$\frac{\partial E_y}{\partial x} - \frac{\partial E_x}{\partial y} = -\frac{1}{c_0}\left[\mu_{zx}\frac{\partial \tilde{H}_x}{\partial t} + \mu_{zy}\frac{\partial \tilde{H}_y}{\partial t} + \mu_{zz}\frac{\partial \tilde{H}_z}{\partial t}\right] \tag{4.12}$$

Similarly, three equations are derived by simplifying equation (4.9) for electric field calculations.

$$\frac{\partial \tilde{H}_z}{\partial y} - \frac{\partial \tilde{H}_y}{\partial z} = \frac{1}{c_0}\left[\epsilon_{xx}\frac{\partial E_x}{\partial t} + \epsilon_{xy}\frac{\partial E_y}{\partial t} + \epsilon_{xz}\frac{\partial E_z}{\partial t}\right] \tag{4.13}$$

$$\frac{\partial \tilde{H}_x}{\partial z} - \frac{\partial \tilde{H}_z}{\partial x} = \frac{1}{c_0}\left[\epsilon_{yx}\frac{\partial E_x}{\partial t} + \epsilon_{yy}\frac{\partial E_y}{\partial t} + \epsilon_{yz}\frac{\partial E_z}{\partial t}\right] \tag{4.14}$$

$$\frac{\partial \tilde{H}_y}{\partial x} - \frac{\partial \tilde{H}_x}{\partial y} = \frac{1}{c_0}\left[\epsilon_{zx}\frac{\partial E_x}{\partial t} + \epsilon_{zy}\frac{\partial E_y}{\partial t} + \epsilon_{zz}\frac{\partial E_z}{\partial t}\right] \tag{4.15}$$

It is always preferable to start with simple equations. Permittivity and permeability tensors are very important for implementation of different types of materials in computer software. Simplified equations are derived by assuming only nonzero diagonal elements in permeability and permittivity tensors.

$$\frac{\partial E_z}{\partial y} - \frac{\partial E_y}{\partial z} = -\frac{\mu_{xx}}{c_0}\left[\frac{\partial \tilde{H}_x}{\partial t}\right] \tag{4.16}$$

$$\frac{\partial E_x}{\partial z} - \frac{\partial E_z}{\partial x} = -\frac{\mu_{yy}}{c_0}\left[\frac{\partial \tilde{H}_y}{\partial t}\right] \tag{4.17}$$

$$\frac{\partial E_y}{\partial x} - \frac{\partial E_x}{\partial y} = -\frac{\mu_{zz}}{c_0}\left[\frac{\partial \tilde{H}_z}{\partial t}\right] \tag{4.18}$$

Finite difference approximations of electromagnetic fields are calculated by considering the blue circle of figure 4.2. Calculated finite difference approximations are applied to equation (4.16).

$$\frac{E_z^{i,j+1,k} - E_z^{i,j,k}}{\Delta y} - \frac{E_y^{i,j,k+1} - E_z^{i,j,k}}{\Delta z} = -\frac{\mu_{xx}^{i,j,k}}{c_0}\left[\frac{\tilde{H}_x^{i,j,k}\Big|_{t+\frac{\Delta t}{2}} - \tilde{H}_x^{i,j,k}\Big|_{t-\frac{\Delta t}{2}}}{\Delta t}\right] \tag{4.19}$$

Finite difference approximations of electromagnetic fields are calculated by considering the blue circle of figure 4.3. Calculated finite difference approximations are applied to equation (4.17).

$$\frac{E_x^{i,j,k+1} - E_x^{i,j,k}}{\Delta z} - \frac{E_z^{i+1,j,k} - E_z^{i,j,k}}{\Delta x} = -\frac{\mu_{yy}^{i,j,k}}{c_0}\left[\frac{\tilde{H}_y^{i,j,k}\Big|_{t+\frac{\Delta t}{2}} - \tilde{H}_y^{i,j,k}\Big|_{t-\frac{\Delta t}{2}}}{\Delta t}\right] \tag{4.20}$$

Finite difference approximations of electromagnetic fields are calculated by considering the blue circle of figure 4.4. Calculated finite approximations are applied to equation (4.18).

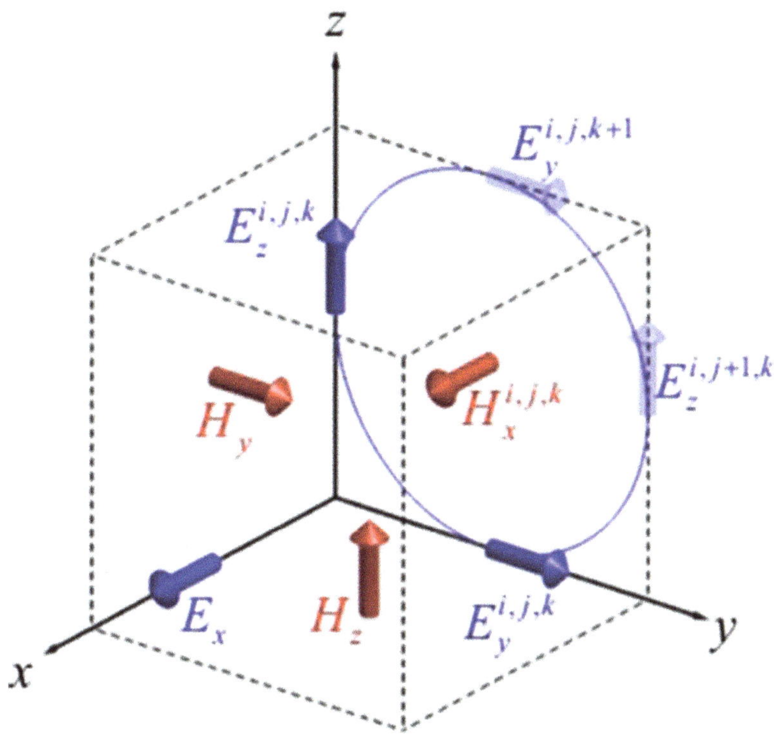

Figure 4.2. Yee grid for finite difference approximations of spatial electric field components and x direction time domain magnetic field. Reprinted with permission from Rumpf (2020) https://empossible.net/wp-content/uploads/2020/01/Lecture-Formulation-of-1D-FDTD.pdf.

$$\frac{E_y^{i+1,j,k+1} - E_y^{i,j,k}}{\Delta x} - \frac{E_x^{i,j+1,k} - E_x^{i,j,k}}{\Delta y} = -\frac{\mu_{zz}^{i,j,k}}{c_0}\left[\frac{\tilde{H}_z^{i,j,k}\Big|_{t+\frac{\Delta t}{2}} - \tilde{H}_z^{i,j,k}\Big|_{t-\frac{\Delta t}{2}}}{\Delta t}\right] \tag{4.21}$$

$$\frac{\partial \tilde{H}_z}{\partial y} - \frac{\partial \tilde{H}_y}{\partial z} = \frac{\epsilon_{xx}}{c_0}\left[\frac{\partial E_x}{\partial t}\right] \tag{4.22}$$

$$\frac{\partial \tilde{H}_x}{\partial z} - \frac{\partial \tilde{H}_z}{\partial x} = \frac{\epsilon_{yy}}{c_0}\left[\frac{\partial E_y}{\partial t}\right] \tag{4.23}$$

$$\frac{\partial \tilde{H}_y}{\partial x} - \frac{\partial \tilde{H}_x}{\partial y} = \frac{\epsilon_{zz}}{c_0}\left[\frac{\partial E_z}{\partial t}\right] \tag{4.24}$$

Finite difference approximations of electromagnetic fields are calculated by considering the blue circle of figure 4.5. Calculated finite difference approximations are applied to equation (4.22).

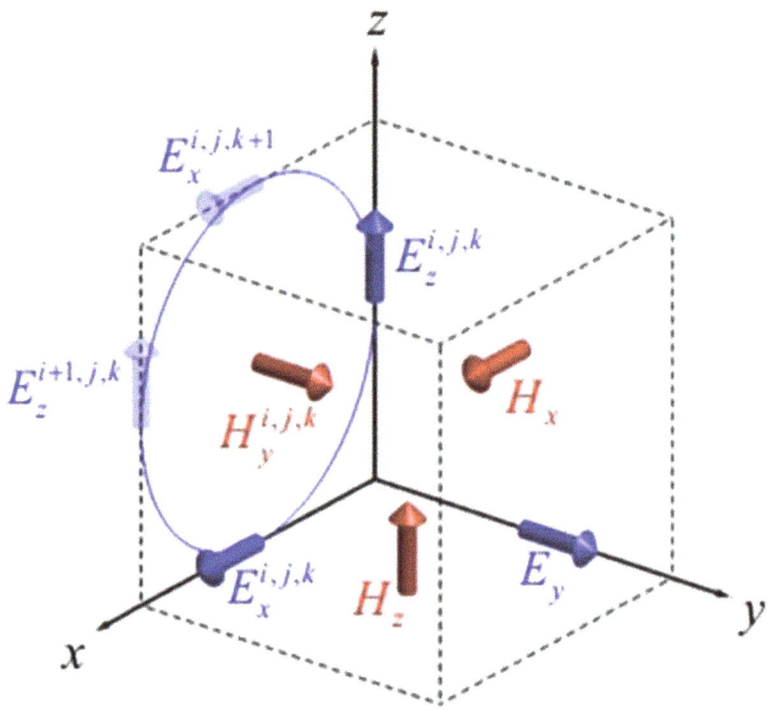

Figure 4.3. Yee grid for finite difference approximations of spatial electric field components and y direction time domain magnetic field. Reprinted with permission from Rumpf (2020) https://empossible.net/wp-content/uploads/2020/01/Lecture-Formulation-of-1D-FDTD.pdf.

$$\frac{\tilde{H}_z^{i,j+1,k}\big|_{t+\frac{\Delta t}{2}} - \tilde{H}_z^{i,j,k}\big|_{t+\frac{\Delta t}{2}}}{\Delta y} - \frac{\tilde{H}_y^{i,j,k+1}\big|_{t+\frac{\Delta t}{2}} - \tilde{H}_y^{i,j,k}\big|_{t+\frac{\Delta t}{2}}}{\Delta z} = \frac{\epsilon_{xx}^{i,j,k}}{c_0}\left[\frac{E_x^{i,j,k}\big|_{t+\Delta t} - E_x^{i,j,k}\big|_t}{\Delta t}\right] \tag{4.25}$$

Finite difference approximations of electromagnetic fields are calculated by considering the blue circle of figure 4.6. Calculated finite difference approximations are applied to equation (4.23).

$$\frac{\tilde{H}_x^{i,j,k+1}\big|_{t+\frac{\Delta t}{2}} - \tilde{H}_x^{i,j,k}\big|_{t+\frac{\Delta t}{2}}}{\Delta z} - \frac{\tilde{H}_z^{i+1,j,k}\big|_{t+\frac{\Delta t}{2}} - \tilde{H}_z^{i,j,k}\big|_{t+\frac{\Delta t}{2}}}{\Delta x} = \frac{\epsilon_{yy}^{i,j,k}}{c_0}\left[\frac{E_y^{i,j,k}\big|_{t+\Delta t} - E_y^{i,j,k}\big|_t}{\Delta t}\right] \tag{4.26}$$

Finite difference approximations of electromagnetic fields are calculated by considering the blue circle of figure 4.7. Calculated finite difference approximations are applied to equation (4.24).

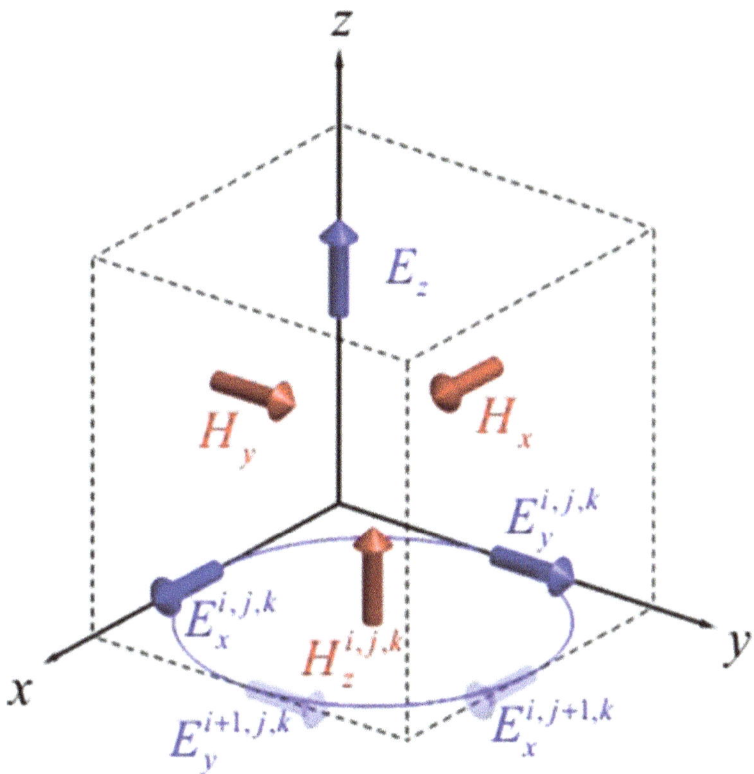

Figure 4.4. Yee grid for finite difference approximations of spatial electric field components and z direction time domain magnetic field. Reprinted with permission from Rumpf (2020) https://empossible.net/wp-content/uploads/2020/01/Lecture-Formulation-of-1D-FDTD.pdf.

$$\frac{\tilde{H}_y^{i+1,j,k}\big|_{t+\frac{\Delta t}{2}} - \tilde{H}_y^{i,j,k}\big|_{t+\frac{\Delta t}{2}}}{\Delta x} - \frac{\tilde{H}_x^{i,j+1,k}\big|_{t+\frac{\Delta t}{2}} - \tilde{H}_x^{i,j,k}\big|_{t+\frac{\Delta t}{2}}}{\Delta y} = \frac{\epsilon_{zz}^{i,j,k}}{c_0}\left[\frac{E_z^{i,j,k}\big|_{t+\Delta t} - E_z^{i,j,k}\big|_t}{\Delta t}\right] \tag{4.27}$$

An FDTD update equation for the x component of magnetic field is derived by simplifying equation (4.19).

$$\tilde{H}_x^{i,j,k}\big|_{t+\frac{\Delta t}{2}} = \tilde{H}_x^{i,j,k}\big|_{t-\frac{\Delta t}{2}} + \frac{c_0 \times \Delta t}{\mu_{xx}^{i,j,k}}\left[\frac{E_z^{i,j+1,k} - E_z^{i,j,k}}{\Delta y} - \frac{E_y^{i,j,k+1} - E_z^{i,j,k}}{\Delta z}\right] \tag{4.28}$$

In the above equation, $\tilde{H}_x^{i,j,k}\big|_{t+\frac{\Delta t}{2}}$ is the x component of magnetic field at time $t + \frac{\Delta t}{2}$ and $\tilde{H}_x^{i,j,k}\big|_{t-\frac{\Delta t}{2}}$ is the x component of magnetic field at time $t - \frac{\Delta t}{2}$. The second term of equation (4.28), $\frac{c_0 \times \Delta t}{\mu_{xx}^{i,j,k}}\left[\frac{E_z^{i,j+1,k} - E_z^{i,j,k}}{\Delta y} - \frac{E_y^{i,j,k+1} - E_z^{i,j,k}}{\Delta z}\right]$ is known as the update term.

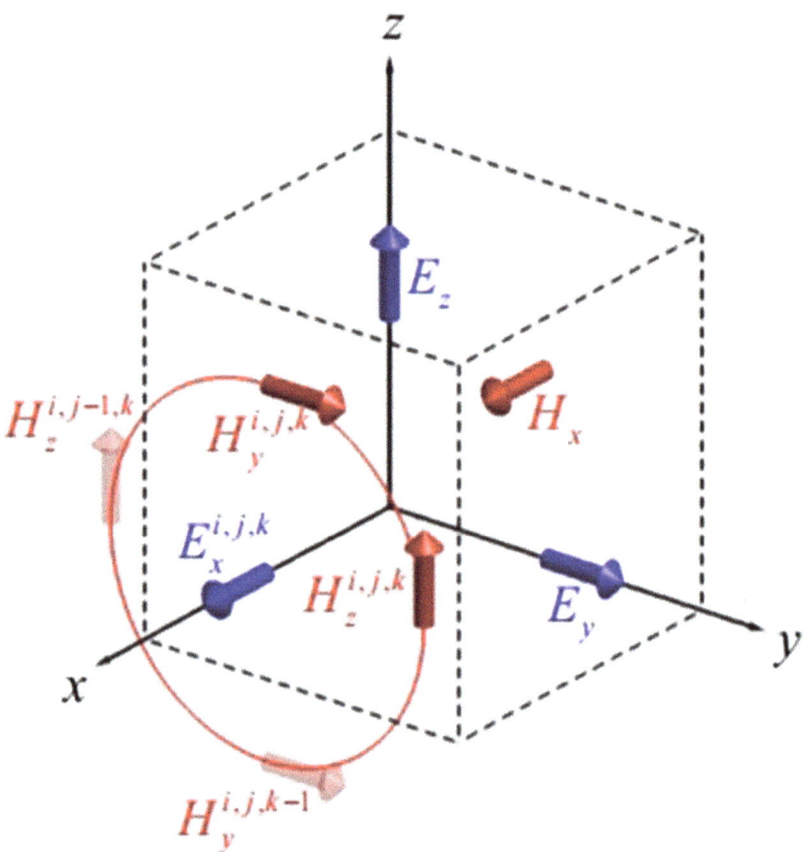

Figure 4.5. Yee grid for finite difference approximations of spatial magnetic field components and x direction time domain electric field. Reprinted with permission from Rumpf (2020) https://empossible.net/wp-content/uploads/2020/01/Lecture-Formulation-of-1D-FDTD.pdf.

Similarly, the FDTD update equation for the y component of the magnetic field is derived by simplifying equation (4.20).

$$\tilde{H}_y^{i,j,k}\Big|_{t+\frac{\Delta t}{2}} = \tilde{H}_y^{i,j,k}\Big|_{t-\frac{\Delta t}{2}} + \frac{c_0 \times \Delta t}{\mu_{yy}^{i,j,k}}\left[\frac{E_x^{i,j,k+1} - E_x^{i,j,k}}{\Delta z} - \frac{E_z^{i+1,j,k} - E_z^{i,j,k}}{\Delta x}\right] \quad (4.29)$$

In the above equation, $\tilde{H}_y^{i,j,k}|_{t+\frac{\Delta t}{2}}$ is the y component of magnetic field at time $t + \frac{\Delta t}{2}$ and $\tilde{H}_y^{i,j,k}|_{t-\frac{\Delta t}{2}}$ is the y component of magnetic field at time $t - \frac{\Delta t}{2}$. The second term of equation (4.29), $\frac{c_0 \times \Delta t}{\mu_{yy}^{i,j,k}}\left[\frac{E_x^{i,j,k+1} - E_x^{i,j,k}}{\Delta z} - \frac{E_z^{i+1,j,k} - E_z^{i,j,k}}{\Delta x}\right]$ is known as the update term. The magnetic field update equation for the z component is derived by following the same procedure.

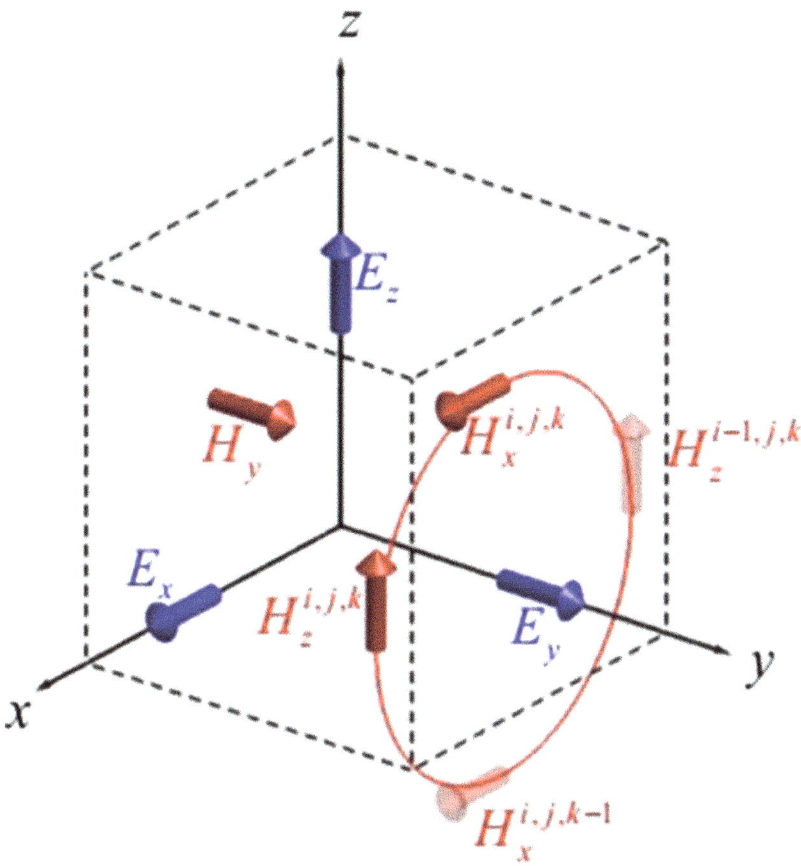

Figure 4.6. Yee grid for finite difference approximations of spatial magnetic field components and y direction time domain electric field. Reprinted with permission from Rumpf (2020) https://empossible.net/wp-content/uploads/2020/01/Lecture-Formulation-of-1D-FDTD.pdf.

$$\tilde{H}_z^{i,j,k}\Big|_{t+\frac{\Delta t}{2}} = \tilde{H}_z^{i,j,k}\Big|_{t-\frac{\Delta t}{2}} + \frac{c_0 \times \Delta t}{\mu_{zz}^{i,j,k}}\left[\frac{E_y^{i+1,j,k+1} - E_y^{i,j,k}}{\Delta x} - \frac{E_x^{i,j+1,k} - E_x^{i,j,k}}{\Delta y}\right] \tag{4.30}$$

Equations (4.28), (4.29) and (4.30) are known as the magnetic field FDTD update equations for the three-dimensional Yee grid. Electric field update equations are derived by following the same procedure as stated above.

$$E_x^{i,j,k}\big|_{t+\Delta t} = E_x^{i,j,k}\big|_t - \frac{c_0 \times \Delta t}{\epsilon_{xx}^{i,j,k}}\left[\frac{\tilde{H}_z^{i,j+1,k}\big|_{t+\frac{\Delta t}{2}} - \tilde{H}_z^{i,j,k}\big|_{t+\frac{\Delta t}{2}}}{\Delta y} - \frac{\tilde{H}_y^{i,j,k+1}\big|_{t+\frac{\Delta t}{2}} - \tilde{H}_y^{i,j,k}\big|_{t+\frac{\Delta t}{2}}}{\Delta z}\right] \tag{4.31}$$

$$E_y^{i,j,k}\big|_{t+\Delta t} = E_y^{i,j,k}\big|_t - \frac{c_0 \times \Delta t}{\epsilon_{yy}^{i,j,k}}\left[\frac{\tilde{H}_x^{i,j,k+1}\big|_{t+\frac{\Delta t}{2}} - \tilde{H}_x^{i,j,k}\big|_{t+\frac{\Delta t}{2}}}{\Delta z} - \frac{\tilde{H}_z^{i+1,j,k}\big|_{t+\frac{\Delta t}{2}} - \tilde{H}_z^{i,j,k}\big|_{t+\frac{\Delta t}{2}}}{\Delta x}\right] \tag{4.32}$$

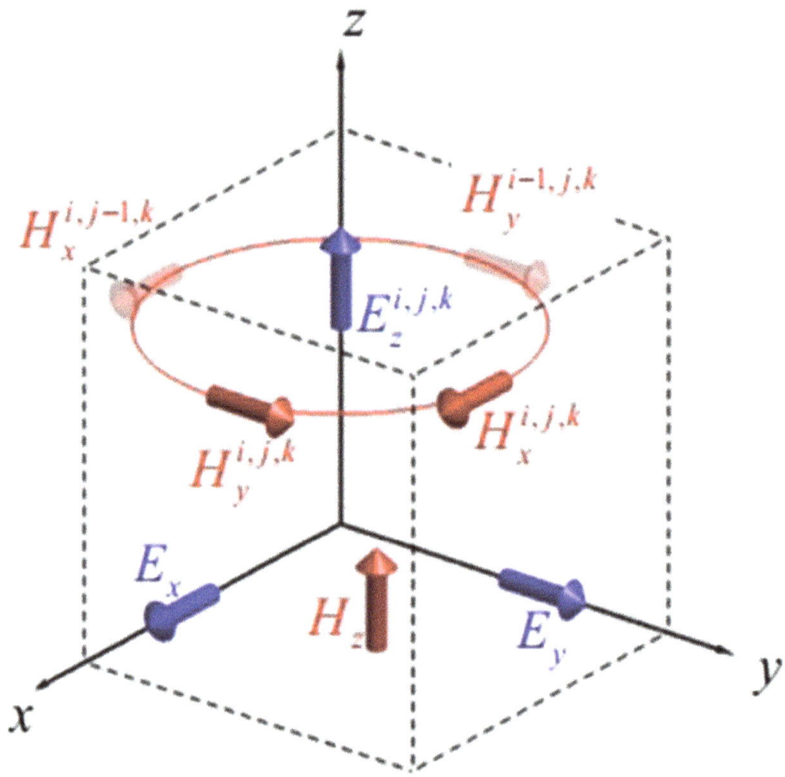

Figure 4.7. Yee grid for finite difference approximations of spatial magnetic field components and z direction time domain electric field. Reprinted with permission from Rumpf (2020) https://empossible.net/wp-content/uploads/2020/01/Lecture-Formulation-of-1D-FDTD.pdf.

$$E_z^{i,j,k}\big|_{t+\Delta t} = E_z^{i,j,k}\big|_t - \frac{c_0 \times \Delta t}{\epsilon_{zz}^{i,j,k}} \left[\frac{\tilde{H}_y^{i+1,j,k}\big|_{t+\frac{\Delta t}{2}} - \tilde{H}_y^{i,j,k}\big|_{t+\frac{\Delta t}{2}}}{\Delta x} - \frac{\tilde{H}_x^{i,j+1,k}\big|_{t+\frac{\Delta t}{2}} - \tilde{H}_x^{i,j,k}\big|_{t+\frac{\Delta t}{2}}}{\Delta y} \right] \tag{4.33}$$

Equations (4.31), (4.32) and (4.33) are known as electric field FDTD update equations for the three-dimensional Yee grid.

4.5 Polarization current density equation derivation for numerical breast phantom region

There are two regions in the modular FDTD approach. Numerical breast phantom and perfectly matched layer (PML) are shown in figure 4.8. The light grey region is used for numerical breast phantom and dark grey region at the boundary is used for perfectly matched layer (PML). Dispersion and polarization are included by using Debye equation for numerical breast phantom region [22]. Equations for PML are needed only at the boundaries. Now, there are two sets of electric field update equations. The first set of electric field update equations are used for the numerical breast phantom region excluding boundaries. The second set of electric field update

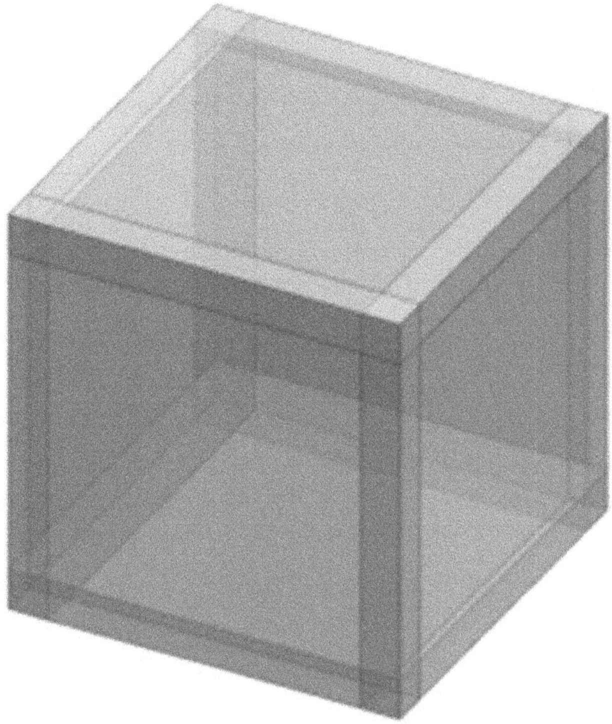

Figure 4.8. Grid for 3D FDTD. Reprinted with permission from Rumpf (2020) https://empossible.net/wp-content/uploads/2020/01/Lecture-The-Perfectly-Matched-Layer.pdf.

equations is used for PML boundaries. The human body tissues are represented by numerical breast phantom region. Polarization current is generated in human body tissues or cells due to applied electromagnetic field. The polarization current density equation is given in equation (4.34). The polarization current density FDTD update equation is used to derive the electric field FDTD update equation. The polarization and dispersion properties of human breast tissues are included by substituting the Debye model into the Ampere's law equation.

$$\nabla \times \vec{H} = \epsilon_0 \epsilon_\infty j\omega \vec{E} + j\omega \epsilon_0 \frac{\Delta\epsilon}{1 + j\omega\tau} \vec{E} + \sigma_s \vec{E} \tag{4.34}$$

In equation (4.34), σ_s is static conductivity. $\Delta\epsilon$ is difference between static permittivity and infinite permittivity. Equation (4.35) given below is obtained by rearranging the above equation.

$$\nabla \times \vec{H} = \epsilon_0 \epsilon_\infty j\omega \vec{E} ++ \sigma_s \vec{E} + j\omega \epsilon_0 \frac{\Delta\epsilon}{1 + j\omega\tau} \vec{E} \tag{4.35}$$

The polarization current density equation is derived after including Debye equation in Ampere's law. The polarization current density is given by equation (4.36).

$$\vec{J}_{\mathrm{p}} = j\omega\epsilon_0 \frac{\Delta\epsilon}{1 + j\omega\tau}\vec{E} \tag{4.36}$$

$\vec{J}_{\mathrm{p}}$ is polarization current density vector and $\vec{E}$ is electric field intensity vector. The above equation is rearranged to derive equation (4.37).

$$\vec{J}_{\mathrm{p}}(1 + j\omega\tau) = j\omega\epsilon_0\Delta\epsilon\vec{E} \tag{4.37}$$

Equation (4.37) is in frequency domain. Time domain representation of the above equation is obtained by applying inverse Fourier transform to it. Equation (4.38) is the time domain representation of equation (4.37).

$$\vec{J}_{\mathrm{p}} + \tau\frac{\partial\vec{J}_{\mathrm{p}}}{\partial t} = \epsilon_0\Delta\epsilon\frac{\partial\vec{E}}{\partial t} \tag{4.38}$$

Now, the above equation is in time domain. Differentiation terms can be obtained by using finite difference approximations in time domain. In order to get equation (4.39), FDTD is applied to the above equation.

$$\frac{\tau}{\Delta t}\vec{J}_{\mathrm{P}}^{t+\Delta t}\left(1 + \frac{\Delta t}{2\tau}\right) = \frac{\tau}{\Delta t}\vec{J}_{\mathrm{P}}^{t}\left(1 - \frac{\Delta t}{2\tau}\right) + \epsilon_0\Delta\epsilon\frac{\vec{E}_{t+\Delta t} - \vec{E}_t}{\Delta t} \tag{4.39}$$

Whatever is the value of time-constant τ, it can be expressed as a multiple of the time step, $\tau = N_t\Delta t$ where N_t does not need to be an integer. In order to get equation (4.40), put $\tau = N_t\Delta t$ and multiply both sides by $\Delta x = \delta$.

$$\delta\vec{J}_{\mathrm{P}}^{t+\Delta t} = \left(\frac{1 - \dfrac{1}{2N_t}}{1 + \dfrac{1}{2N_t}}\right)\delta\vec{J}_{\mathrm{P}}^{t} + \left(\frac{\epsilon_0\Delta\epsilon\delta}{N_t\Delta t\cdot\left(1 + \dfrac{1}{2N_t}\right)}\right)(\vec{E}_{t+\Delta t} - \vec{E}_t) \tag{4.40}$$

The first coefficient of polarization current density at time t is $mj1$, its value is given as in equation (4.41).

$$mj1 = \frac{1 - \dfrac{1}{2N_t}}{1 + \dfrac{1}{2N_t}} \tag{4.41}$$

In equation (4.41), relaxation time constant is given by $\tau = N_t\Delta t$. The second coefficient $mj2$ is given as an equation (4.42).

$$mj2 = \frac{\epsilon_0\Delta\epsilon\Delta x}{N_t\Delta t\cdot\left(1 + \dfrac{1}{2N_t}\right)} \tag{4.42}$$

Equation (4.43) is obtained by substituting equations (4.41) and (4.42) into equation (4.40).

$$\delta \vec{J}_{\mathrm{P}}^{t+\Delta t} = (mj1)\delta \vec{J}_{\mathrm{P}}^{t} + (mj2)(\vec{E}_{t+\Delta t} - \vec{E}_{t}) \tag{4.43}$$

Equation (4.44) is obtained by using equation (4.43). Equation (4.44) is used to get the electric field update equations in the next section.

$$\delta \vec{J}_{\mathrm{P}}^{t+\frac{\Delta t}{2}} = \frac{\delta \vec{J}_{\mathrm{P}}^{t+\Delta t} + \delta \vec{J}_{\mathrm{P}}^{t}}{2} = 1/2[(1 + mj1)\delta \vec{J}_{\mathrm{P}}^{t} + mj2(\vec{E}_{t+\Delta t} - \vec{E}_{t})] \tag{4.44}$$

4.6 Electric field update equation derivation for numerical breast phantom region

The Debye equation is substituted in Ampere's law to express dispersion and polarization of human body tissues. Equation (4.45) is Ampere's law after substituting the Debye model into it.

$$\nabla \times \vec{H} = \epsilon_0 \epsilon_\infty j\omega \vec{E} + j\omega \epsilon_0 \frac{\Delta \epsilon}{1 + j\omega\tau} \vec{E} + \sigma_{\mathrm{s}} \vec{E} \tag{4.45}$$

Equation (4.45) is in frequency domain. It is converted into time domain by applying inverse Fourier transform to it. Equation (4.46) given below represents the time domain equivalent of equation (4.45).

$$\nabla \times \vec{H}_{t+\frac{\Delta t}{2}} = \epsilon_0 \epsilon_\infty \frac{\partial \vec{E}}{\partial t} + \sigma_{\mathrm{s}} \vec{E} + \vec{J}_{\mathrm{P}}^{t+\frac{\Delta t}{2}} \tag{4.46}$$

Equation (4.46) is now approximated by applying finite difference time domain to it. Equation (4.47) is obtained by applying FDTD and multiplying both sides by $\Delta x = \delta$.

$$\delta \nabla \times \vec{H}_{t+\frac{\Delta t}{2}} = \delta \epsilon_0 \epsilon_\infty \frac{\vec{E}_{t+\Delta t} - \vec{E}_{t}}{\Delta t} + \delta \sigma_{\mathrm{s}} \frac{\vec{E}_{t+\Delta t} + \vec{E}_{t}}{2} + \delta \vec{J}_{\mathrm{P}}^{t+\frac{\Delta t}{2}} \tag{4.47}$$

Equation (4.44) is substituted for the term $\delta J_{\mathrm{P}}^{t+\frac{\Delta t}{2}}$ in the above equation (4.47).

$$\begin{aligned} \delta \nabla \times \vec{H}_{t+\frac{\Delta t}{2}} = \delta \epsilon_0 \epsilon_\infty \frac{\vec{E}_{t+\Delta t} - \vec{E}_{t}}{\Delta t} + \delta \sigma_{\mathrm{s}} \frac{\vec{E}_{t+\Delta t} + \vec{E}_{t}}{2} + \\ 1/2[(1 + mj1)\delta \vec{J}_{\mathrm{P}}^{t} + mj2(\vec{E}_{t+\Delta t} - \vec{E}_{t})] \end{aligned} \tag{4.48}$$

Equation (4.48) is simplified and rearranged to get equation (4.49).

$$\frac{\delta\epsilon_0\epsilon_\infty}{\Delta t}\left(1+\frac{\sigma_s\Delta t}{2\epsilon_0\epsilon_\infty}+\frac{\Delta t\cdot mj2}{2\delta\epsilon_0\epsilon_\infty}\right)\vec{E}_{t+\Delta t}$$
$$=\frac{\delta\epsilon_0\epsilon_\infty}{\Delta t}\left(1-\frac{\sigma_s\Delta t}{2\epsilon_0\epsilon_\infty}+\frac{\Delta t\cdot mj2}{2\delta\epsilon_0\epsilon_\infty}\right)\vec{E}_t \tag{4.49}$$
$$+\frac{\delta}{\eta_0}\nabla\times\vec{H}_{t+\frac{\Delta t}{2}}-\frac{1}{2}(1+mj1)\delta\vec{J}_{\mathrm{P}}^{t}$$

The electric field update equation (4.50) is obtained by rearranging the terms of equation (4.49).

$$\vec{E}_{t+\Delta t}=\frac{\left(1-\frac{\sigma_s\Delta t}{2\epsilon_0\epsilon_\infty}+\frac{\Delta t\cdot mj2}{2\delta\epsilon_0\epsilon_\infty}\right)}{\left(1+\frac{\sigma_s\Delta t}{2\epsilon_0\epsilon_\infty}+\frac{\Delta t\cdot mj2}{2\delta\epsilon_0\epsilon_\infty}\right)}\vec{E}_t+\frac{c_0\Delta t}{2\delta\epsilon_\infty\left(1+\frac{\sigma_s\Delta t}{2\epsilon_0\epsilon_\infty}+\frac{\Delta t\cdot mj2}{2\delta\epsilon_0\epsilon_\infty}\right)} \tag{4.50}$$
$$\cdot\left(2\delta\nabla\times\vec{H}_{t+\frac{\Delta t}{2}}-\eta_0(1+mj1)\delta\vec{J}_P^{t}\right)$$

By substituting $\frac{\left(1-\frac{\sigma_S\Delta t}{2\epsilon_0\epsilon_\infty}+\frac{\Delta t\cdot mj2}{2\delta\epsilon_0\epsilon_\infty}\right)}{\left(1+\frac{\sigma_S\Delta t}{2\epsilon_0\epsilon_\infty}+\frac{\Delta t\cdot mj2}{2\delta\epsilon_0\epsilon_\infty}\right)}=me1$ and $\frac{c_0\Delta t}{2\delta\epsilon_\infty\left(1+\frac{\sigma_S\Delta t}{2\epsilon_0\epsilon_\infty}+\frac{\Delta t\cdot mj2}{2\delta\epsilon_0\epsilon_\infty}\right)}=me2$

$$\vec{E}_{t+\Delta t}=me1\cdot\vec{E}_t+me2\cdot\left[\left(2\Delta x\cdot\nabla\times\vec{H}_{t+\frac{\Delta t}{2}}\right)-\left(\eta_0\cdot(1+mj1)\cdot\Delta x\cdot\vec{J}_P^{t}\right)\right] \tag{4.51}$$

$$me1=\frac{1-\frac{\sigma_s\Delta t}{2\epsilon_0\epsilon_\infty}+\frac{mj2\cdot\Delta t}{2\epsilon_0\epsilon_\infty\Delta x}}{1+\frac{\sigma_s\Delta t}{2\epsilon_0\epsilon_\infty}+\frac{mj2\cdot\Delta t}{2\epsilon_0\epsilon_\infty\Delta x}} \tag{4.52}$$

In equation (4.52), Δt is time step. Coefficient $me2$ is given by equation (4.53).

$$me2=\frac{c_0\Delta t}{2\Delta x\cdot\epsilon_\infty\left(1+\frac{\sigma_s\Delta t}{2\epsilon_0\epsilon_\infty}+\frac{mj2\cdot\Delta t}{2\epsilon_0\epsilon_\infty\Delta x}\right)} \tag{4.53}$$

Equations (4.41), (4.42) and (4.43) are implemented and updated for x, y and z components of the polarization current density vector. The polarization current density vector is updated before updating electric field vector. Equations (4.51), (4.52) and (4.53) are implemented and updated for x, y, z components of the electric field vector.

4.7 Derivation of electric field update equations for PML region

PML is required at grid boundaries to avoid reflection of microwave signals in FDTD. Artificial losses in x direction are given below [22]. PML is shown in figure 4.9 at different boundaries. PML is placed on six boundaries as shown in figure 4.9. Electric field update equations for PML are shown in this section of the book.

$$S_x = \begin{bmatrix} \left(1 + \frac{\sigma_x}{j\omega\epsilon_0}\right)^{-1} & 0 & 0 \\ 0 & \left(1 + \frac{\sigma_x}{j\omega\epsilon_0}\right) & 0 \\ 0 & 0 & \left(1 + \frac{\sigma_x}{j\omega\epsilon_0}\right) \end{bmatrix} \tag{4.54}$$

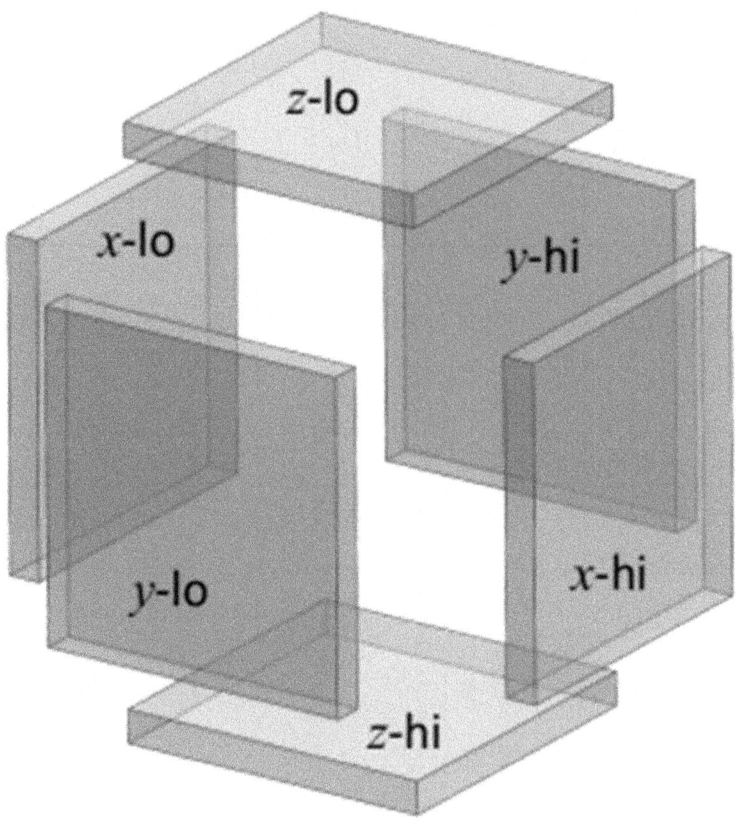

Figure 4.9. PML boundaries for 3D FDTD. Reprinted with permission from Rumpf (2020) https://empossible.net/wp-content/uploads/2020/01/Lecture-The-Perfectly-Matched-Layer.pdf.

In equation (4.54), σ_x is given by equation (4.55).

$$\sigma_x = \frac{0.5\epsilon_0}{\Delta t}\left(\frac{x}{L_x}\right)^3 \tag{4.55}$$

In equation (4.55), L_x is the length of PML in the x direction. x is the particular cell number of PML. Artificial losses in the Y direction are given by equation (4.56).

$$S_y = \begin{bmatrix} \left(1 + \frac{\sigma_y}{j\omega\epsilon_0}\right) & 0 & 0 \\ 0 & \left(1 + \frac{\sigma_y}{j\omega\epsilon_0}\right)^{-1} & 0 \\ 0 & 0 & \left(1 + \frac{\sigma_y}{j\omega\epsilon_0}\right) \end{bmatrix} \tag{4.56}$$

In equation (4.56), L_y is length of PML in the z direction. z is particular cell number of PML. Artificial losses in Z direction are given by equation (4.57).

$$S_z = \begin{bmatrix} \left(1 + \frac{\sigma_z}{j\omega\epsilon_0}\right) & 0 & 0 \\ 0 & \left(1 + \frac{\sigma_z}{j\omega\epsilon_0}\right) & 0 \\ 0 & 0 & \left(1 + \frac{\sigma_z}{j\omega\epsilon_0}\right)^{-1} \end{bmatrix} \tag{4.57}$$

Artificial losses in all three directions can be combined as shown by equation (4.58).

$$[S] = [S_x][S_y][S_z] \tag{4.58}$$

Ampere's law equation can be written to incorporate artificial losses in all directions as shown by equation (4.59).

$$\nabla \times \vec{H} = j\omega[S]\vec{D} \tag{4.59}$$

We write equation (4.60) for the x component of equation (4.59) after substituting $[S]$ into it.

$$\begin{aligned} &j\omega\left(1 + \frac{\sigma_x}{j\omega\epsilon_0}\right)^{-1}\left(1 + \frac{\sigma_y}{j\omega\epsilon_0}\right)\left(1 + \frac{\sigma_z}{j\omega\epsilon_0}\right)D_x \\ &= \left[\frac{\partial H_z}{\partial y} - \frac{\partial H_y}{\partial z}\right] \end{aligned} \tag{4.60}$$

Equation (4.61) is obtained by substituting $\left[\frac{\partial H_z}{\partial y} - \frac{\partial H_y}{\partial z}\right] = (CH)_x$ and rearranging the terms of equation (4.60).

$$j\omega\left(1 + \frac{\sigma_y}{j\omega\epsilon_0}\right)\left(1 + \frac{\sigma_z}{j\omega\epsilon_0}\right)D_x = \left(1 + \frac{\sigma_x}{j\omega\epsilon_0}\right)(CH)_x \tag{4.61}$$

Equation (4.62) is obtained by simplifying equation (4.61).

$$j\omega D_x + \frac{\sigma_y + \sigma_z}{\epsilon_0}D_x + \frac{\sigma_y \sigma z}{j\omega\epsilon_0^2}D_x = (CH)_x + \frac{\sigma_x}{j\omega\epsilon_0}(CH)_x \tag{4.62}$$

Equation (4.63) is obtained by applying inverse Fourier transform to equation (4.62).

$$\begin{aligned}\frac{\partial}{\partial t}D_x + \frac{\sigma_y + \sigma_z}{\epsilon_0}D_x + \frac{\sigma_y \sigma z}{\epsilon_0^2}\int_{-\infty}^{t} D_x \mathrm{d}\tau = (CH)_x \\ + \frac{\sigma_x}{\epsilon_0}\int_{-\infty}^{t} (CH)_x \mathrm{d}\tau\end{aligned} \tag{4.63}$$

Equation (4.64) is obtained by applying FDTD to equation (4.63).

$$\begin{aligned}\frac{D_x^{t+\Delta t} - D_x^t}{\Delta t} + \frac{\sigma_y + \sigma_z}{\epsilon_0}\frac{D_x^{t+\Delta t} + D_x^t}{2} + \frac{\sigma_y \sigma_z \Delta t}{\epsilon_0^2}\left[\frac{D_x^{t+\Delta t} + D_x^t}{4} + \sum_{T=0}^{t-\Delta t} D_x\right] \\ = c_0(CH)_x + \frac{c_0\sigma_x}{\epsilon_0}\sum_{T=0}^{t-\frac{\Delta t}{2}}(CH)_x\end{aligned} \tag{4.64}$$

Equation (4.65) is obtained by rearranging terms of equation (4.64).

$$\begin{aligned}D_x^{t+\Delta t} = \frac{\left(\frac{1}{\Delta t} - \frac{\sigma y + \sigma z}{2\epsilon_0} - \frac{\sigma y \cdot \sigma z \cdot \Delta t}{4\epsilon_0^2}\right)}{\left(\frac{1}{\Delta t} + \frac{\sigma y + \sigma z}{2\epsilon_0} + \frac{\sigma y \cdot \sigma z \cdot \Delta t}{4\epsilon_0^2}\right)}D_x^t + \frac{c_0 \cdot CH_x}{\left(\frac{1}{\Delta t} + \frac{\sigma y + \sigma z}{2\epsilon_0} + \frac{\sigma y \cdot \sigma z \cdot \Delta t}{4\epsilon_0^2}\right)} \\ + \frac{c_0 \cdot \Delta t \cdot \sigma x}{\left(\frac{1}{\Delta t} + \frac{\sigma y + \sigma z}{2\epsilon_0} + \frac{\sigma y \cdot \sigma z \cdot \Delta t}{4\epsilon_0^2}\right) \cdot \epsilon_0}(Ich)_x - \frac{\Delta t \cdot \sigma y \cdot \sigma z \cdot ID x}{\left(\frac{1}{\Delta t} + \frac{\sigma y + \sigma z}{2\epsilon_0} + \frac{\sigma y \cdot \sigma z \cdot \Delta t}{4\epsilon_0^2}\right) \cdot \epsilon_0^2}\end{aligned} \tag{4.65}$$

$$\vec{D}_{t+\Delta t} = mdx1 \cdot \vec{D}_t + mdx2 \cdot (\nabla \times \vec{H})_x + mdx3 \cdot (\mathrm{Ich})_x + mdx4 \cdot (\mathrm{ID})_x \tag{4.66}$$

In equation (4.66), $\vec{D}_{t+\Delta t}$ is electric field density (x component) at next time step, $\vec{D}_t$ is electric field density (x component) at previous time step, $(\nabla \times \vec{H})_x$ is x component of curl of vector H. $(\mathrm{Ich})_x$ is the x component of integration of curl of vector H. $(\mathrm{ID})_x$ is the x component of integration of electric field density vector D. Coefficient $mdx0$ is given by equation (4.5).

$$mdx0 = \frac{1}{\Delta t} + \frac{\sigma_y + \sigma_z}{2\epsilon_0} + \frac{\sigma_y \cdot \sigma_z \cdot \Delta t}{4\epsilon_0^2} \tag{4.67}$$

In equation (4.67), σ_y and σ_z are conductivity in y and z directions, respectively. These conductivity values are nonzero only in the PML region. Coefficient $mdx1$ is given by equation (4.6).

$$mdx1 = \frac{1}{mdx0}\left(\frac{1}{\Delta t} - \frac{\sigma_y + \sigma_z}{2\epsilon_0} - \frac{\sigma_y \cdot \sigma_z \cdot \Delta t}{4\epsilon_0^2}\right) \tag{4.68}$$

Coefficient $mdx2$ is given by equation (4.69).

$$mdx2 = \frac{c_0}{mdx0} \tag{4.69}$$

In equation (4.69), c_0 is speed of light. Coefficient $mdx3$ is given by equation (4.8).

$$mdx3 = \frac{c_0 \cdot \Delta t \cdot \sigma_x}{mdx0 \cdot \epsilon_0} \tag{4.70}$$

In equation (4.70), σ_x is the x component of conductivity. Coefficient $mdx4$ is given by equation (4.71).

$$mdx4 = -\frac{\Delta t \cdot \sigma_y \cdot \sigma_z}{mdx0 \cdot \epsilon_0^2} \tag{4.71}$$

Equations (4.66) to (4.71) are implemented for x, y and z components of electric field density vector D in PML region. The electric field in the PML region is updated by using the simple relation between electric field density and electric field intensity. Electric field can be updated by using equation (4.72).

$$E_x = \frac{D_x}{\epsilon_{xx}} \tag{4.72}$$

Electric field update equations in y and z directions are obtained by repeating the above procedure.

4.8 Magnetic field update equations

The human body is nonmagnetic, so only one set of FDTD equations is required throughout the grid. Faraday's law with loss matrix s is given by equation (4.73).

$$\nabla \times \vec{\tilde{E}} = -j\omega[\mu_r][s]\vec{H} \tag{4.73}$$

Equation (4.74) is obtained by applying the same procedure as the electric field update equation derivation

$$H_x^{t+\frac{\Delta t}{2}} = \frac{\left(\frac{1}{\Delta t} - \frac{\sigma_y + \sigma_z}{2\epsilon_0} - \frac{\sigma_y \cdot \sigma_z \cdot \Delta t}{4\epsilon_0^2}\right)}{\left(\frac{1}{\Delta t} + \frac{\sigma_y + \sigma_z}{2\epsilon_0} + \frac{\sigma_y \cdot \sigma_z \cdot \Delta t}{4\epsilon_0^2}\right)} H_x^{t-\frac{\Delta t}{2}} - \frac{c_0 \cdot CE_x}{\mu_{xx}\left(\frac{1}{\Delta t} + \frac{\sigma_y + \sigma_z}{2\epsilon_0} + \frac{\sigma_y \cdot \sigma_z \cdot \Delta t}{4\epsilon_0^2}\right)} - \frac{c_0 \cdot \Delta t \cdot \sigma_x}{\mu_{xx}\left(\frac{1}{\Delta t} + \frac{\sigma_y + \sigma_z}{2\epsilon_0} + \frac{\sigma_y \cdot \sigma_z \cdot \Delta t}{4\epsilon_0^2}\right) \cdot \epsilon_0} (\mathrm{Ice})_x - \frac{\Delta t \cdot \sigma_y \cdot \sigma_z \cdot \mathrm{IH}_x}{\left(\frac{1}{\Delta t} + \frac{\sigma_y + \sigma_z}{2\epsilon_0} + \frac{\sigma_y \cdot \sigma_z \cdot \Delta t}{4\epsilon_0^2}\right) \cdot \epsilon_0^2} \tag{4.74}$$

$$\vec{H}_{t+\frac{\Delta t}{2}} = mhx1 \cdot \vec{H}_{t-\frac{\Delta t}{2}} + mhx2 \cdot \left(\nabla \times \vec{E}\right)_x + mhx3 \cdot (\mathrm{Ice})_x + mdx4 \cdot (\mathrm{IH})_x \tag{4.75}$$

In equation (4.75), $\vec{H}_{t+\frac{\Delta t}{2}}$ is magnetic field intensity (x component) at future time step, $\vec{H}_{t-\frac{\Delta t}{2}}$ is magnetic field intensity (x component) at previous time step, $(\nabla \times \vec{E})_x$ is x component of the curl of electric field vector E. $(\mathrm{Ice})_x$ is the x component of integration of the curl of electric field vector E. $(\mathrm{IH})_x$ is x component of integration of magnetic field intensity vector H. Coefficient $mhx0$ is given by equation (4.76).

$$mhx0 = \frac{1}{\Delta t} + \frac{\sigma_y + \sigma_z}{2\epsilon_0} + \frac{\sigma_y \cdot \sigma_z \cdot \Delta t}{4\epsilon_0^2} \tag{4.76}$$

In equation (4.76), σ_y and σ_z are conductivity in y and z directions, respectively. These conductivity values are nonzero only in the PML region. Coefficient $mhx1$ is given by equation (4.77).

$$mhx1 = \frac{1}{mhx0}\left(\frac{1}{\Delta t} - \frac{\sigma_y + \sigma_z}{2\epsilon_0} - \frac{\sigma_y \cdot \sigma_z \cdot \Delta t}{4\epsilon_0^2}\right) \tag{4.77}$$

Coefficient $mhx2$ is given by equation (4.78).

$$mhx2 = -\frac{c_0}{mhx0 \cdot \mu_{xx}} \tag{4.78}$$

In equation (4.78), c_0 is speed of light. Coefficient $mhx3$ is given by equation (4.79).

$$mhx3 = -\frac{c_0 \cdot \Delta t \cdot \sigma_x}{mhx0 \cdot \epsilon_0 \mu_{xx}} \tag{4.79}$$

In equation (4.79), σ_x is the x component of conductivity. Coefficient $mhx4$ is given by equation (4.80).

$$mhx4 = -\frac{\Delta t \cdot \sigma_y \cdot \sigma_z}{mhx0 \cdot \epsilon_0^2} \tag{4.80}$$

Equations (4.75) to (4.80) are implemented for x, y and z components of magnetic field intensity vector H.

4.9 Steps for FDTD implementation

FDTD implementation steps are given below.

1. Define all FDTD related parameters.
2. Set all electromagnetic fields to zero.
3. Set all integration terms to zero.
4. Implement numerical breast phantom on the grid.
5. Calculate the coefficients of electric and magnetic fields for update equations (including PML at the boundaries).
6. Implement main FDTD loop.
7. Update curl of electric field components.
8. Update magnetic field related integration terms
9. Update magnetic field using update equations.
10. Implement electric field source.
11. Update curl of magnetic field components.
12. Update electric field related integration terms
13. Update electric field using update equations.
14. Implement magnetic field source.
15. Apply Fourier transform to get the electric field components in frequency domain.
16. Visualize electromagnetic fields.
17. Complete all iterations of main FDTD loop.

4.10 Simulation parameters

Debye parameters are given for different breast tissues in table 5.1. These values are valid for 0.5 GHz to 20 GHz. Two major types of tissues are considered in class 3 numerical breast phantom in order to maintain simplicity. Coronal cross-sections of numerical breast phantom with $\Delta\epsilon$ original profile are shown in figure 4.10. The malignant tumor is assumed within the fibro-glandular tissues. Five frequencies 0.5, 1, 1.5, 2 and 2.5 GHz are considered for 3D FDTD simulation.

4.11 Results

Electric field components are calculated inside numerical breast phantom by using FDTD simulation in MATLAB. A numerical breast phantom dielectric profile as shown in the figure 4.10, is used in the simulation. Electric fields after 200, 400, 600 and 800 iterations are recorded and shown in figures 4.11, 4.12, 4.13 and 4.14 respectively. Electric field is applied as a narrow Gaussian pulse to cover the band of interest (500 MHz to 2.5 GHz). There is clear observation from figures 4.11 and 4.12 that the electric field increases up to 400 iterations. One can easily verify from figures 4.13 and 4.14 that the electric field decreases after 400 iterations. Now, a malignant tumour is added to the numerical breast phantom. The electric field is calculated with the cancer inside the breast phantom. The electric field after 200 iterations is shown in figure 4.15. Comparison of figure 4.11 with figure 4.15 clearly demonstrates the capability of FDTD as a forward problem solver. The electric field in cancerous tissues of figure 4.15 is different from the electric field of

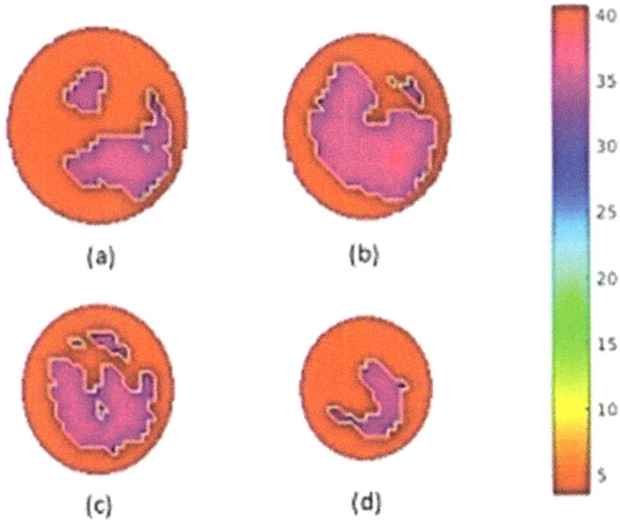

Figure 4.10. Coronal cross-section of class 3 breast phantom with original profile of $\Delta\epsilon$ at (a) 1.5 cm; (b) 3 cm; (c) 4.5 cm; (d) 6 cm. (Dark pink dot of (b) indicates malignant tumour tissues.) Reprinted with permission from [32].

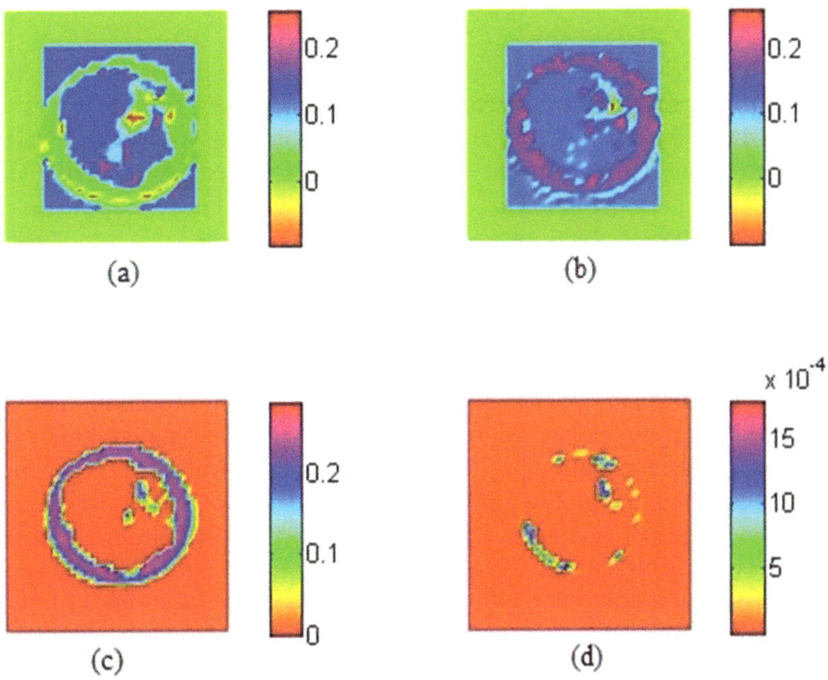

Figure 4.11. Electric field in class 3 numerical breast phantom (without cancer) after 200 iterations at (a) 1.5 cm; (b) 3 cm; (c) 4.5 cm; (d) 6 cm. Reprinted with permission from [32].

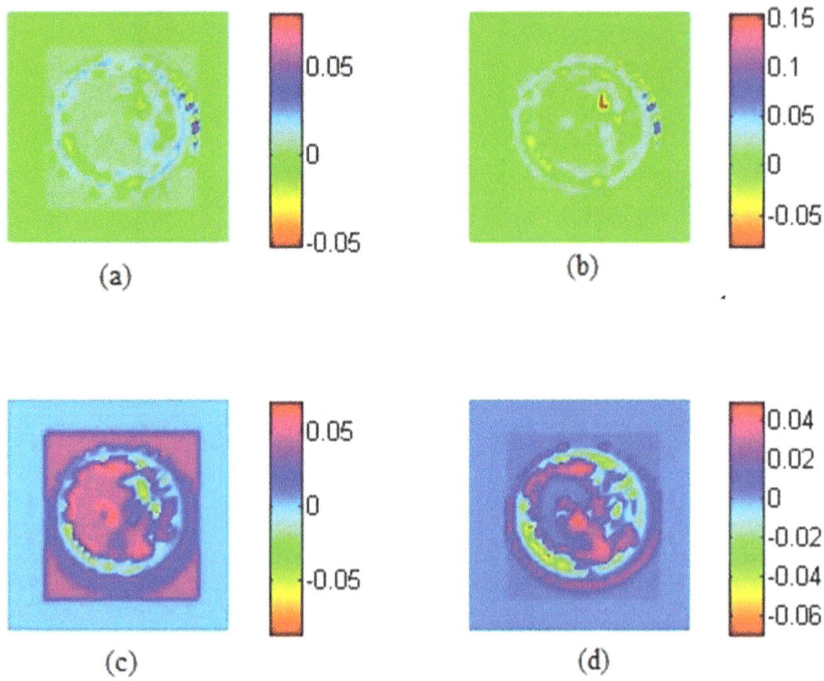

Figure 4.12. Electric field in class 3 numerical breast phantom (without cancer) after 400 iterations at (a) 1.5 cm; (b) 3 cm; (c) 4.5 cm; (d) 6 cm. Reprinted with permission from [32].

figure 4.11. It can be observed from figure 4.15 that the electric field inside the numerical breast phantom is affected due to inclusion of cancerous tissues.

Normalized reflected power versus frequency graph is shown by figure 4.16. It is quite obvious from figure 4.16 that the normalized reflected power varies with the direction of wave propagation. This effect is caused due to the heterogeneous nature of the numerical breast phantom.

4.12 Summary

Derivation of FDTD equations using Yee grid is shown in detail. It is very easy to grasp the derivation and implementation concepts from this section. The Debye model is used to express polarization and dispersion effects of human breast tissues. Electric field update equations are derived using a modular FDTD approach. Magnetic field update equations are derived for the whole structure because of nonmagnetic nature of human body. Using FDTD method, electric field can be obtained very efficiently in heterogeneous numerical breast phantom. It is very easy to include dispersion and polarization properties of breast tissues in 3D FDTD.

The electric field distribution is different in malignant breast tissues as compared to electric field in healthy breast tissues. 3D FDTD is suitable for computation of electric field in the heterogeneous numerical breast phantom. Normalized reflected power varies with direction of wave propagation in the heterogeneous numerical breast phantom.

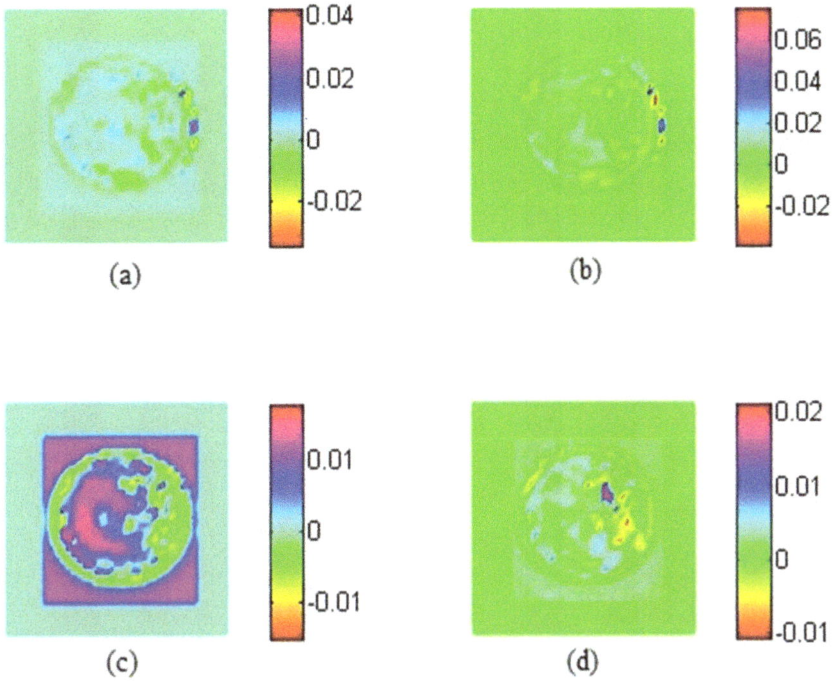

Figure 4.13. Electric field in class 3 numerical breast phantom (without cancer) after 600 iterations at (a) 1.5 cm; (b) 3 cm; (c) 4.5 cm; (d) 6 cm. Reprinted with permission from [32].

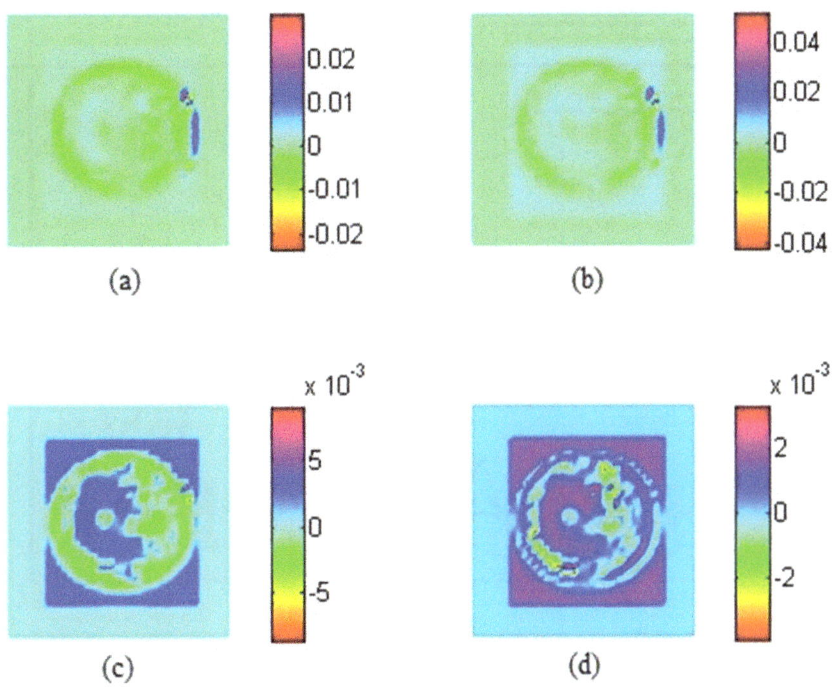

Figure 4.14. Electric field in class 3 numerical breast phantom (without cancer) after 800 iterations at (a) 1.5 cm; (b) 3 cm; (c) 4.5 cm; (d) 6 cm. Reprinted with permission from [32].

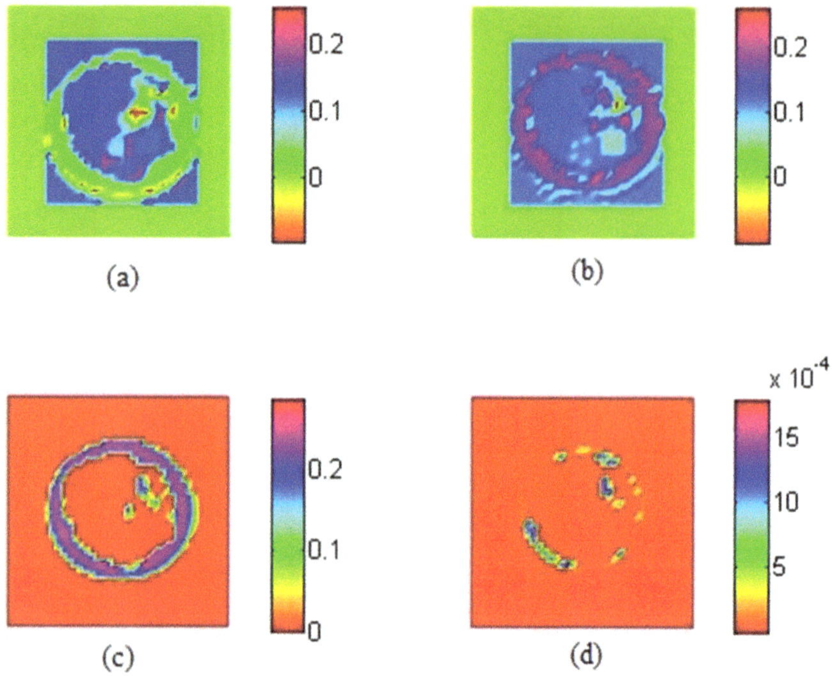

Figure 4.15. Electric field in class 3 numerical breast phantom (with cancer) after 200 iterations at (a) 1.5 cm; (b) 3 cm; (c) 4.5 cm; (d) 6 cm. Reprinted with permission from [32].

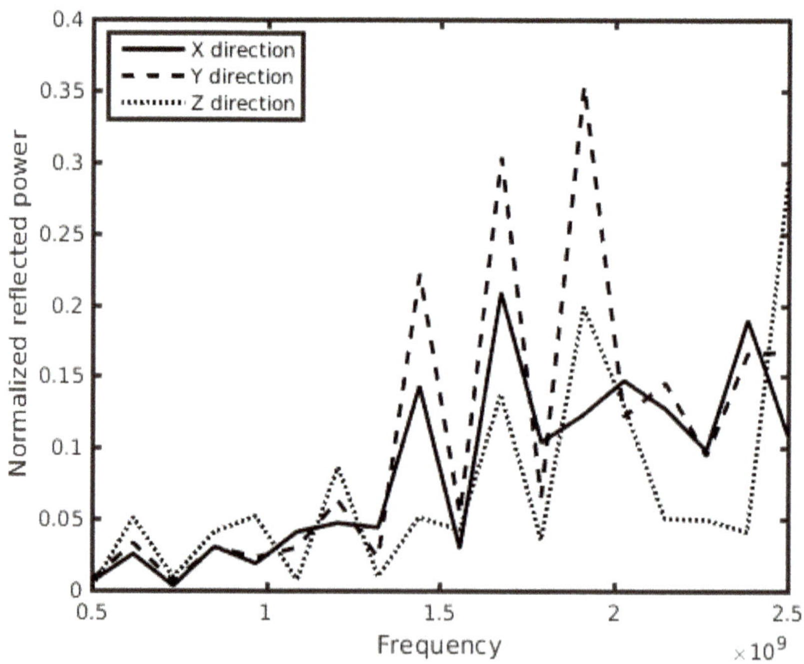

Figure 4.16. Normalized reflected power versus frequency for different directions. Reprinted with permission from [32].

References

[1] Yee K 1966 Numerical solution of initial boundary value problems involving Maxwell's equations in isotropic media *IEEE Trans. Antennas Propag.* **14** 302–7

[2] Jin J-M 2015 *The Finite Element Method in Electromagnetics* (New York: Wiley)

[3] Harrington R F 1987 The method of moments in electromagnetics *J. Electromagn. Waves Appl.* **1** 181–200

[4] Gibson W C 2014 *The Method of Moments in Electromagnetics* (London: Chapman and Hall/CRC)

[5] Keller J B 1962 Geometrical theory of diffraction *J. Opt. Soc. Am.* **52** 116–30

[6] Balanis C A 1999 *Advanced Engineering Electromagnetics* (New York: Wiley)

[7] Ling H, Chou R and Lee S W 1986 Shooting and bouncing rays: calculating RCS of an arbitary cavity *IEEE Antennas and Propagation Society, AP-S Int. Sympos. (Digest)* (Piscataway, NJ: Institute of Electrical and Electronics Engineers Inc.) pp 293–6

[8] Ling H, Chou R-C and Lee S-W 1989 Shooting and bouncing rays: calculating the RCS of an arbitrarily shaped cavity *IEEE Trans. Antennas Propag.* **37** 194–205

[9] Yee K 1966 Numerical solution of initial boundary value problems involving Maxwell's equations in isotropic media *IEEE Trans. Antennas Propag.* **14** 302–7

[10] Taflove A 1980 Application of the finite-difference time-domain method to sinusoidal steady-state electromagnetic-penetration problems *IEEE Trans. Electromagn. Compat.* **22** 191–202

[11] Okonievski M, Mrozowski M and Stuchly M A 1997 Simple treatment of multi-term dispersion in FDTD *IEEE Microw. Guided Wave Lett.* **7** 121–3

[12] Hagness S C, Taflove A and Bridges J E 1998 Two-dimensional FDTD analysis of a pulsed microwaved confocal system for breast cancer detection: fixed-focus and antenna-array sensors *IEEE Trans. Antennas Propag.* **45** 1470–9

[13] Hagness S C, Taflove A and Bridges J E 1999 Three-dimensional FDTD analysis of a pulsed microwaved confocal system for breast cancer detection: design of an antenna-array element *IEEE Trans. Antennas Propag.* **47** 783–91

[14] Bond E J, Li X, Hagness S C and Van Veen B D 2003 Microwave imaging via space-time beam-forming for early detection of breast cancer *IEEE Trans. Antennas Propag.* **51** 1690–705

[15] Li X, Davis S K, Hagness S C, Van der Weide D W and Van Veen B D 2004 Microwave imaging via space-time beam-forming: Experimental investigation of tumour detection in multilayer breast phantoms *IEEE Trans. Microw. Theory Techn.* **52** 1856–65

[16] Kosmas P and Rappaport C 2005 Time reversal with FDTD method for microwave breast cancer detection *IEEE Trans. Microwave Theory and Techniques* **53** 2317–22

[17] Guo B, Jian L and Zmuda H 2006 A new FDTD formulation for wave propagation in biological media with Cole-Cole model *IEEE Microw. Wirel. Compon. Lett.* **16** 633–5

[18] Kosmas P and Rappaport C 2006 FDTD-basedtime reversal for microwave breast cancer detection:Localization in three dimensions *IEEE Trans. Microw. Theory Techn.* **54** 1921–7

[19] Kosmas P and Rappaport C 2006 A matched fllter FDTD-based time reversal approach for microwave breast cancer detection *IEEE Trans. Antennas Propag.* **54** 1257–64

[20] Kang K, Chu X, Dilmaghani R and Ghavami M 2007 Low-complexity Cole–Cole expression for modelling human biological tissues in FDTD method *Electron. Lett.* **43** 143–4

[21] Gedney S D 1996 An anisotropic perfectly matched layer-absorbing medium for the truncation of FDTD lattices *IEEE Trans. Antennas Propag.* **44** 1630–9

[22] Schneider J B 2010 *Understanding the Finite-Difference Time-Domain Method* pp 33–8 http://www.eecs.wsu.edu/schneidj/ufdtd

[23] Taflove A and Hagness S C 2000 *Computational Electrodynamics: The Finite-difference Time-domain Method* (Boston, MA: Artech House) pp 81–105

[24] Moll J, Bauer C and Krozer V 2013 Microwave-based tumor localization in moderate heterogeneous breast tissue *2013 14th International Radar Symposium (IRS)* vol 2 (Piscataway, NJ: IEEE) pp 877–84

[25] Moll J, Sarafianou M, Kelly T N, Krozer V and Craddock I J 2014 Radar-based tumor localization in heterogeneous breast tissue using a 3D permittivity model *Antennas and Propagation (EuCAP), 2014 8th European Conference* (Piscataway, NJ: IEEE) pp 1288–91

[26] Yin T and Ali F H 2015 Adaptive combining via correlation exploration for ultrawideband breast cancer imaging *IEEE Antennas Wirel. Propag. Lett.* **14** 587–90

[27] Song H, Xiao X, Wang Z and Kikkawa T 2015 UWB microwave breast cancer detection with MRI-derived 3-D realistic numerical breast model *2015 IEEE Int. Symp. Antennas and Propagation & USNC/URSI National Radio Science Meeting* 544–5

[28] Mirza A F, Abdulsalam F, Asif R, Dama Y A S, Abusitta M M, Elmegri F, Abd-Alhameed R A, Noras J M and Qahwaji R 2015 Breast cancer detection using 1D, 2D, and 3D FDTD numerical methods *2015 IEEE Int. Conf. on Computer and Information Technology; Ubiquitous Computing and Communications; Dependable, Autonomic and Secure Computing; Pervasive Intelligence and Computing (CIT/IUCC/DASC/PICOM)* (Piscataway, NJ: IEEE) pp 1042–5

[29] Wang F, Arslan T and Wang G 2017 Breast cancer detection with microwave imaging system using wearable conformal antenna arrays *2017 Int. Conf. on Imaging Systems and Techniques (IST)* (Piscataway, NJ: IEEE) pp 1–6

[30] Kwon S and Lee S 2013 Instantaneous microwave imaging with time-domain measurements for breast cancer detection *Electron. Lett.* **49** 639–41

[31] Lecture-5-Formulation of FDTD of 1D FDTD available at https://empossible.net/wp-content/uploads/2019/08/Lecture-5-Formulation-of-1D-FDTD.pdf

[32] Patel H N 2019 Microwave imaging for breast cancer detection using 3D level set based optimization, FDTD method and method of moments *PhD Dissertation* Dhirubhai Ambani Institute of Information and Communication Technology

Chapter 5

3D level set based optimization

A single frequency has limited imaging information about healthy and malignant tissues of the breast. The multiple frequency inverse scattering problem is formulated for breast cancer detection by using microwave imaging. The breast imaging problem is converted into matrices and cost function is also calculated for this formulation. 3D level set based evolution and optimization approaches for the solution of inverse scattering problems are described. Single and double 3D level set function based problem formulations are given with the implementation steps. The effects of Tikhonov and total variation (TV) regularization on breast image reconstruction are evaluated through simulation. The performance of TV regularization is found to be better than Tikhonov regularization.

5.1 Multiple frequency inverse scattering problem formulation

5.2 Introduction

Multiple frequency inclusion in the inverse scattering problem improves computational efficiency and accuracy of a microwave imaging system. Numerical breast phantom, antenna placement and Debye model are required for multiple frequency inverse scattering problem formulation. Numerical breast phantom and antenna placement are given in appendix A for a breast cancer detection system. Zastrow *et al* have developed an anatomically realistic numerical breast phantom with accurate dielectric properties in [1]. The Debye model is used to model polarization and dispersion properties of human breast tissues. Derivation of Debye model is given in appendix B1. Lazebnik *et al* have developed highly accurate Debye models for normal and malignant breast tissue dielectric properties in 0.5–20GHz frequency range [2]. Experimental approximation of human breast tissue properties by using improved Debye model is proposed by Khuda *et al* in [3]. Average dielectric

doi:10.1088/978-0-7503-2592-9ch5

property analysis and bulk dielectric permittivity estimation for breast tissues are given in [4] and [5], respectively. Winters *et al* have proposed multiple frequency inverse scattering problem in [6]. Shea *et al* have also used multiple frequency inverse scattering problem formulation of Winters *et al* in [7]. Irishina has proposed antenna placement for a 2D microwave breast imaging system in [8]. Colgan *et al* have used multiple frequency inverse scattering problem formulation for a 3D level set technique in [9]. Our work on multiple frequency inverse scattering problem formulation is described in [10–12].

5.3 Problem formulation

Multiple frequency inverse scattering problem formulation for human breast tissues requires the Debye model. The Debye model is incorporated in the system of scattered field equations. Antenna placement surrounding the breast in appendix A2 is used to formulate the multiple frequency inverse scattering problem. Scattered fields at antenna locations are calculated by using equation (5.1).

$$\vec{E}^{s}(\vec{r}) = \iiint G(\vec{r}, \vec{r}^{'}) \cdot \vec{J}(\vec{r}^{'})\, dv' \tag{5.1}$$

In equation (5.1), $\vec{E}^{s}(\vec{r})$ is scattered electric field at antenna locations $\vec{r}$, Green's function of homogeneous background medium is $G(\vec{r}, \vec{r}^{'})$, and $\vec{J}(\vec{r}^{'})$ is polarization current density. Equation (5.2) is obtained by substituting polarization current density into equation (5.1).

$$\vec{E}^{s}(\vec{r}) = \omega^2\mu \iiint G(\vec{r}, \vec{r}^{'}) \cdot \vec{E}_t(\vec{r}^{'})[\epsilon(\vec{r}^{'}) - \epsilon^{b}(\vec{r})]dr' \tag{5.2}$$

In equation (5.2), $\epsilon(\vec{r}^{'}) - \epsilon^{b}(\vec{r})$ is contrast in permittivity with respect to homogeneous background medium, $\vec{E}_t(\vec{r}^{'})$ is total electric field intensity at location $\vec{r}^{'}$. A single-pole Debye model of equation (5.3) is substituted in equation (5.2).

$$\epsilon(\omega) = \epsilon_\infty + \frac{\Delta\epsilon}{1 + j\omega\tau} + \frac{\sigma_s}{j\omega\epsilon_0} \tag{5.3}$$

In equation (5.3), ϵ_∞ is infinite frequency permittivity, $\Delta\epsilon$ is difference between static permittivity (ϵ_s) and infinite frequency permittivity (ϵ_∞), and σ_s is static conductivity. τ is relaxation time constant with 15 ps value for all breast tissues. Relaxation time constant is assumed to be spatially invariant. Approximation of equation (5.2) is obtained by using procedure of [6, 7]. Numerical breast phantom is represented by K voxels after discretization. There are 40 antennas surrounding the breast, as shown in appendix A2. Each antenna works as a transceiver. One antenna transmits microwave signal on the breast and other antennas receive scattered microwave signal due to different breast tissues. This process is repeated for each antenna present in the system. Let us consider there are N antennas in the system. F is the number of frequencies. Ideally there are N^2F measurements possible. There are only $M = (N(N - 1)/2)F$ measurements possible after removing redundancy. There are $N - 1$ receivers when the first antenna transmits. There are $N - 2$ receivers when the second antenna transmits. By this way, there are channels among transmitters and receivers. By considering N antennas, M number of channels, F number of frequencies, and K voxels, equation (5.4) is obtained from equation (5.2).

$$\begin{bmatrix} \mathrm{Re}(A_1^{\infty}) & \mathrm{Re}(A_1^{\Delta}) & \mathrm{Re}(A_1^{\sigma}) \\ \mathrm{Im}(A_1^{\infty}) & \mathrm{Im}(A_1^{\Delta}) & \mathrm{Im}(A_1^{\sigma}) \\ & \vdots & \\ \mathrm{Re}(A_M^{\infty}) & \mathrm{Re}(A_M^{\Delta}) & \mathrm{Re}(A_M^{\sigma}) \\ \mathrm{Im}(A_M^{\infty}) & \mathrm{Im}(A_M^{\Delta}) & \mathrm{Im}(A_M^{\sigma}) \end{bmatrix} \begin{bmatrix} \delta(\epsilon_\infty) \\ \delta(\Delta\epsilon) \\ \delta(\sigma_\mathrm{s}) \end{bmatrix} = \begin{bmatrix} \mathrm{Re}(E_1^\mathrm{s}) \\ \mathrm{Im}(E_1^\mathrm{s}) \\ \vdots \\ \mathrm{Re}(E_M^\mathrm{s}) \\ \mathrm{Im}(E_M^\mathrm{s}) \end{bmatrix} \tag{5.4}$$

In equation (5.4), $\delta(\epsilon_\infty) = (\epsilon_\infty)_k - (\epsilon_\infty)_\mathrm{b}$, is the difference between kth voxel's infinite frequency permittivity and background medium's infinite frequency permittivity, $\delta(\Delta\epsilon) = (\Delta\epsilon)_k - (\Delta\epsilon)_\mathrm{b}$ and $\delta(\sigma_\mathrm{s}) = (\sigma_\mathrm{s})_k - (\sigma_\mathrm{s})_\mathrm{b}$ are defined the same as above. Re(·) and Im(·) represent real part and imaginary part, respectively. By comparing equation (5.4) with $A\epsilon = b$, sizes of A, ϵ and b are $2MF \times 3K$, $3K \times 1$ and $2MF \times 1$ respectively. There are a total of $2MF$ equations, and $3K$ unknowns. Let's consider an example with 40 antennas, 18 frequencies, and 64 000 voxels. There are 28 080 equations and 192 000 unknowns in our system. It means this approximated linear system of equation (5.4) is under-determined. In equation (5.4), each element of matrix A is represented by equation (5.5) and the scattered fields column vector of the right-hand side is given by equation (5.6). In equation (5.5), $a_k^p(\omega_1) = \omega_1^2\mu\epsilon_0 \cdot E_y^t(\vec{r}_j|\vec{r}_m, \omega_1) \cdot \mathrm{IG}_y(\vec{r}_n|\vec{r}_j, \omega_1)$ and $C_\infty(\omega) = 1$, $C_\Delta(\omega) = (1 + j\omega\tau)^{-1}$, $C_\sigma(\omega) = (j\omega\epsilon_0)^{-1}$. $E_y^t(\vec{r}_j|\vec{r}_m, \omega_l)$ is the y direction electric field present at the jth voxel location due to the transmitter at location $\vec{r}_m$ for angular frequency ω_l, $\mathrm{IG}_y(\vec{r}_n|\vec{r}_j, \omega_l)$ is the y direction component of the integration of the Green's function at angular frequency ω_l, where, $\vec{r}_n$, p and k represent receiver location, particular channel number and total number of voxels respectively. The scattered electric field matrix of equation (5.4) is known due to forward simulation. The left-hand side matrix A of equation (5.4) is also known. Permittivity contrast profile column matrix is only unknown in equation (5.4).

$$A_\mathrm{p}^\mathrm{e} = \begin{bmatrix} C_\mathrm{e}(\omega_1)[a_1^\mathrm{p}(\omega_1) \ldots\ldots a_k^\mathrm{p}(\omega_1)] \\ \vdots \\ C_\mathrm{e}(\omega_F)[a_1^\mathrm{p}(\omega_F) \ldots\ldots a_k^\mathrm{p}(\omega_F)] \end{bmatrix} \tag{5.5}$$

$$E_\mathrm{p}^\mathrm{s} = \begin{bmatrix} E_y^t(\vec{r}_n|\vec{r}_m, \omega_1) - E_y^i(\vec{r}_n|\vec{r}_m, \omega_1) \\ \vdots \\ E_y^t(\vec{r}_n|\vec{r}_m, \omega_F) - E_y^i(\vec{r}_n|\vec{r}_m, \omega_F) \end{bmatrix} \tag{5.6}$$

$$C(\epsilon) = \frac{1}{2}\sum_{f=1}^{F}\sum_{n=1}^{M}|E_{\mathrm{m}}^{\mathrm{s}}(\vec{r}_n, \omega_f) - E_{\mathrm{r}}^{\mathrm{s}}(\vec{r}_n, \omega_f, \epsilon(\vec{r}^{\,'}))|^2 \tag{5.7}$$

In equation (5.7), $C(\epsilon)$ is cost function, $E_{\mathrm{m}}^{\mathrm{s}}(\vec{r}_n, \omega_f)$ is known scattered field (measured) at location $\vec{r}_n$ for frequency ω_f, $E_{\mathrm{r}}^{\mathrm{s}}(\vec{r}_n, \omega_f, \epsilon(\vec{r}^{\,'}))$ is the reconstructed scattered field at location $\vec{r}_n$ for frequency ω_f and dielectric profile $\epsilon(\vec{r}^{\,'})$, F is the number of frequencies, M is the number of measurements (channels), $\vec{r}_n$ is receiver location, ω_f is angular frequency. Now, cost function is represented in residual form by using equation (5.8).

$$C(\epsilon) = \frac{1}{2}\sum_{i=1}^{FM}|R_i|^2 \tag{5.8}$$

The cost function of equation (5.8) is minimized in the next section.

5.4 Review of previous work

In 1988, level set method was proposed for the first time by Osher and Sethian as propagating fronts for algorithms based on Hamilton–Jacobi formulation [13]. Level set method is very good at topology reconstruction due to its automatic merging and breaking property. Better shape and dielectric properties reconstruction are provided by 3D level set based optimization for microwave breast imaging. Most of the traditional optimization techniques do not include shape reconstruction. 3D level set function based methods avoid this limitation of traditional optimization techniques. Simultaneous reconstruction of dielectric properties and shape are both provided by 3D level set based optimization methods. Values of dielectric properties and shape are both reconstructed by minimizing cost function for Debye parameters and level set functions. This problem is quite challenging due to the ill-posed system matrix and the noisy scattered fields data make. Regularization is very effective to solve the ill-posed and noisy problem.

Osher and Fedkiw have proposed level set methods for different applications in [14]. Santosa has proposed a novel level set based evolution and optimization approaches for inverse problems in [15]. Single 3D level set function based breast classification is implemented by Colgan *et al* in [16]. Classical reviews on level set methods for inverse problems are described in [17–19].

Human breast complex permittivity profile reconstruction is always challenging in three dimensions. Shape and value reconstructions are both important in three dimensions. Shape reconstruction is not involved in most of the current optimization techniques. It is considered as a major drawback in 3D reconstruction. This limitation is avoided using 3D level set functions. Novel 3D level set based optimization is used to reconstruct values as well as shape of complex permittivity profile. Debye parameter values and 3D level set functions are updated to minimize cost function. Ill-posed system matrix and noisy scattered fields data make 3D reconstruction very challenging. Regularization is used in 3D level set based optimization to overcome the above challenges. Osher *et al* have solved the Hamilton–Jacobi equation by using moving fronts with curvature dependent speed in [13]. Now, their work is recognized as level set methods. The algorithm proposed by Osher *et al* handles topology merging and breaking naturally which makes it attractive for shape reconstruction. Osher *et al* have proposed level set method with fast marching method and extension velocity in [14]. Their level set methods are used widely in many fields of science, engineering and technology now. Santosa has proposed level set based evolution and optimization approaches for inverse problems with deconvolution and diffraction screen reconstruction examples in [15].

Dorn *et al* have proposed an efficient two-step shape reconstruction method for electromagnetic cross-borehole tomography using adjoint fields and level set in [20]. In this method, the shape of an obstacle is reconstructed by applying adjoint fields and level set to an initial guess. Finite difference time domain (FDTD) is used twice per iteration to solve Helmholtz equations. Dorn *et al* have considered only shape reconstruction of the object by using known permittivity values inside the object. This level set method is the method of asymptotic regularization, which has been developed for ill-posed problems in Hilbert spaces. They have shown regularizing properties of the level set method with the discrepancy principle as a stopping criteria. Ferraye *et al* have proposed a shape reconstruction of the obstacle for electromagnetic tomography using level set method based on contour deformations with frequency hopping technique in [21]. In this approach, automatic merging and breaking capability is used for the shape reconstruction inverse scattering problem.

A very good survey of level set method for inverse problems is done in [17–19]. The survey includes general level set method formulation for the following areas:

1. Geometry based inverse and optimization problems.
2. Level set methods based evolving interfaces.
3. Shape calculus by using level set method.
4. Level set methods based shape optimization.
5. Level set method for ill-posed problems.

A general framework for the above topics is given nicely with several open issues in [17, 18]. Recent techniques which have a level set based representation of shapes for solving inverse scattering problems are given in [19]. Electromagnetic scattering by using different popular models, for example TM-polarized and TE-polarized waves, Maxwell's equations, impedance tomography, a transport equation or its diffusion approximation are described with topological derivatives and shape sensitivity analysis in this work. Various techniques are proposed with realistic application examples in two and three dimensions for incorporating regularization into the shape inverse scattering problem.

Aghasi *et al* have proposed reconstruction of obstacles by using parametric level set method in [22]. General level set evolution equations are derived for an unknown obstacle reconstruction. A significantly lower dimensional problem is obtained by applying the appropriate form of parametric level set function. Radial basis function is used to make the parametric level set which provides a 'narrow-banding' advantage such that the number of unknowns are reduced at each step of the evolution by using this approach. The performance of this approach is tested in diffuse optical tomography, electrical impedance tomography and x-ray computed tomography.

Semerci *et al* have proposed a novel polychromatic dual-energy processing algorithm, which can detect and characterize objects embedded in the background [23]. In this paper, level set based characteristic function of the object is used with a number of regularization techniques for addressing both the physical properties of the object and the prior information. The proposed approach gives zero characteristic function in the absence of an object. So, it can be viewed as simultaneously solving both characterization and detection problems. Level set is defined parametrically by using radial basis functions with a Gauss–Newton algorithm for cost minimization. Numerical results show that the algorithm successfully detects objects. It also finds objects' shape and location with reconstruction of the background. A modified level set method (MLSM) is proposed to reconstruct a 2D object's shape and electrical properties simultaneously in [24]. Eskandari *et al* have proposed an evolution strategy to reconstruct complex permittivity and shape of a 2D object. As the cost function is minimized iteratively, the initial guesses about the complex permittivity and shape of the target object converge to their values. L_1 and L_2 norms are added to cost function as regularization terms. Sudden changes in the shape of the object are prevented by a curvature-based regularization. Fluctuations in the object's parameters are reduced by Laplacian based regularization. The capabilities of MLSM in microwave imaging are evaluated by using different synthetic data sets. Two objects separated by a distance of one-fifteenth of a wavelength can be reconstructed completely using MLSM. Targets of different relative permittivity can be retrieved with less than 10% error by using this method. Reconstruction of the immersed one-tenth wavelength targets in highly contrasting domains is considered as an important feature of this method. These features of MLSM are precious in distinguishing malignant tissues from normal tissues.

Irishina *et al* have proposed a level set based evolution strategy in two broad steps for early breast cancer detection using microwave imaging [27]. In the first step, location and size of tumor is found, whereas in the second step, dielectric property of the tumor is determined. The level set method of [27] is verified by a 2D numerical breast phantom. The tumor characterization may fail for very small hidden breast tumours in the presence of strong noise [27]. Irishina *et al* have proposed a level set based strategy for microwave imaging based early breast cancer detection in [28, 8]. The level set based solution has advantages over traditional pixel based approaches when reconstruction of size, shape and static permittivity value of hidden tumor is crucial. Level set based strategy is useful for correct estimation of interfaces between fibro-glandular and fatty tissues. The level set based proposed strategy of [28, 8] is able to detect and characterize small tumors successfully. In order to reconstruct correct shape, size and location of the tumor an initial guess of tumor permittivity value is required.

Reconstructed difference permittivity ($\Delta\epsilon$) profile of a class 3 numerical breast phantom by using conjugate gradient method is shown in figure 5.1 [26]. Results of

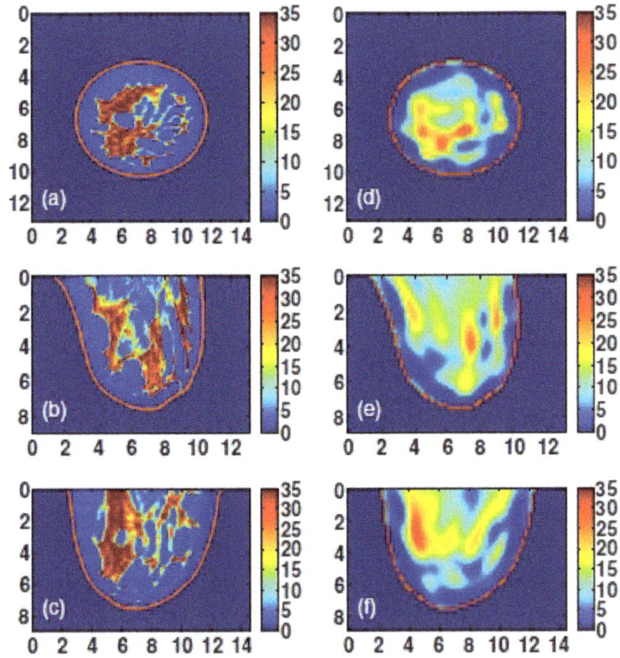

Figure 5.1. Class 3 phantom:(a)–(c) exact and (d)–(f) reconstructed profile of $\Delta\epsilon$ shown in coronal (x–y, top row), sagittal (y–z, middle row), and axial (x–z, bottom row) cross-sections. Reprinted from [26] by permission from John Wiley & Sons, copyright 2010.

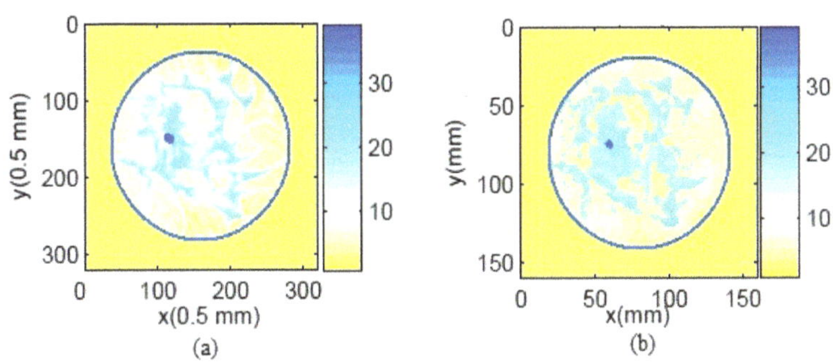

Figure 5.2. Comparison of permittivity profiles in less dense breast. (a) Original permittivity profile. (b) Reconstructed permittivity profile at the end of the four-stage algorithm [8].

figure 5.1 clearly show that the shape is not reconstructed well by using conjugate gradient method. Some important results of [8] are shown below. figure 5.2 shows a comparison of permittivity profiles in a less dense breast. figure 5.3 shows comparison of permittivity profiles in a more dense breast. Figures 5.2 and 5.3 show promising results of a level set based four-stage inversion method [8]. figure 5.4 shows original and reconstructed permittivity profiles when there is no tumor. Figure 5.5 shows original and reconstructed permittivity profiles when there are two tumors. The above results clearly show robustness of the algorithm proposed in [8].

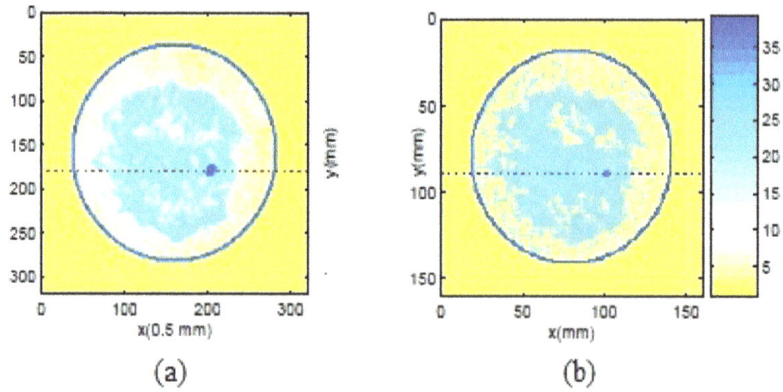

Figure 5.3. Comparison of permittivity profiles in high dense breast. (a) Original permittivity profile. (b) Reconstructed permittivity profile at the end of the four-stage algorithm [8].

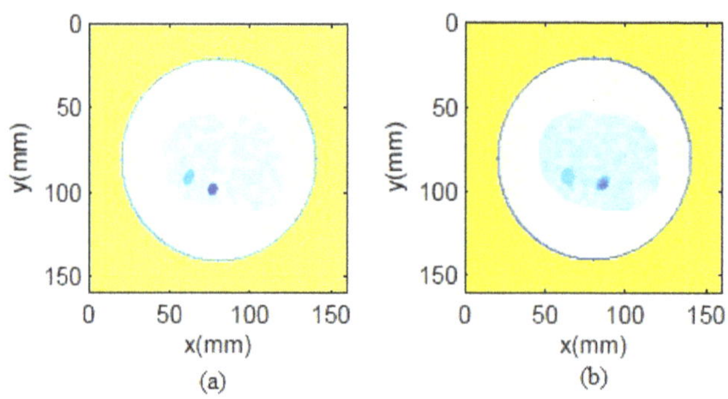

Figure 5.4. Comparison of permittivity profiles without tumour. (a) Original permittivity profile. (b) Reconstructed permittivity profile at the end of the four-stage algorithm [8].

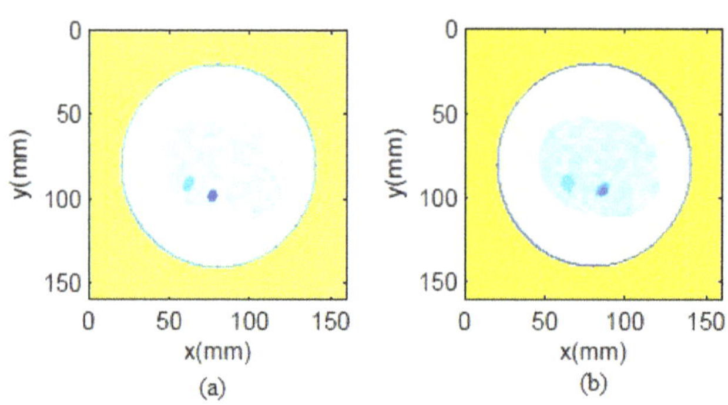

Figure 5.5. Comparison of permittivity profiles with two tumour. (a) Original permittivity profile. (b) Reconstructed permittivity profile at the end of the four-stage algorithm [8].

Colgan *et al* have proposed 3D level set based optimization for microwave breast imaging in [16]. Breast density classification is proposed using single-level set function. The level set based adjoint method requires two FDTD simulations per iteration. The level set method of [16] is computationally efficient as compared to the

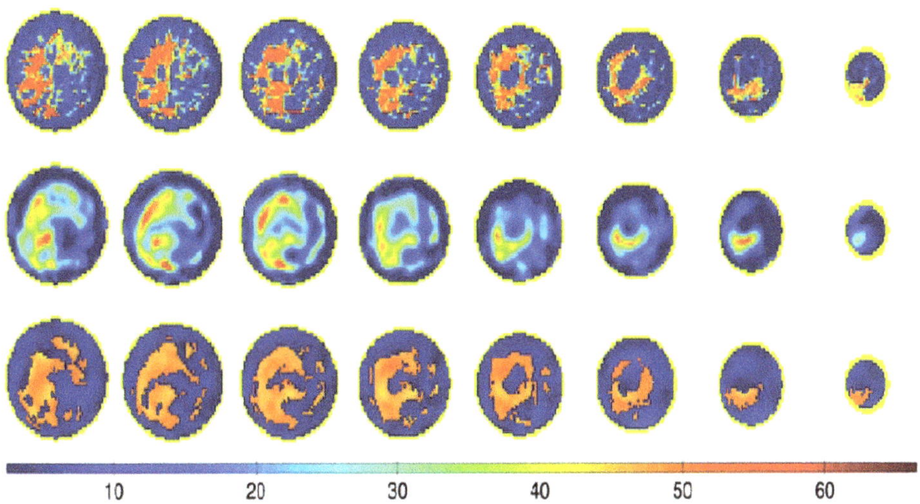

Figure 5.6. Coronal cross-section of static permittivity profiles in class 3 breast phantom. Top row shows original permittivity profiles. Middle row shows reconstructed permittivity profiles by using 3D Distorted born iterative method (DBIM). Bottom row shows reconstructed permittivity profiles by using 3D level set based optimization. The coronal cross-sections are taken every 8 mm. Copyright (1990) IEEE. Reprinted, with permission, from [39].

adjoint method of Dorn *et al* because it requires a single FDTD simulation per iteration. Figure 5.6 shows promising results of level set based optimization by using a single-level set function [16]. Results of figure 5.6 clearly show that the performance of 3D level set optimization is better than 3D distorted born iterative method (DBIM).

5.5 Theoretical foundations

There are two approaches for a level set based solution of inverse problems. Evolution and optimization are two well-known approaches used for level set based optimization of inverse problems [15]. G is a characteristic set of interest with its boundary function $\psi(r)$.

$$\partial G = \{r \colon \psi(r) = 0\} \tag{5.9}$$

The level set approach is used to generate a sequence of functions $\phi_n(r)$ such that the below given condition is satisfied.

$$G_n = G \tag{5.10}$$

Complex permittivity reconstruction is achieved by solving the inverse scattering problem. Let's take ϵ as an unknown permittivity profile. Equation (5.11) gives the relationship of $\phi(r)$ with ϵ.

$$\epsilon(r) = \begin{cases} \epsilon_{\text{int}} & \text{for } \{r \colon \psi(r) < 0\} \\ \epsilon_{\text{ext}} & \text{for } \{r \colon \psi(r) > 0\} \end{cases} \tag{5.11}$$

In equation (5.11), $\epsilon(r) = \epsilon_{\mathrm{int}}$ whenever function $\psi(r)$ is negative, $\epsilon(r) = \epsilon_{\mathrm{ext}}$ whenever function $\psi(r)$ is positive. Advantages of representing ϵ as function $\psi(r)$ are given below.

- *A priori* assumptions are not needed for the topology of G. Several disconnected subregions can be part of G. G may be multiple times connected.
- There is no requirement of *a priori* assumptions related to the nature of G.

Equation (5.11) makes the linear inverse problem nonlinear due to dependence of ϵ on ψ. In equation (5.11), $\psi(r)$ is found such that $A\epsilon = y$, where A and y are known. If $\psi(r)$ is changed by a small variation $\delta\psi(r)$ then r is changed by δr. This variation results in the new region denoted by G'. If variation of the equation $\psi(r)$ is equal to 0, then

$$\delta\psi + \nabla\psi \cdot \delta r = 0 \tag{5.12}$$

In figure 5.7, the unit outward normal at r is given by equation (5.13).

$$n(r) = \frac{\nabla\psi(r)}{|\nabla\psi(r)|} \tag{5.13}$$

The inner product of $\delta\epsilon$ with a test function $f(x)$ is given by equation (5.14).

$$\langle \delta\epsilon, f \rangle := \int_{R^2} \delta\epsilon(r) f(r) \mathrm{d}r = \int_{G \cap G'} \delta\epsilon(r) f(r) \mathrm{d}r \tag{5.14}$$

The value of $\delta\epsilon(r)$ is equal to $\epsilon_{\mathrm{int}} - \epsilon_{\mathrm{ext}}$ with plus or minus sign. Inner product is simplified to equation (5.15) for infinitesimal $\delta\epsilon$.

$$\langle \delta\epsilon, f \rangle := \int_{\partial G} (\epsilon_{\mathrm{int}} - \epsilon_{\mathrm{ext}}) \delta r \cdot n(r) f(r) \mathrm{d}s(r) \tag{5.15}$$

where $\mathrm{d}s(r)$ is the incremental arc length. $\delta\epsilon$ is given by equation (5.16).

$$\delta\epsilon = (\epsilon_{\mathrm{int}} - \epsilon_{\mathrm{ext}}) \frac{\nabla\phi(r)}{|\nabla\phi(r)|} \cdot \delta r \tag{5.16}$$

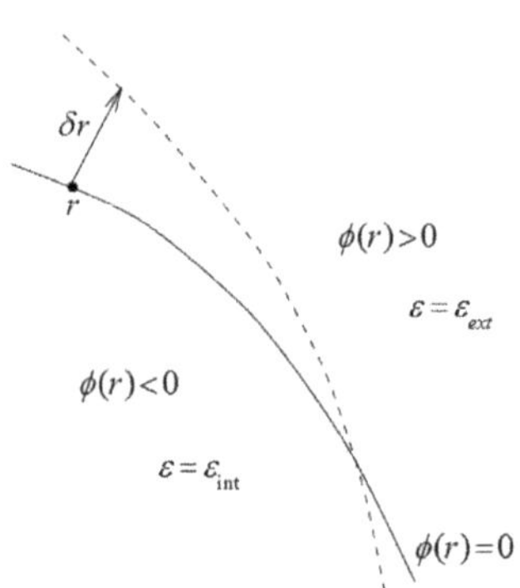

Figure 5.7. The variations of the curve r: $\phi(r) = 0$ under variation $\delta\phi(r)$. Source: [38] and [15].

The dot product in the above equation includes correct sign for $\delta\epsilon$. $\delta\epsilon$ will have the same sign as $(\epsilon_{\text{int}} - \epsilon_{\text{ext}})$ at the point r. The opposite sign will be there if the normal component of δr is in the opposite direction of the normal.

5.5.1 Evolution approach

The evolution equation for $\phi(r)$ is obtained to solve the inverse scattering or obstacle problem in this approach. According to the property of the evolution equation, as time t tends to infinity the function $\psi(r)$ is evolved such that the associated $\epsilon(r)$ is the solution to the inverse problem. If t represents time, then level set function ψ depends on both r and t.

$$\partial G(t) = \{r: \psi(r, t) = 0\} \tag{5.17}$$

Therefore, an evolving region is associated with $\psi(r, t)$. The cost function of equation (5.18) is to be minimized in the least square sense.

$$S(\epsilon) = \frac{1}{2}\|A\epsilon - y\|_2^2 \tag{5.18}$$

The minimal requirement for the variation of $\psi(r, t)$ is that $S(\epsilon)$ be a decreasing function of t. Let's assume that each point $r \in \partial G(t)$ moves perpendicular to the surface. The variation of δr satisfies equation (5.19).

$$\delta r = \beta(r, t)\frac{\nabla\psi}{|\nabla\psi|} \tag{5.19}$$

In equation (5.19), $\beta(r, t)$ is viewed as the velocity of the surface at r. Equation (5.20) is obtained by substituting equation (5.19) into equation (5.16).

$$\delta\epsilon = (\epsilon_{\text{int}} - \epsilon_{\text{ext}})\beta(r, t) \tag{5.20}$$

The directional derivative of the function $S(\epsilon)$ in the direction $\delta\epsilon$ is given by

$$\delta S(\epsilon) = \langle J^T(\epsilon)(A\epsilon - y), \delta\epsilon\rangle \tag{5.21}$$

where $J(\epsilon)$ is Jacobian of $A\epsilon$ at ϵ. Equation (5.22) is obtained by substituting equation (5.20) into equation (5.21).

$$\delta S(\epsilon) = \int_{\partial G(t)} [J^T(\epsilon)(A\epsilon - y)](\epsilon_{\text{int}} - \epsilon_{\text{ext}})\beta(r, t)\, \mathrm{d}s(r) \tag{5.22}$$

Assuming that $\epsilon_{\text{int}} > \epsilon_{\text{ext}}$, the natural choice of $\beta(r, t)$ is given by equation (5.23).

$$\beta(r, t) = -J^T(\epsilon)(A\epsilon - y) \tag{5.23}$$

Equation (5.24) for $\delta\psi(x, t)$ is determined by using equations (5.12) and (5.19).

$$\delta\psi = -\nabla\psi \cdot \delta r = -\nabla\psi \cdot \left(\beta(r, t)\frac{\nabla\psi}{|\nabla\psi|}\right) = -\beta(r, t)|\nabla\psi| \tag{5.24}$$

Any $\beta(r, t)$ satisfying equation (5.23) produces $\delta\psi$ which will reduce $S(\epsilon)$. This leads to the equation of $\delta\psi$.

$$\delta\psi = [J^T(\epsilon)(A\epsilon - y)]|\nabla\psi| \tag{5.25}$$

This initial value problem for $\psi(r, t)$ is a Hamilton–Jacobi system as shown by equations (5.26) and (5.27).

$$\frac{\partial\psi}{\partial t} = [J^T(\epsilon)(A\epsilon - y)]|\nabla\psi| \tag{5.26}$$

$$\psi(r, 0) = \psi_0(r) \tag{5.27}$$

It is observed that the evolutionary approach has the following characteristics.

1. The evolution is such that $S(\epsilon)$ is non-increasing; that is $\frac{\partial}{\partial t}S(\epsilon) \leqslant 0$.
2. If a solution ϵ exists, then at the solution $A\epsilon = y$, so that $\frac{\partial\psi}{\partial t} = 0$ at the solution.
3. It can be viewed as the evolution in the steepest descent direction for the residual of $S(\epsilon)$.

This evolution approach can be used to find a solution of inverse problems.

5.5.2 Optimization approach

In the optimization approach, it is the sequence of surfaces $\psi_k(r)$ whose associated function $\epsilon(r)$ represents descent directions for the functional $S(\epsilon)$. It is convenient to use the notation given below for this purpose.

$$\partial G_k = \{r\colon \psi_k(r) = 0\} \tag{5.28}$$

Consider $\psi_k(r)$ as an initial point in this approach. An update $\delta\psi(r)$ is needed to generate $\psi_{k+1}(r)$. The Gauss–Newton approach is used to minimize $S(\epsilon)$. The descent update is given by $\delta\epsilon'$, where

$$J^T(\epsilon)J(\epsilon)\delta\epsilon' = J^T(\epsilon)(y - A\epsilon) \tag{5.29}$$

Equation (5.29) is an update for ϵ. Now our task is to find the associated update for ψ. Equation (5.20) is rewritten as follows.

$$\delta\epsilon = (\epsilon_{\text{int}} - \epsilon_{\text{ext}})\beta(r) \tag{5.30}$$

For $\delta\epsilon'$, equation (5.30) can be written as equation (5.31)

$$\delta\epsilon' = (\epsilon_{\text{int}} - \epsilon_{\text{ext}})\beta(r) \tag{5.31}$$

Equation (5.32) can be obtained by rearranging equation (5.31).

$$\beta(r) = \frac{\delta\epsilon'}{(\epsilon_{\text{int}} - \epsilon_{\text{ext}})} \tag{5.32}$$

The natural choice for $\beta(r)$ is to extend the above relation to all points on R^3. An update for $\delta\psi(r)$ is given by equation (5.33).

$$\delta\psi(r) = -\frac{\delta\epsilon'}{(\epsilon_{\text{int}} - \epsilon_{\text{ext}})}|\nabla\psi_k(r)| \tag{5.33}$$

It can be shown that this is the descent direction for $S(\epsilon)$. Equation (5.32) is substituted in equation (5.22) to get.

$$\delta S(\epsilon) = -\int_{\partial G_k} [J^T(\epsilon)(A\epsilon - y)]\delta\epsilon' \mathrm{d}s(r) \tag{5.34}$$

Equation (5.35) is obtained by substituting $\delta\epsilon'$ value of equation (5.29) in equation (5.34).

$$\delta S(\epsilon) = -\int_{\partial G_k} [J^T(\epsilon)(A\epsilon - y)][J^T(\epsilon)J(\epsilon)]^{-1}J^T(\epsilon)(y - A\epsilon)\, rmds(r) \tag{5.35}$$

The above equation is negative if $J^T(\epsilon)J(\epsilon) > 0$. Therefore, the variation $\delta\psi(r)$ corresponds to a variation in $S(\epsilon)$ that is negative. Gauss–Newton algorithm for the inverse problem is given below.

1. Choose $\psi_0(r)$; set $k = 0$.
2. Compute associated ϵ; if $S(\epsilon)>$ tolerance, do
   (i) Compute $J(\epsilon)^T J(\epsilon)\delta\epsilon' = J^T(\epsilon)(y - A\epsilon)$.
   (ii) Compute $\delta\psi(r) = -\frac{\delta\epsilon'}{(\epsilon_{\text{int}} - \epsilon_{\text{ext}})}|\nabla\psi_k(r)|$.
   (iii) Set $k = k + 1$, update $\psi_{k+1}(r) = \psi_k(r) + \delta\psi(r)$.

This algorithm is implemented to find a solution of the inverse problem.

5.6 Single 3D level set function based optimization

The single 3D level set function based optimization is described in [16]. Reviews of level set methods for different types of inverse problems are described in [17–19]. Electromagnetic tomography for shape reconstruction is proposed by using adjoint and level set methods in [20]. The contour deformation based inverse scattering method using frequency hopping technique is given in [21]. The parametric level set method for inverse problems is described in [20, 21]. MLSM for simultaneous microwave imaging and parameter estimation is given in [24]. The single-level set function is shown in figure 5.8. Figure 5.8 shows the level set function which distinguishes two different regions in 2D. A scenario of figure 5.8 is given as an equation.

$$\epsilon(r) = \epsilon^{\text{fib}}(r)H(\phi(r)) + \epsilon^{\text{fat}}(r)(1 - H(\phi(r))) \tag{5.36}$$

In equation (5.36), $\phi(r)$ is level set function, $H(\cdot)$ is the unit step function, ϵ^{fib} is the complex permittivity of the fibro-glandular tissues, ϵ^{fat} is the complex permittivity of the fatty tissues. Region $\phi > 0$ is represented by $H(\phi)$ and region $\phi \leqslant 0$ is represented by $1 - H(\phi)$. Equations (5.37) and (5.38) represent linear relationships among Debye parameters [16].

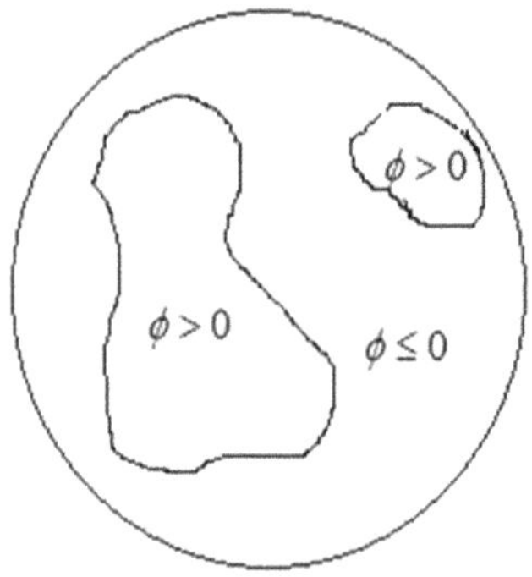

Figure 5.8. Level set function to distinguish two different regions. Source: [38].

$$\epsilon_\infty = 0.326\,5\epsilon_s + 1.632\,6 \tag{5.37}$$

$$\sigma_s = 0.015\,1\epsilon_s - 0.036\,5 \tag{5.38}$$

The above equations are used to reduce the number of unknowns per voxel. Now, cost function of equation (5.8) is minimized in level set based optimization. The adjoint solution of level set optimization is computationally heavy. This computational cost is avoided by calculating the Jacobian matrix. The Jacobian matrix of cost function equation (5.8) is calculated using equation (5.39) [16].

$$G_r(r|r')\circ E_r^t(r') = J(\epsilon) \tag{5.39}$$

In equation (5.39), $G_r(r|r')$ is the $MF \times K$ Green's function matrix, $E_r^t(r')$ is the $MF \times K$ total field matrix, where M, F and K are number of measurements, number of frequencies and number of voxels, respectively. The Jacobian matrix is an element-by-element product of Green's function matrix and total field matrix. Each row of the Jacobian matrix is the Frechet derivative of the residuals with respect to complex permittivity ϵ. Green function calculations are given in [16, 25, 26]. The Frechet derivative of the cost function is calculated by using equation (5.40) [16].

$$\nabla C(\epsilon) = J^T(\epsilon)R(\epsilon) \tag{5.40}$$

In equation (5.40), size of $J^T(\epsilon)$ is $K \times MF$ and size of residual is $MF \times 1$. The size of partial derivative of cost function with respect to ϵ is $K \times 1$. This method of calculating Frechet derivative reduces computational complexity as compared to adjoint method [16, 20]. Only single FDTD simulation is required at every iteration in this method. Therefore, it reduces computational burden by half at every iteration. The partial derivative of equation (5.36) with respect to ϕ is computed by using equation (5.41) [16].

$$\frac{\partial \epsilon}{\partial \phi} = (\epsilon^{\text{fib}}(r) - \epsilon^{\text{fat}}(r))\delta(\phi(r)) \tag{5.41}$$

The partial derivative of equation (5.36) with respect to static permittivity of fibroglandular tissues ϵ_s^{fib} is computed by using equation (5.42) [16].

$$\frac{\partial \epsilon}{\partial \epsilon_s^{\text{fib}}} = H(\phi(r))\frac{\partial \epsilon^{\text{fib}}}{\partial \epsilon_s^{\text{fib}}} \tag{5.42}$$

The partial derivative of equation (5.36) with respect to static permittivity of fatty tissues ϵ_s^{fat} is computed by using equation (5.43) [16].

$$\frac{\partial \epsilon}{\partial \epsilon_s^{\text{fat}}} = (1 - H(\phi(r)))\frac{\partial \epsilon^{\text{fat}}}{\partial \epsilon_s^{\text{fat}}} \tag{5.43}$$

The partial derivative of cost function with respect to level set function ϕ is calculated by using equation (5.44) [16].

$$\frac{\partial C}{\partial \phi} = \nabla C(\epsilon)\frac{\partial \epsilon}{\partial \phi} \tag{5.44}$$

The partial derivative of cost function with respect to ϵ_s^{fib} is computed by using equation (5.45) [16].

$$\frac{\partial C}{\partial \epsilon_s^{\text{fib}}} = \nabla C(\epsilon)\frac{\partial \epsilon}{\partial \epsilon_s^{\text{fib}}} \tag{5.45}$$

The partial derivative of cost function with respect to ϵ_s^{fat} is computed by using equation (5.46) [16].

$$\frac{\partial C}{\partial \epsilon_s^{\text{fat}}} = \nabla C(\epsilon)\frac{\partial \epsilon}{\partial \epsilon_s^{\text{fat}}} \tag{5.46}$$

The partial derivatives obtained above are used to implement gradient based descent optimization approach as shown below [16].

$$\phi^{n+1} = \phi^n - \alpha_\phi \frac{\partial C}{\partial \phi} \tag{5.47}$$

$$(\epsilon_s^{\text{fib}})^{n+1} = (\epsilon_s^{\text{fib}})^n - \alpha_{\epsilon_s}^{\text{fib}} \frac{\partial C}{\partial \epsilon_s^{\text{fib}}} \tag{5.48}$$

$$(\epsilon_s^{\text{fat}})^{n+1} = (\epsilon_s^{\text{fat}})^n - \alpha_{\epsilon_s}^{\text{fat}} \frac{\partial C}{\partial \epsilon_s^{\text{fat}}} \tag{5.49}$$

where n is the iteration number. The step sizes are α_ϕ, $\alpha_{\epsilon_s}^{\text{fib}}$, and $\alpha_{\epsilon_s}^{\text{fat}}$ are individually chosen. *A priori* information related to breast tissues is useful in deciding the above parameters.

5.7 Two 3D level set function based optimization

Shape and dielectric property reconstruction are both important in 3D reconstructions [8, 27, 28]. 3D level set based optimization is more suitable for 3D reconstruction because it can reconstruct shape and dielectric property simultaneously. Two-level set functions are used in figure 5.9 to identify four different

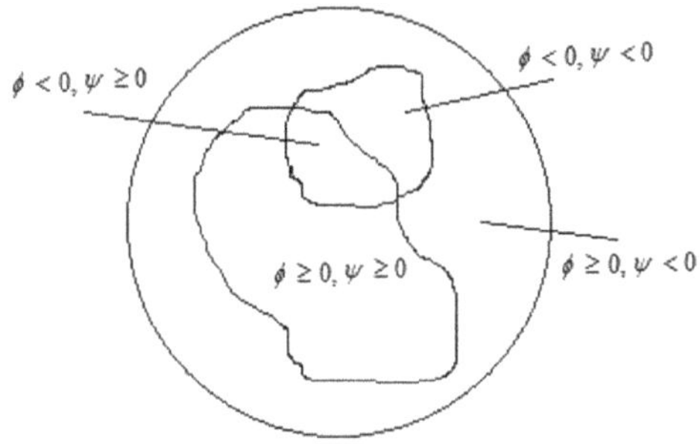

Figure 5.9. Application of two-level set functions to distinguish four different regions (in 2D). Source: [38].

regions. In figure 5.9, $\phi \geqslant 0$, $\psi \geqslant 0$, $\phi \geqslant 0$, $\psi < 0$, $\phi < 0$, $\psi \geqslant 0$ and $\phi < 0$, $\psi < 0$ represent healthy fatty tissues, healthy fibro-glandular tissues, malignant fatty tissues and malignant fibro-glandular tissues, respectively. A scenario of figure 5.9 is expressed as equation (5.50).

$$\epsilon(r) = \epsilon^{\text{tum}}(1 - H(\phi)) + H(\phi)[\epsilon^{\text{fib}}H(\psi) + \epsilon^{\text{fat}}(1 - H(\psi))] \tag{5.50}$$

In equation (5.50), ϵ^{tum}, ϵ^{fib} and ϵ^{fat} are complex permittivity of tumour, fibro-glandular and fatty tissues, respectively, $H()$ is unit step or heavy-side function. ϵ^{tum}, ϵ^{fib} and ϵ^{fat} are expressed in terms of the single-pole Debye model. In equation (5.50), ϕ and ψ are two-level set functions. 3D level set based optimization starts with an initial guess about the solution. A signed distance function of initial guess is required. Steps to calculate signed distance function are given below.

- Find the edges of the initial guess.
- Find the positive distance inside the edge boundary.
- Find the negative distance outside the edge boundary.
- Normalize the distance.

Signed distance function is between −1 and 1 after performing the above steps. Now, this signed distance function is updated using iterative optimization approach. Equations (5.37) and (5.38) represent linear relationships among Debye parameters. A partial derivative of equation (5.8) (cost function) with respect to permittivity is given below.

$$\frac{\partial C}{\partial \epsilon} = J^T(\epsilon)R(\epsilon) \tag{5.51}$$

In equation (5.51), $J^T(\epsilon)$ is the transpose of the Jacobian matrix, $R(\epsilon)$ is residual. The Jacobian matrix is calculated by element-wise multiplication of Green's function matrix with total electric field matrix [16, 25, 26]. A partial derivative of cost function with respect to level set function ϕ is calculated by using equation (5.52).

$$\frac{\partial C}{\partial \phi} = \frac{\partial C}{\partial \epsilon}\frac{\partial \epsilon}{\partial \phi} \tag{5.52}$$

In equation (5.52), a second partial derivative is calculated by taking the partial derivative of equation (5.50) with respect to level set function ϕ.

$$\frac{\partial C}{\partial \phi} = J^T(\epsilon)R(\epsilon) \cdot \delta(\phi)(\epsilon^{\text{fib}}H(\psi) + \epsilon^{\text{fat}}(1 - H(\psi)) - \epsilon^{\text{tum}}) \tag{5.53}$$

Similarly, a partial derivative of cost function with respect to level set function ψ is calculated by using equation (5.54).

$$\frac{\partial C}{\partial \psi} = \frac{\partial C}{\partial \epsilon}\frac{\partial \epsilon}{\partial \psi} \tag{5.54}$$

In equation (5.54), a second partial derivative is calculated by taking the partial derivative of equation (5.50) with respect to level set function ψ.

$$\frac{\partial C}{\partial \psi} = J^T(\epsilon)R(\epsilon) \cdot (H(\phi)\delta(\psi)(\epsilon^{\text{fib}} - \epsilon^{\text{fat}})) \tag{5.55}$$

A partial derivative of cost function with respect to fibro-glandular tissue's static permittivity is given by equation (5.56).

$$\frac{\partial C}{\partial \epsilon_s^{\text{fib}}} = \frac{\partial C}{\partial \epsilon}\frac{\partial \epsilon}{\partial \epsilon^{\text{fib}}}\frac{\partial \epsilon^{\text{fib}}}{\partial \epsilon_s^{\text{fib}}} \tag{5.56}$$

A second partial derivative of equation (5.56) is calculated by taking the partial derivative of equation (5.50) with respect to ϵ^{fib}. A third partial derivative of equation (5.56) is calculated using two steps. In the first step, equations (5.37) and (5.38) are substituted in equation (5.3). In the second step, a partial derivative of the resultant equation is taken with respect to ϵ_s^{fib}. Equation (5.57) is obtained by substituting the partial derivatives in equation (5.56).

$$\frac{\partial C}{\partial \epsilon_s^{\text{fib}}} = J^T(\epsilon)R(\epsilon) \cdot H(\phi)H(\psi)\frac{\partial \epsilon^{\text{fib}}}{\partial \epsilon_s^{\text{fib}}} \tag{5.57}$$

A partial derivative of cost function with respect to fatty tissue's static permittivity is given by equation (5.58).

$$\frac{\partial C}{\partial \epsilon_s^{\text{fat}}} = \frac{\partial C}{\partial \epsilon}\frac{\partial \epsilon}{\partial \epsilon^{\text{fat}}}\frac{\partial \epsilon^{\text{fat}}}{\partial \epsilon_s^{\text{fat}}} \tag{5.58}$$

Equation (5.59) is obtained after calculating the second and third partial derivatives of equation (5.58).

$$\frac{\partial C}{\partial \epsilon_s^{\text{fat}}} = J^T(\epsilon)R(\epsilon) \cdot H(\phi)(1 - H(\psi))\frac{\partial \epsilon^{\text{fat}}}{\partial \epsilon_s^{\text{fat}}} \tag{5.59}$$

Now, four update equations are derived using equations (5.53), (5.55), (5.57) and (5.59).

$$\phi^{n+1} = \phi^n - \alpha_\phi \frac{\partial C}{\partial \phi} \tag{5.60}$$

$$\psi^{n+1} = \psi^{n} - \alpha_{\psi}\frac{\partial C}{\partial \psi} \tag{5.61}$$

$$(\epsilon_{s}^{\text{fib}})^{n+1} = (\epsilon_{s}^{\text{fib}})^{n} - \alpha_{\epsilon_{s}^{\text{fib}}}\frac{\partial C}{\partial \epsilon_{s}^{\text{fib}}} \tag{5.62}$$

$$(\epsilon_{s}^{\text{fat}})^{n+1} = (\epsilon_{s}^{\text{fat}})^{n} - \alpha_{\epsilon_{s}^{\text{fat}}}\frac{\partial C}{\partial \epsilon_{s}^{\text{fat}}} \tag{5.63}$$

The algorithm cannot converge to a solution for larger values of step size. It becomes slower due to smaller step size. Equations (5.60), (5.61), (5.62) and (5.63) are updated using a four-stage reconstruction strategy and frequency hopping [16, 8]. The four-stage reconstruction strategy used in thesis is modified to reduce computations. The first stage is an initial guess of class 3 numerical breast phantom internal structure. The second stage is reconstruction of breast tissues' shapes and dielectric profiles by using equations (5.61), (5.62) and (5.63). In the third stage, tumor location and shape are reconstructed by using equations (5.60) and (5.61). In the last stage, tumor permittivity value is decided by using equation (5.60).

5.7.1 3D level set based regularized optimization

In the case of an inverse scattering problem solution using ill-posed system matrix and noise affected measurements, regularization is very useful [29–31]. The need for regularization is quite clear from figure 5.10. Numerical breast phantom and antenna placement of figure 5.10 are described in appendices A1 and A2, respectively. Sizes of system matrix A, permittivity column vector x or ϵ and scattered electric field column vector b are $2MF \times 3K$, $3K \times 1$ and $2MF \times 1$ respectively. Additive white Gaussian noise n is added to scattered electric field vector b. Tikhonov and total variation regularization techniques are evaluated in this section. Details of both techniques are given in [31].

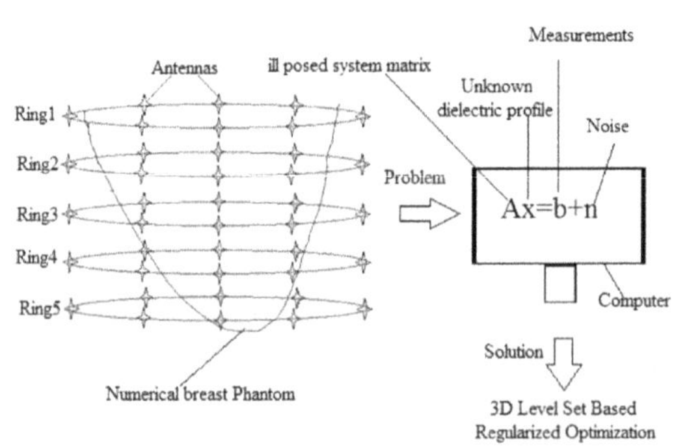

Figure 5.10. Block diagram of practical microwave breast imaging system. Source: [38].

5.7.1.1 Tikhonov regularization

Tikhonov regularization is a very well-known technique. Cost function is updated to include the regularization term. Now, cost function of equation (5.64) is obtained by adding the Tikhonov regularization term in equation (5.8).

$$C(\epsilon) = \frac{1}{2}\left(\sum_{i=1}^{FM}|R_i|^2 + \lambda\|X_1\|^2\right) \tag{5.64}$$

In equation (5.64), λ is regularization parameter, and $\|X_1\|$ is L_2 norm of column vector X_1. Column vector X_1 contains static permittivity values for all voxels. Two things are achieved by regularization: first, a small residue is obtained with an accurate solution. Second, a small solution is achieved such that the perturbation does not affect it much. A partial derivative of cost function with respect to the unknown parameter is given by equation (5.65).

$$\frac{\partial C}{\partial \epsilon} = J^T(\epsilon)R(\epsilon) + \lambda X_1 \tag{5.65}$$

In equation (5.65), $J^T(\epsilon)$ is the transpose of the Jacobian matrix. It is element-by-element multiplication of Green's function matrix and total electric field matrix, $R(\epsilon)$ is residual.

5.7.1.2 Total variation regularization

Tikhonov regularization performs well in the situation where the solution has smooth changes. It will not perform well in the case where the solution has abrupt changes. The total variation regularization term is defined as shown in equation (5.66).

$$TV(X) = \sum_{j=1}^{n-1}|X_{j+1} - X_j| = \|L_1X\|_1 \tag{5.66}$$

In equation (5.66), $\|L_1X\|_1$ is L^1 norm of $\|L_1X\|$. L_1 is a derivative matrix as shown by equation (5.67).

$$L_1 = \begin{bmatrix} -1 & 1 & 0 & \cdot & \cdot & 0 \\ 0 & -1 & 1 & 0 & \cdot & 0 \\ 0 & 0 & -1 & 1 & 0 & \cdot \\ \cdot & \cdot & 0 & \cdot & \cdot & \cdot \\ \cdot & \cdot & \cdot & \cdot & \cdot & \cdot \\ \cdot & \cdot & \cdot & 0 & -1 & 1 \\ 0 & 0 & 0 & 0 & 0 & -1 \end{bmatrix} \tag{5.67}$$

Now, equation (5.68) is obtained by replacing Tikhonov regularization term with total variation regularization term.

$$C(\epsilon) = \frac{1}{2}\sum_{i=1}^{FM}|R_i|^2 + \lambda\|L_1X\|_1 \tag{5.68}$$

L_1 norm is non-differentiable. In order to obtain the partial derivative, diagonal matrix W is used. Equation (5.69) is obtained by using the procedure of [31].

$$\frac{\partial C}{\partial \epsilon} = J^T(\epsilon)R(\epsilon) + \lambda L_1^T W L_1 x \tag{5.69}$$

$W_{j,j} = 1/|x_{j+1} - x_j|$, where $(x_{j+1} - x_j)$ is the jth element of vector L_1x. Tolerance can be set on values of W to accommodate non differentiability of L_1 norm.

$$w_{j,j} = \begin{cases} \dfrac{1}{|X_{j+1} - X_j|} & , |X_{j+1} - X_j| \geqslant \epsilon \\ \dfrac{1}{\epsilon} & , |X_{j+1} - X_j| < \epsilon \end{cases} \tag{5.70}$$

Diagonal matrix W is calculated by using equation (5.70) in the iterative process. Cost function and its partial derivative with respect to permittivity are changed to include regularization.

5.7.2 Steps for 3D level set based optimization implementation

Level set based optimization implementation steps are given below.

1. Convert system in matrix form ($A\epsilon = b$).
2. Calculate scattered electric field vector b using known ϵ values.
3. Add noise to scattered electric field ($\hat{b} = b + n$).
4. Identify different regions to be reconstructed.
5. Decide number of level set functions to be used.
6. Start with the initial guess about ϵ.
7. Calculate signed distance function.
8. Calculate initial cost function ($C(\epsilon)$).
9. Calculate total electric field using 3D FDTD.
10. Calculate Jacobian matrix ($J(\epsilon)$).
11. Calculate required partial derivatives of cost function.
12. Update all equations such that the cost function is minimized.
13. If stopping criteria is satisfied then stop, else repeat steps 8 to 13 by using reconstructed results of current iteration.

The above steps are implemented to reconstruct static permittivity values and shapes of breast tissues by minimizing cost function.

5.8 Simulation parameters

Values of Debye parameters are given for different breast tissues in table 5.1 [25, 26]. These values are valid for 0.5GHz to 3 GHz. For simplicity, only two major types of tissues are considered in class 3 numerical breast phantom [32, 33]. Five frequencies 0.5, 1, 1.5, 2 and 2.5 GHz are considered in the microwave breast imaging system simulation. Static permittivity values are found by adding $\Delta\epsilon$ to ϵ_∞. These static permittivity values are used in simulation. In microwave breast imaging using 3D

Table 5.1. Values of Debye parameters for different breast tissues. Source: [38].

Tissues	ϵ_∞	$\Delta\epsilon$	σ_s (s m^{-1})
Adipose (fatty)	4.09	3.54	0.084 2
Fibro-glandular	18.6	35.6	0.817
Skin	15.3	24.8	0.741
Tumour (assumed)	23.2	41	0.93
Immersion (Surrounding) medium	2.6	0	0

level set based optimization, a human breast is immersed in an oil based surrounding medium because it matches the average dielectric properties of the human breast. RMSE in complex permittivity is calculated by using equation (5.71).

$$\text{RMSE} = \sqrt{\frac{\sum_{i=1}^{K}((\epsilon_s)_i - (\widehat{\epsilon_s})_i)^2}{K}} \tag{5.71}$$

In equation (5.71), $(\epsilon_s)_i$ is an original static permittivity value of the ith cell. $(\hat{\epsilon_s})_i$ is reconstructed permittivity value of ith cell. K is total number of cells used in the breast phantom.

5.9 Results

Inverse scattering problem is solved for two regularization schemes to compare performance of both. Signal-to-noise ratio (SNR) is 20 dB for all reconstructions. The original profile of static permittivity (ϵ_s) with a 2 cm × 2 cm × 2 cm tumor is shown in figure 5.11.

Now, the original static permittivity profile of figure 5.11 is used in simulation. A reconstructed profile of static permittivity without regularization is shown in figure 5.12. By comparing figure 5.12 with figure 5.11, it is clear that the reconstruction without regularization results in poor static permittivity profile. The size and shape parameters of the reconstructed tumor are different as compared to the original tumor. Reconstructed profiles of static permittivity (ϵ_s) with Tikhonov and TV regularization schemes are shown in figures 5.13 and 5.14 respectively.

By comparing figure 5.13 with figure 5.12, it is clear that the reconstruction with Tikhonov regularization results in a better static permittivity profile than reconstruction without regularization. By comparing figure 5.14 with figures 5.12 and 5.13, it is clear that the reconstruction with TV regularization results in a better static permittivity profile than all other reconstructions.

The original profile of static permittivity (ϵ_s) with 1 cm × 1 cm × 1 cm tumor is shown in figure 5.15. A reconstructed profile of static permittivity without regularization is shown in figure 5.16. By comparing figure 5.15 with figure 5.16, it is clear that the reconstruction of small tumor parameters is very difficult without regularization. Reconstructed profiles of static permittivity (ϵ_s) with Tikhonov and

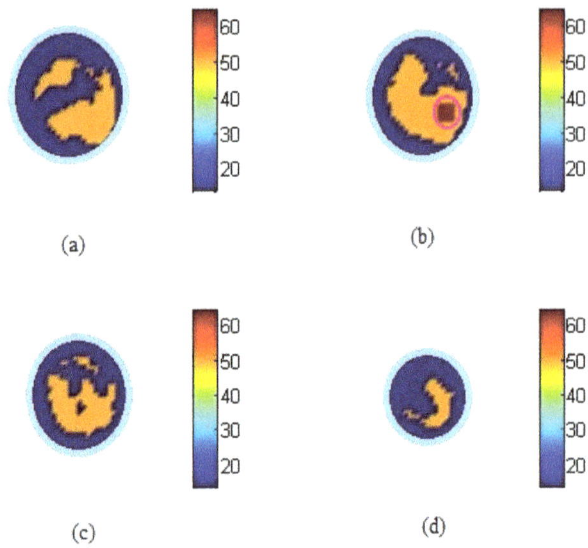

Figure 5.11. Coronal cross-section of original static permittivity (ϵ_s) profile at (a) 1.5 cm; (b) 3 cm; (c) 4.5 cm; (d) 6 cm. (Brown dot in (b) represents a 2 cm × 2 cm × 2 cm tumor.) Source: [38].

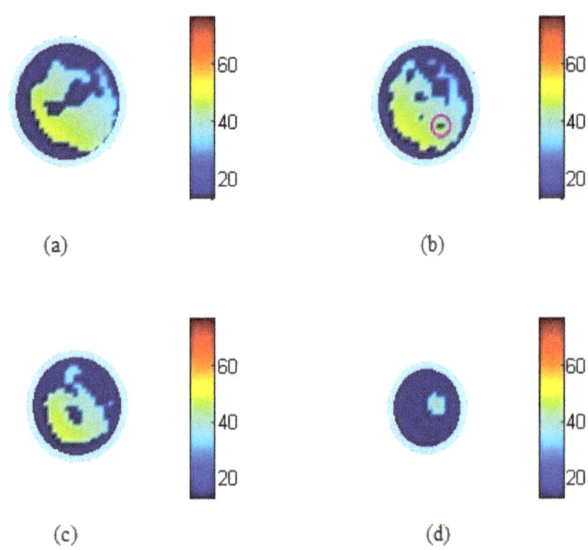

Figure 5.12. Coronal cross-section of reconstructed static permittivity (ϵ_s) profile without regularization at (a) 1.5 cm; (b) 3 cm; (c) 4.5 cm; (d) 6.5 cm. (Brown dot in (b) represents tumor.) Source: [38].

TV regularization schemes are shown in figure 5.17 and figure 5.18 respectively. By comparing figure 5.17 with figure 5.13, it is clear that the reconstruction of small tumor parameters is difficult with Tikhonov regularization. Figure 5.18 shows that the reconstruction of small tumor parameters is very good with TV regularization.

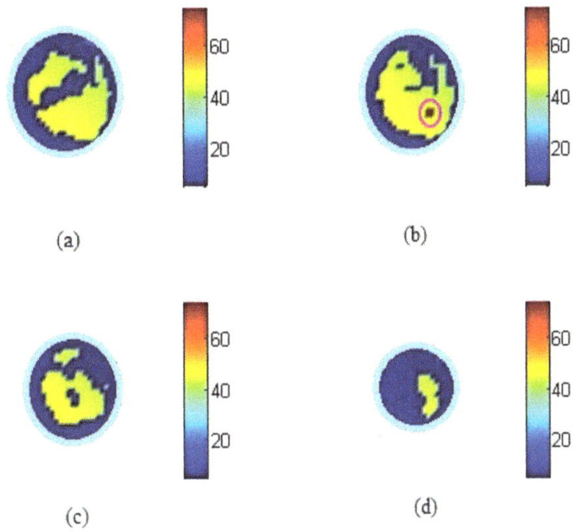

Figure 5.13. Coronal cross-section of reconstructed static permittivity (ϵ_s) profile with Tikhonov regularization at (a) 1.5 cm; (b) 3 cm; (c) 4.5 cm; (d) 6.5 cm. (Brown dot in (b) represents tumor.) Source: [38].

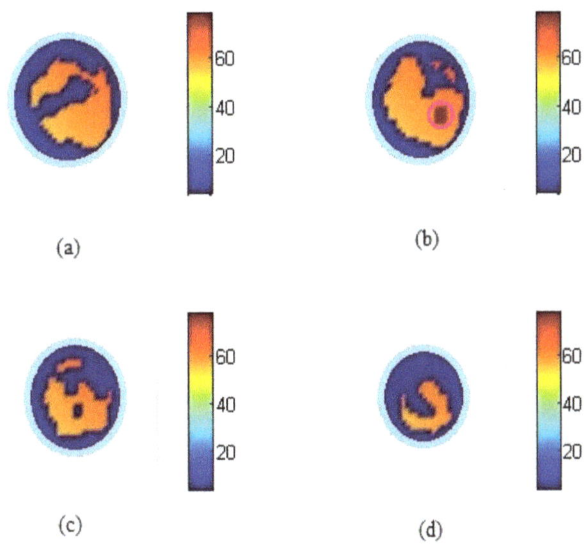

Figure 5.14. Coronal cross-section of reconstructed static permittivity (ϵ_s) profile with TV regularization at (a) 1.5 cm; (b) 3 cm; (c) 4.5 cm; (d) 6.5 cm. (Brown dot in (b) represents tumor.) Source: [38].

The original profile of static permittivity (ϵ_s) with 0.5 cm × 0.5 cm × 0.5 cm tumor is shown in figure 5.19. A reconstructed profile of static permittivity without regularization is shown in figure 5.20. By comparing figure 5.20 with figure 5.19, it is clear that the reconstruction of very small tumor parameters is impossible without regularization. Reconstructed profiles of static permittivity (ϵ_s) with Tikhonov and TV regularization schemes are shown in figures 5.21 and 5.22

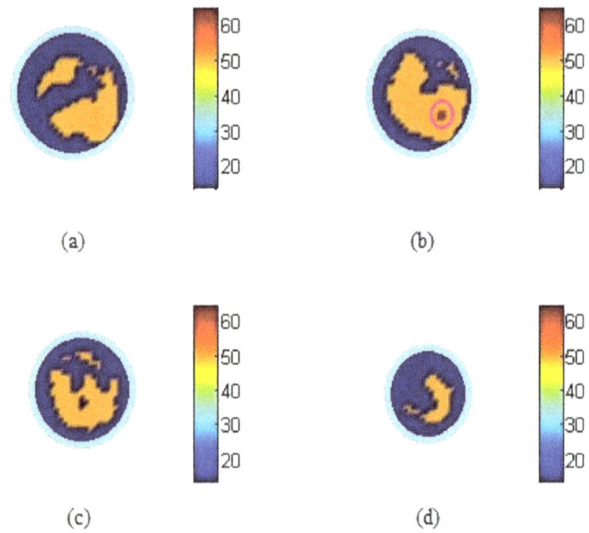

Figure 5.15. Coronal cross-section of original static permittivity (ϵ_s) profile at (a) 1.5 cm; (b) 3 cm; (c) 4.5 cm; (d) 6.5 cm. (Brown dot in (b) represents 1 cm × 1 cm × 1 cm tumor.) Source: [38].

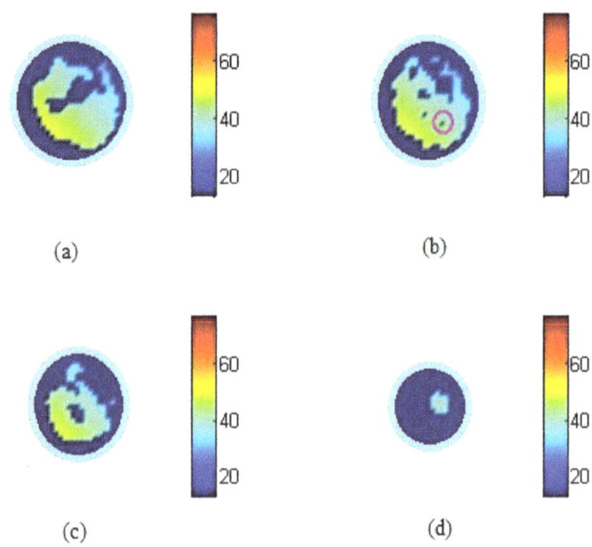

Figure 5.16. Coronal cross-section of reconstructed static permittivity (ϵ_s) profile without regularization at (a) 1.5 cm; (b) 3 cm; (c) 4.5 cm; (d) 6.5 cm. (Brown dot in (b) represents tumor.) Source: [38].

respectively. By comparing figure 5.21 with figure 5.19, it is clear that the reconstruction of very small tumor parameters is almost impossible with Tikhonov regularization. By comparing figure 5.22 with figure 5.19, it is clear that the reconstruction of very small tumor parameters is difficult with TV regularization. Location of a very small tumor is not properly detected with TV regularization.

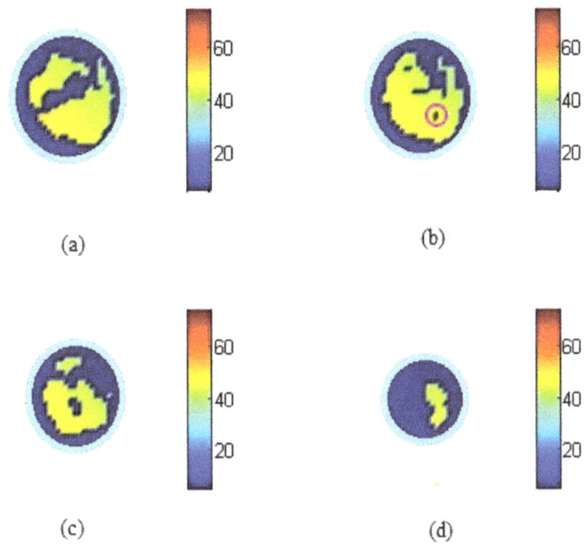

Figure 5.17. Coronal cross-section of reconstructed static permittivity (ϵ_s) profile with Tikhonov regularization at (a) 1.5 cm; (b) 3 cm; (c) 4.5 cm; (d) 6.5 cm. (Brown dot in (b) represents tumor.) Source: [38].

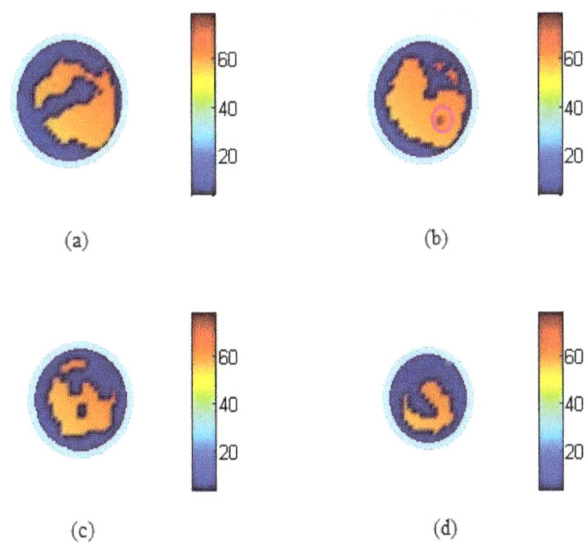

Figure 5.18. Coronal cross-section of reconstructed static permittivity (ϵ_s) profile with TV regularization at (a) 1.5 cm; (b) 3 cm; (c) 4.5 cm; (d) 6.5 cm. (Brown dot in (b) represents tumor.) Source: [38].

A root mean square error (RMSE) versus SNR graph is shown in figure 5.23 for three cases. A cost function versus number of iterations graph is shown in figure 5.24. RMSE values clearly show that the performance of total variation regularization is better than the Tiknonov regularization. Comparison of different algorithms are

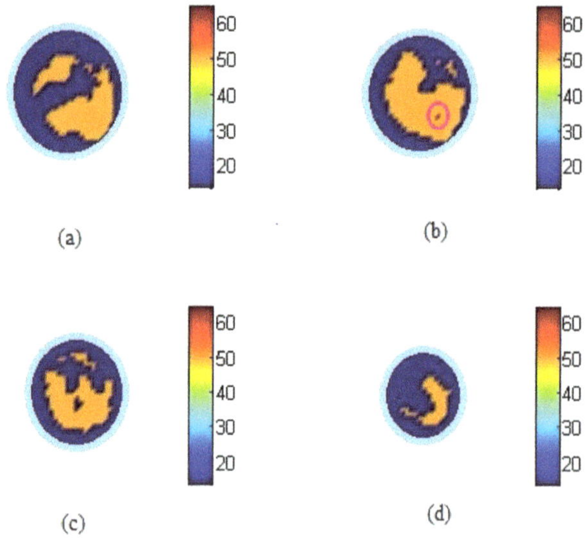

Figure 5.19. Coronal cross-section of original static permittivity (ϵ_s) profile at (a) 1.5 cm; (b) 3 cm; (c) 4.5 cm; (d) 6.5 cm. (Brown dot in (b) represents 0.5 cm × 0.5 cm × 0.5 cm tumor.) Source: [38].

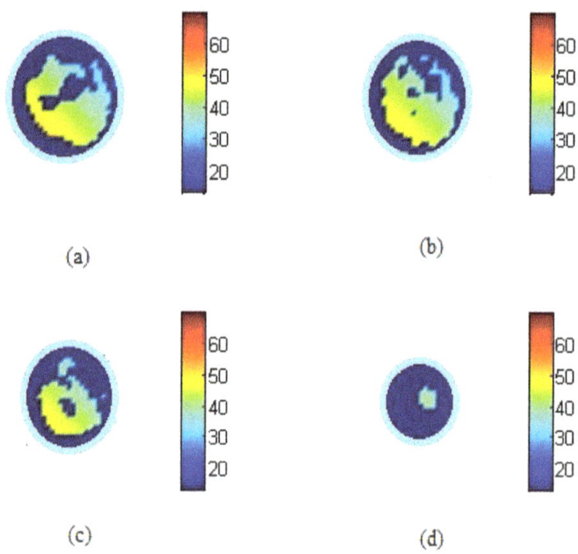

Figure 5.20. Coronal cross-section of reconstructed static permittivity (ϵ_s) profile without regularization at (a) 1.5 cm; (b) 3 cm; (c) 4.5 cm; (d) 6.5 cm. Source: [38].

given below. Details of Gauss–Newton, conjugate gradient and genetic algorithms are given in [11, 26, 34–12]. Table 5.2 clearly shows that the performance of 3D level set method is better than all other methods. 3D level set method has a shape optimization feature which results in less error as compared to other methods.

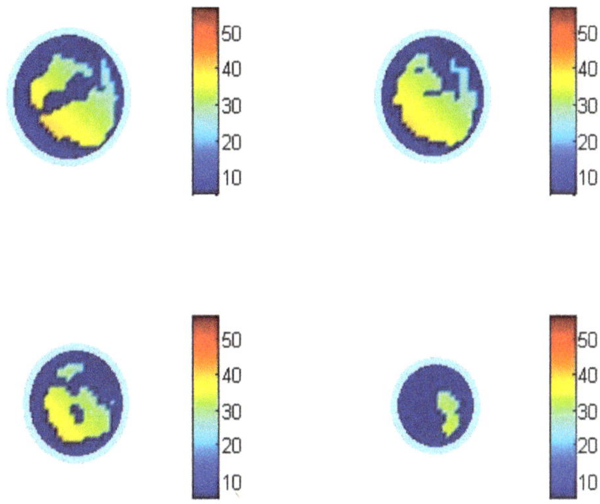

Figure 5.21. Coronal cross-section of reconstructed static permittivity (ϵ_s) profile with Tikhonov regularization at (a) 1.5 cm; (b) 3 cm; (c) 4.5 cm; (d) 6.5 cm. Source: [38].

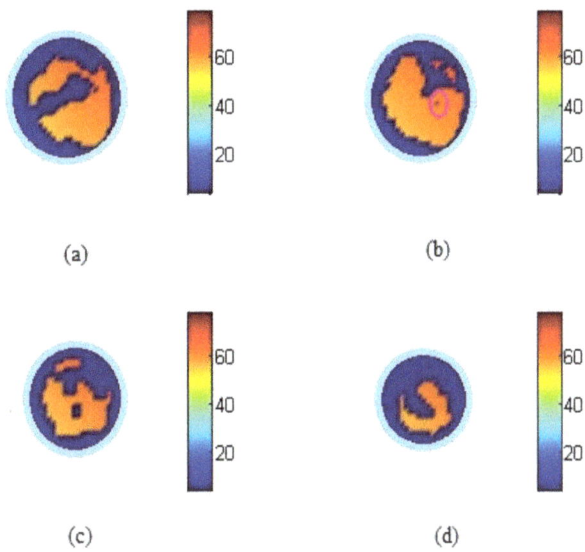

Figure 5.22. Coronal cross-section of reconstructed static permittivity (ϵ_s) profile with TV regularization at (a) 1.5 cm; (b) 3 cm; (c) 4.5 cm; (d) 6.5 cm. (Brown dot in (b) represents tumor.) Source: [38].

5.10 Summary

3D level set based evolution and optimization approaches are described with a mathematical framework for inverse scattering problems. Characteristics of evolution approach are discussed with implementation details. The Gauss–Newton based optimization algorithm is described with steps for implementation. Four update equations are derived for the two-level set functions based optimization approach

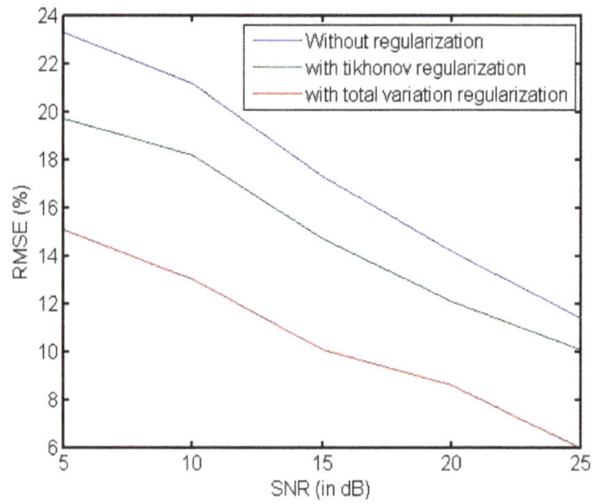

Figure 5.23. RMSE in static permittivity (ϵ_s) versus SNR. Source: [38].

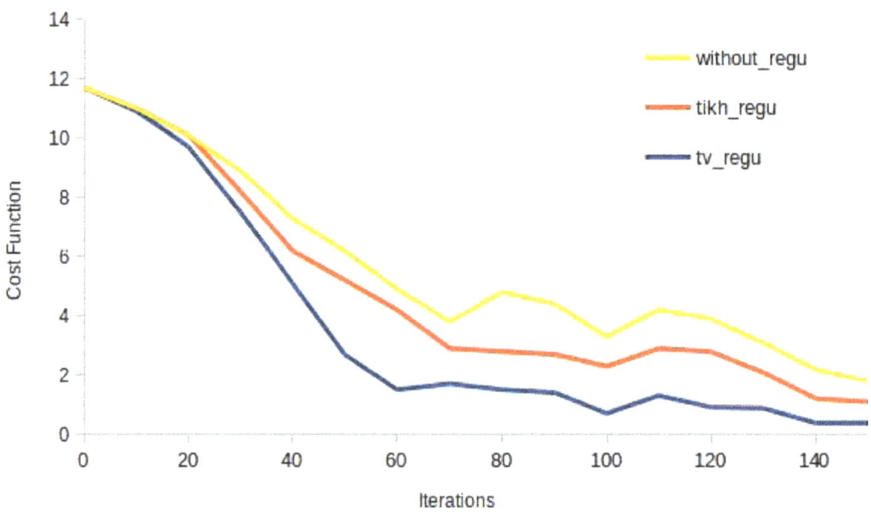

Figure 5.24. Cost versus number of iterations. Source: [38].

which can detect healthy and malignant breast tissues. Tikhonov and TV regularization schemes are used to improve performance of 3D level set based optimization. Shape, size and location detection of breast tumour is possible by using 3D level set based methods.

Tikhonov regularization improves reconstruction results but its performance degrades for very small breast tumor size. The performance of TV regularization is better than Tikhonov regularization for medium, small and very small breast tumors. TV regularization reconstructs shape and size of a very small tumor but it fails to reconstruct its exact location. Total variation regularization performs

Table 5.2. Comparison of RMSE for different algorithms. Source: [38].

Methods	RMSE (%)
Gauss–Newton	24.14
Conjugate gradient method	21.62
Genetic algorithm	17.71
Level set method	12.43

better than Tikhonov regularization because there are abrupt changes in the solution. Oscillations in cost function minimization are reduced by using regularization schemes, which makes convergence faster.

3D level set based optimization with TV regularization is very effective for 5 dB to 25 dB SNR. In this work, 20 dB SNR is required for better microwave image reconstruction and breast tumour detection. Shape and dielectric properties are both reconstructed simultaneously in 3D level set based regularized optimization.

References

[1] Zastrow E, Davis S K, Lazebnik M, Kelcz F, Van Veen B D and Hagness S C 2008 Development of anatomically realistic numerical breast phantoms with accurate dielectric properties for modelling microwave interactions with the human breast *IEEE Trans. Biomed. Eng.* **55** 2792–800

[2] Lazebnik M, Okoniewski M, Booske J H and Hagness S C 2007 Highly accurate Debye models for normal and malignant breast tissue dielectric properties at microwave frequencies *IEEE Microw. Wirel. Compon. Lett.* **17** 822–4

[3] Khuda I, Khatun S, Reza K J, Rahman M M and Fakir M M 2013 Improved Debye model for experimental approximation of human breast tissue properties at 6 GHz ultra-wideband centre frequency *Int. J. Eng. Technol.* **5** 4708–17

[4] Garrett J D and Fear E C 2015 Average dielectric property analysis of complex breast tissue with microwave transmission measurements *Sensors* **15** 1199–216

[5] Bourqui J and Fear E C 2016 System for bulk dielectric permittivity estimation of breast tissues at microwave frequencies *IEEE Trans. Microw. Theory Techn.* **64** 3001–9

[6] Winters D W, Shea J D, Kosmas P, Van Veen B D and Hagness S C 2009 Three-dimensional microwave breast imaging: dispersive dielectric properties estimation using patient-specific basis functions *IEEE Trans. Med. Imaging* **28** 969–81

[7] Shea J D, Kosmas P, Hagness S C and Van Veen B D 2010 Three-dimensional microwave imaging of realistic numerical breast phantoms via a multiple-frequency inverse scattering technique *Med. Phys.* **37** 4210–26

[8] Irishina N 2009 Microwave medical imaging using level set techniques *PhD Thesis* University of Carlos

[9] Colgan T J, Hagness S C and Van Veen B D 2015 A 3-D level set method for microwave breast imaging *IEEE Trans. Biomed. Eng.* **62** 2526–34

[10] Patel H N and Ghodgaonkar D K 2017 Study of effect of numerical breast phantom heterogeneity on dielectric profile reconstruction using microwave imaging *Prog. Electromagn. Res.* M **58** 135–45

[11] Patel H N and Ghodgaonkar D K 2017 3D level set based optimization of inverse scattering problem for microwave breast imaging *IEEE MTT-S Int. Microwave Bio Conf. (Gothenburg, Sweden, 15–17 May 2017)* 1–4

[12] Patel H N and Ghodgaonkar D K 2019 Application of 3D level set based optimization in microwave breast imaging for cancer detection *Level Set Method in Medical Imaging Segmentation* (Boca Raton, FL: CRC Press)

[13] Osher S and Sethian J A 1988 Fronts propagating with curvature-dependent speed: algorithms based on Hamilton-Jacobi formulations *J. Comput. Phys.* **79** 12–49

[14] Osher S and Fedkiw R 2003 *Level set methods and dynamic implicit surfaces, Applied Mathematical Sciences* (New York: Springer) pp 1–142

[15] Santosa F 1996 A level-set approach for inverse problems involving obstacles *ESAIM Control Optim. Calc. Var.* **1** 17–33

[16] Colgan T J, Hagness S C and Van Veen B D 2015 A 3-D level set method for microwave breast imaging *IEEE Trans. Biomed. Eng.* **62** 2526–34

[17] Burger M 2001 A level set method for inverse problems *Inverse Probl.* **17** 1327

[18] Burger M and Osher S J 2005 A survey on level set methods for inverse problems and optimal design *Eur. J. Appl. Math.* **16** 263–301

[19] Dorn O and Lesselier D 2006 Level set methods for inverse scattering *Inverse Probl.* **22** 1–79

[20] Dorn O, Miller E L and Rappaport C M 2000 A shape reconstruction method for electromagnetic tomography using adjoint fields and level sets *Inverse Probl.* **16** 1119

[21] Ferraye R, Dauvignac J Y and Pichot C 2003 An inverse scattering method based on contour deformations by means of a level set method using frequency hopping technique *IEEE Trans. Antennas Propag.* **51** 1100–13

[22] Aghasi A, Kilmer M and Miller E L 2011 Parametric level set methods for inverse problems *SIAM Journal on Imaging Sciences* **4** 618–50

[23] Semerci O and Miller E L 2012 A parametric level-set approach to simultaneous object identification and background reconstruction for dual-energy computed tomography *IEEE Trans. Image Process.* **21** 2719–34

[24] Eskandari M R, Dehmollaian M and Safian R 2016 Simultaneous microwave imaging and parameter estimation using modified level-set method *IEEE Trans. Antennas Propag.* **64** 3554–64

[25] Winters D W, Shea J D, Kosmas P, Van Veen B D and Hagness S C 2009 Three-dimensional microwave breast imaging: dispersive dielectric properties estimation using patient-specific basis functions *IEEE Trans. Med. Imaging* **28** 969–81

[26] Shea J D, Kosmas P, Hagness S C and Van Veen B D 2010 Three-dimensional microwave imaging of realistic numerical breast phantoms via a multiple-frequency inverse scattering technique *Med. Phys.* **37** 4210–26

[27] Irishina N, Dorn O and Miguel M 2008 A level set evolution strategy in microwave imaging for early breast cancer detection *Comput. Math. Appl.* **56** 607–18

[28] Irishina N, Moscoso M and Dorn O 2009 Microwave imaging for early breast cancer detection using a shape-based strategy *IEEE Trans. Biomed. Eng.* **56** 1143–53

[29] Hua P, Woo E J, Webster J G and Tompkins W J 1991 Iterative reconstruction methods using regularization and optimal current patterns in electrical impedance tomography *IEEE Trans. Med. Imaging* **10** 621–8

[30] Zhang H, Huang J, Ma J, Bian Z, Feng Q, Lu H, Liang Z and Chen W 2014 Iterative reconstruction for X-ray computed tomography using prior-image induced nonlocal regularization *IEEE Trans. Biomed. Eng.* **61** 2367–78

[31] Zhao S and Al-Qadi I L 2017 Development of regularization methods on simulated ground-penetrating radar signals to predict thin asphalt overlay thickness *Signal Process.* **132** 261–71
[32] Zastrow E, Davis S K, Lazebnik M, Kelcz F, Van Veen B D and Hagness S C 2008 Development of anatomically realistic numerical breast phantoms with accurate dielectric properties for modelling microwave interactions with the human breast *IEEE Trans. Biomed. Eng.* **55** 2792–800
[33] Lazebnik M, Okoniewski M, Booske J H and Hagness S C 2007 Highly accurate Debye models for normal and malignant breast tissue dielectric properties at microwave frequencies *IEEE Microw. Wirel. Compon. Lett.* **17** 822–4
[34] Stang J P 2008 A 3D active microwave imaging system for breast cancer screening *PhD Thesis* Duke University
[35] Zaeytijd J D, Franchois A, Eyraud C and Geffrin J 2007 Full-wave three-dimensional microwave imaging with a regularized Gauss–Newton method-theory and experiment *IEEE Trans. Antennas Wave Propag.* **55** 3279–92
[36] Park C S and Jeong B S 1999 Reconstruction of a high contrast and large object by using the hybrid algorithm combining a Levenberg-Marquardt algorithm and a genetic algorithm *IEEE Trans. Magn.* **35** 1582–5
[37] Rubaek T, Meaney P M, Meincke P and Paulsen K D 2007 Nonlinear microwave imaging for breast-cancer screening using Gauss–Newton's method and the CGLS inversion algorithm *IEEE Trans. Antennas Propag.* **55** 2320–31
[38] Patel H N 2019 Microwave imaging for breast cancer detection using 3D level set based optimization, FDTD method and method of moments *PhD Dissertation* Dhirubhai Ambani Institute of Information and Communication Technology
[39] Bocquet B J, Van de Velde C, Mamouni A, Leroy Y, Giaux G, Delannoy J and Delvalee D 1990 Microwave radiometric imaging at 3 GHz for the exploration of breast tumors *IEEE Trans. Microw. Theory Tech.* **38** 791–3

Hardik N Patel, Deepak K Ghodgaonkar and Jasjit S Suri

Chapter 6

Method of moments

The method of moments based formulation is described for the inverse scattering problem for breast cancer detection by using microwave imaging. The electric field integral equation is derived and converted into matrices by using method of moment. Mathematical breast models are constructed and used in this approach. Symmetry present in this electromagnetic inverse scattering problem has been exploited by applying group theory. Inverse scattering problem has been formulated and solved by applying the Levenberg–Marquardt algorithm. In order to mimic experimental data, noise is added to the simulated data. Now, the reconstruction problem is solved by optimizing the inverse scattering problem through the Levenberg–Marquardt algorithm.

6.1 Theoretical background

Frequency domain methods were used extensively in microwave breast imaging before the rise of time domain methods. Method of moments is one of the most used techniques in electromagnetic scattering and imaging problems. Electric field integral equation (EFIE) is solved in method of moments for complex permittivity estimation. Matrix formation and inversion time should be reduced to allow a large number of cells in the breast model. This is achieved by symmetry exploitation using group theory which improves computational efficiency of the imaging system.

EFIE is solved by using method of moments to find the scattered electric field due to human breast models. Additive white Gaussian noise is added to this electric field vector. The matrix formed by method of moments is ill-posed due to presence of a large number of buried cells in inverse scattering formulation [1]. Ill-posed system matrix and noise are two major challenges in the solution of the inverse scattering problem. The Levenberg–Marquardt method is used to solve the above challenges. The effects of total volume, multiple view, symmetry and number of cells on

doi:10.1088/978-0-7503-2592-9ch6

complex permittivity reconstruction are investigated in this chapter. The effect of saline and air as surrounding medium on complex permittivity reconstruction is evaluated for microwave breast imaging system. Consider a biological body with an arbitrary shape with dielectric parameters. It is illuminated by an incident electromagnetic wave, as shown in figure 6.1. The current gets induced in the body due to incident electromagnetic wave which in turn generates scattered electric field. This scattered electric field can be calculated by replacing the body with an equivalent free space current density given by equation (6.1).

$$J_{\mathrm{eq}}(r) = (\sigma(r) + j\omega[\epsilon(r) - \epsilon_0])E(r) = \tau(r)E(r) \tag{6.1}$$

In equation (6.1), $J_{\mathrm{eq}}(r)$ is an equivalent induced current density, $\sigma(r)$ is the conductivity of a biological body at location r, ω is a frequency in radian, $\epsilon(r)$ is permittivity of the biological body at r, $E(r)$ is total electric field generated inside the body at location r. The first and second terms of equation (6.1) are the conduction current density and polarization current density, respectively. Equations (6.2) and (6.3) are derived by using Maxwell's equations.

$$\nabla \times E^{\mathrm{s}} = -J_{\mathrm{eq}} - j\omega H^{\mathrm{s}} \tag{6.2}$$

Equation (6.2) is Faraday's law in frequency domain and it is also known as one of Maxwell's equations in frequency domain. E^{s} is a scattered electric field, H^{s} is a scattered magnetic field. Spatial rotation of scattered electric field generates a time varying magnetic field scattered magnetic field.

$$\nabla \times H^{\mathrm{s}} = j\omega E^{\mathrm{s}} \tag{6.3}$$

Equation (6.2) is Ampere's law in frequency domain and it is also known as one of Maxwell's equations in frequency domain. Spatial rotation of scattered magnetic

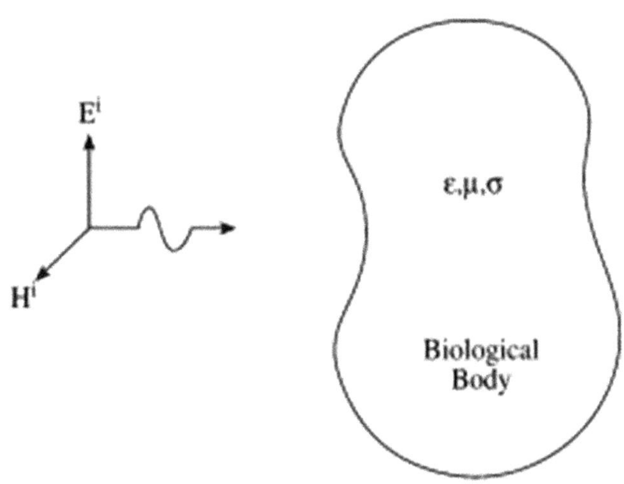

Figure 6.1. Arbitrary shape biological body illuminated by plane electromagnetic wave. Source: [23].

field generates time varying scattered electric field. Equation (6.4) is obtained by applying curl to both sides of equation (6.2) and simplifying it after that.

$$\nabla \times \nabla \times E^{s} - K_0^2 E^{s} = -j\omega\mu_0 J_{eq} \tag{6.4}$$

Equation (6.5) is obtained by applying curl to both sides of equation (6.3) and simplifying it after that.

$$\nabla \times \nabla \times H^{s} - K_0^2 H^{s} = \nabla \times J_{eq} \tag{6.5}$$

where $k_0^2 = \omega^2\mu_0\epsilon_0$. The solutions of equations (6.4) and (6.5) are given by equations (6.6) and (6.7), respectively.

$$E^{s} = -j\omega\left[1 + \frac{1}{k_0^2}\nabla\nabla\cdot\right]A \tag{6.6}$$

$$H^{s} = -j\omega\frac{1}{\mu_0}\nabla \times A \tag{6.7}$$

where A is given by equation (6.8).

$$A = \mu_0 \int_v G_0(r, r')J_{eq}(r')dv' \tag{6.8}$$

The scalar Green's function is given by equation (6.9).

$$G_0(r, r') = \frac{e^{-jk_0(r-r')}}{4\pi|r - r'|} \tag{6.9}$$

In equation (6.6), $\nabla\nabla \cdot A = \nabla(\nabla \cdot A)$. E^{s} and H^{s} depend on equivalent current density. J_{eq} is an infinite elementary source at r' pointed in the x direction so that

$$J_{eq} = \delta(r - r')a_x \tag{6.10}$$

Vector potential can be obtained by substituting equation (6.10) into equation (6.8).

$$A = \mu_0 G_0(r, r')a_x \tag{6.11}$$

$G_0(r, r')$ is the electric field produced by the elementary source so it should satisfy

$$\nabla \times \nabla \times G_{0x}(r, r') - k_0^2 G_{0x}(r, r') = -j\omega\mu_0\delta(r, r') \tag{6.12}$$

Solution of equation (6.12) is given by equation (6.13).

$$G_{0x}(r, r') = -j\omega\mu_0\left(1 + \frac{1}{k^2}\nabla\nabla\cdot\right)G_0(r, r') \tag{6.13}$$

$G_{0x}(r, r')$ is known as a free space vector Green's function with a source pointed in the x direction. Similarly $G_{0y}(r, r')$ and $G_{0z}(r, r')$ corresponding to source pointed in y and z direction can also be used. Now dyadic Green's function is given with three elements in equation (6.14).

$$G_0(r, r') = G_{0x}(r, r')a_x + G_{0y}(r, r')a_y + G_{0z}(r, r')a_z \tag{6.14}$$

The above equation is also known as free space dyadic Green's function. It is also a solution of the dyadic differential equation.

$$\nabla \times \nabla \times G_0(r, r') - k_0^2 G_0(r, r') = \tilde{I}\delta(r - r') \tag{6.15}$$

where $\tilde{I}$ is unit dyad defined as

$$\tilde{I} = a_x a_x + a_y a_y + a_z a_z \tag{6.16}$$

$G_0(r, r')$ is used to calculate electric field at a field point r due to infinitesimal source present at r'. Equation (6.17) can be derived from equations (6.4) and (6.15).

$$E^{\mathrm{s}}(r) = -j\omega\mu_0 \int G_0(r, r')J_{\mathrm{eq}}(r')\,\mathrm{d}v' \tag{6.17}$$

$G_0(r, r')$ has a singularity of the order $|r - r'|^3$, the integral of equation (6.17) diverges if the field point r is inside the volume v of this body or source region. This problem can be avoided by excluding a small volume surrounding the field point, then considering the small volume tends to zero. As shown in equation (6.18), principal value and correction terms are included to get the correct solution.

$$E^{\mathrm{s}}(r) = PV \int J_{\mathrm{eq}}(r)G(r, r')\,\mathrm{d}v' + [E^{\mathrm{s}}(r)]_{\mathrm{correction}} \tag{6.18}$$

The correction term of the above equation is $-\frac{J_{\mathrm{eq}}(r)}{j3\omega\epsilon_0}$. The total electric field inside the body is the sum of the incident field E^{i} and scattered E^{s}

$$E(r) = E^{\mathrm{i}}(r) + E^{\mathrm{s}}(r) \tag{6.19}$$

Combining equations (6.1), (6.18) and (6.19) gives the desired equation for total electric field $E(r)$.

$$\left[1 + \frac{\tau(r)}{3j\omega\epsilon_0}\right]E(r) - PV\int_v \tau(r')E(r)\cdot G(r, r')\,\mathrm{d}v' = E^{\mathrm{i}}(r) \tag{6.20}$$

In the above equation, $\tau(r) = \sigma(r) + j\omega[\epsilon(r) - \epsilon_0]$ and incident electric field E^{i} are known. Only the total electric field inside an arbitrary shaped body is unknown.

The inner product of equation (6.20) can be represented in the matrix form as shown by equation (6.21).

$$E(r)\cdot G(r, r') = \begin{bmatrix} G_{xx}(r, r') & G_{xy}(r, r') & G_{xz}(r, r') \\ G_{yx}(r, r') & G_{yy}(r, r') & G_{yz}(r, r') \\ G_{zx}(r, r') & G_{zy}(r, r') & G_{zz}(r, r') \end{bmatrix} \begin{bmatrix} E_x(r') \\ E_y(r') \\ E_z(r') \end{bmatrix} \tag{6.21}$$

If $c1 = x$, $c2 = y$, $c3 = z$ then the symmetric dyad of Green's function can be shown by equation (6.22).

$$G_{c_pc_q} = -j\omega\mu_0\left[\delta_{pq} + \frac{1}{k_0^2}\frac{\partial^2}{\partial c_q \partial c_p}\right]G_0(r, r'), \tag{6.22}$$

where p, $q = 1, 2, 3$. Now by applying method of moments, the whole body is partitioned into N discrete cells to transform equation (6.20).

$E(r)$ and $\tau(r)$ are assumed to be constant within each cell. If the center of each cell is denoted by r_m then

$$\left[1 + \frac{\tau(r)}{3j\omega\epsilon_0}\right]E_{c_p}(r_m) - \sum_{q=1}^{3}\left[\sum_{q=1}^{3}\tau(r_n)PV\int_{v_m} G_{c_pc_q}(r_m, r')\mathrm{d}v'\right]E_{x_q}(r_n) = E^{\mathrm{i}}_{c_p}(r_m) \tag{6.23}$$

If $G_{c_pc_q}$ is an $N \times N$ matrix with elements

$$G^{mn}_{c_pc_q} = \tau(r_n)PV\int_{v_n} G_{c_pc_q}(r_m, r')\mathrm{d}v' - \delta_{pq}\delta_{mn}\left[1 + \frac{\tau(r)}{3j\omega\epsilon_0}\right] \tag{6.24}$$

where $m, n = 1, 2, \ldots, N$ and $p, q = 1, 2, 3$. Let E_{c_p} and $E^{\mathrm{i}}_{c_p}$ be the column matrices with elements.

$$E_{c_p} = \begin{bmatrix} E_{c_p}(r_1) \\ \vdots \\ E_{c_p}(r_N) \end{bmatrix} \tag{6.25}$$

$$E^{\mathrm{i}}_{c_p} = \begin{bmatrix} E^{\mathrm{i}}_{c_p}(r_1) \\ \vdots \\ E^{\mathrm{i}}_{c_p}(r_N) \end{bmatrix} \tag{6.26}$$

$3N$ simultaneous equations can be obtained for E_x, E_y and E_z at the centers of N cells by point matching technique and method of moments. These simultaneous equations can be written in the matrix form as shown by equation (6.27).

$$[G][E] = -[E^{\mathrm{i}}] \tag{6.27}$$

where $[G]$ is a $3N \times 3N$ matrix and $[E]$ and $[E^{\mathrm{i}}]$ are 3N column matrices. Incident electric field column vector $[E^{\mathrm{i}}]$ is known but electric field $[E]$ is to be determined by calculating elements of $[G]$. $G_{c_pc_q}$ is continuous in volume v_n and the principal value operation can be dropped. Now, equation (6.24) can be represented as equation (6.28).

$$G^{mn}_{c_pc_q} = \tau(r_n)\int_{v_n} G_{c_pc_q}(r_m, r')\mathrm{d}v' \tag{6.28}$$

where $m \neq n$. By applying first approximation.

$$G_{c_pc_q}^{mn} = \tau(r_n)G_{c_pc_q}(r_m, r')\Delta v_n \tag{6.29}$$

where $m \neq n$ and Δv_n is the volume of cell v_n. By using equations (6.13) and (6.22) in equation (6.29).

$$G_{c_pc_q}^{mn} = \frac{-j\omega\mu k_0 \Delta v_n \tau(r_n)\exp(-j\alpha_{mn})}{4\pi\alpha_{mn}^3} \left[(\alpha_{mn} - 1 - j\alpha_{mn})\delta_{pq} + \cos(\theta_{c_p}^m n)\cos(\theta_{c_q}^m n)(3 - \alpha_{mn}^2 + 3j\alpha_{mn})\right] \tag{6.30}$$

where $m \neq n$, $\alpha_{mn} = k_0 R_{mn}$, $R_{mn} = |r_m - r_n|$, $\cos(\theta_{c_p}^{mn}) = \frac{c_p^m - c_p^n}{R_{mn}}$, $\cos(\theta_{c_q}^{mn}) = \frac{c_q^m - c_q^n}{R_{mn}}$, $r_m = (c1^m, c2^m, c3^m)$, $r_n = (c1^n, c2^n, c3^n)$

The approximation in equation (6.30) produces sufficient results provided N is large. Integration of equation (6.28) can be obtained numerically for greater accuracy. Equation (6.31) is obtained for the diagonal terms

$$G_{c_pc_q}^{mn} = \tau(r_n)PV\int_{v_n} G_{c_pc_q}(r_n, r')\mathrm{d}v' - \delta_{pq}\delta_{mn}\left[1 + \frac{\tau(r)}{3j\omega\epsilon_0}\right] \tag{6.31}$$

In order to evaluate the above integral, a cell is approximated by an equal volume sphere of radius a_n centered at r_n.

$$\Delta v = \frac{4}{3}\pi a_n^3. \tag{6.32}$$

Equation (6.33) is derived after lengthy calculation.

$$G_{c_pc_q}^{nn} = \delta_{pq}\left[\frac{-2j\omega\mu_0\tau(r_n)}{3K_0^3}(\exp(-jk_0a_n)(1 + jk_0a_n) - 1) - \left(1 + \frac{\tau(r_n)}{3j\omega\epsilon_0}\right)\right] \tag{6.33}$$

where $m = n$. Numerical implementation of integration is preferable for better accuracy.

6.2 Problem formulation

Low power microwave signals are transmitted by antennas onto the breast. These incident signals interact with numerical breast tissues. As a result of this interaction, microwave signals get scattered, lost and transmitted through the breast model. Scattered electric field at observation point $\vec{r}$ is calculated by equation (6.34).

$$\vec{E}^s(\vec{r}) = \iiint G(\vec{r}, \vec{r}')J(\vec{r}')\mathrm{d}v' \tag{6.34}$$

Green's function $G(\vec{r}, \vec{r}')$ and polarization current density $J(\vec{r}')$ are substituted in equation (6.34) to obtain equation (6.35).

$$\vec{E}^{s}(\vec{r}) = k_{\epsilon}^{2} \iiint (\epsilon_r(\vec{r}') - 1)\vec{E}(\vec{r}')\left[I + \frac{\nabla\nabla}{k_{\epsilon}^{2}}\right]\frac{e^{-jk_{\epsilon}R}}{4\pi R}dv' \tag{6.35}$$

In equation (6.35), $E(\vec{r}')$ is total electric field at source point $\vec{r}'$, $\nabla\nabla$ is dyadic, R is the distance between observation point and source point, and k_{ϵ} is a wave number of the immersion (surrounding) medium. The relationship between total electric field, incident electric field and scattered electric field is given by equation (6.36).

$$\vec{E}(\vec{r}) = \vec{E}^{i}(\vec{r}) + \vec{E}^{s}(\vec{r}) \tag{6.36}$$

Equation (6.37) is obtained by substituting equation (6.35) in equation (6.36).

$$-\vec{E}^{i}(\vec{r}) = k_{\epsilon}^{2} \iiint (\epsilon_r(\vec{r}') - 1)\vec{E}(\vec{r}')\left[I + \frac{\nabla\nabla}{k_{\epsilon}^{2}}\right]\frac{e^{-jk_{\epsilon}R}}{4\pi R}dv' - \vec{E}(\vec{r}) \tag{6.37}$$

Now, the body is divided into N cells by applying the procedure of the above section. The matrix form of equation (6.38) is obtained by applying method of moments to equation (6.37) [1–4].

$$-\vec{E}^{i} = (A_1 R^{\epsilon} - I)\vec{E} \tag{6.38}$$

Volume integral of Green's function is solved as per the procedure of the previous section to obtain A_1. It has dimensions of $3N \times 3N$. R^{ϵ} is a complex permittivity matrix with size of $3N \times 3N$. $\vec{E}^{i}$ is incident electric field matrix in the absence of the body and it has size of $3N \times 1$. $\vec{E}$ is electric field inside the body with size of $3N \times 1$. Equation (6.1) is obtained by writing $(A_1 R^{\epsilon} - I) = A$ in equation (6.38).

$$-\vec{E}^{i} = A\vec{E} \tag{6.39}$$

A matrix form of equation (6.40) is obtained by applying method of moments to equation (6.35) [1–4].

$$\vec{E}^{s} = B_1 R^{\epsilon}\vec{E} \tag{6.40}$$

Volume integral of Green's function is solved by using the procedure of the previous section to obtain B_1. It has size of $3N \times 3N$. $\vec{E}^{s}$ is scattered electric field matrix with size of $3N \times 1$. Equation (6.41) is obtained by writing $B_1 R^{\epsilon} = B$ in equation (6.40).

$$\vec{E}^{s} = B\vec{E} \tag{6.41}$$

By applying source, incident electric field matrix of equation (6.39) is obtained. Matrix A of equation (6.39) is obtained by applying volume integral to Green's function. Total electric field inside the body is the only unknown in equation (6.39). Now, electric field inside body of N cells is calculated by inverting matrix A of equation (6.39). Now matrix B and matrix E of equation (6.41) are known. Scattered electric fields at receiver locations are calculated using equation (6.41). This process is known as the forward problem. In the inverse problem, R^{ϵ} is the only unknown in equation (6.40). The process of obtaining matrix R^{ϵ} using equation (6.40) is known as the inverse problem.

6.3 Computation reduction using group theory

6.3.1 Human breast models

Human breast models are designed to verify the solution of the inverse scattering problem. A human breast model in its simplest form is shown in figure 6.2 and has 16 cells. It is easy to understand group theory by using this model. Figures 6.3 and 6.4 show top and bottom layers of numerical breast model, respectively. Both layers have cell and receiver numbers as shown in figures 6.3 and 6.4. Complex permittivity is assigned to each cell center according to breast anatomy. Complex permittivity is calculated by using equation (6.4).

$$\epsilon_{\mathrm{r}}^{*}(\omega) = \epsilon_{\mathrm{r}} - j\frac{\sigma}{\omega\epsilon_0} \tag{6.42}$$

In equation (6.42), ϵ_{r}, σ, ϵ_0 and ω are relative permittivity, conductivity, absolute permittivity, and angular frequency, respectively.

A breast model with 64 cells is designed to add complexity to the simple 16 cell breast model. A two-dimensional view of the 64 cell breast model is shown in figure 6.5 with volume of 512 cm^3. The nipple is represented by layer 1. Skin, milk ducts, fatty tissues, and fibro-glandular tissues are represented by layer 2. Skin, fatty tissues, fibro-glandular tissues, and lobules are represented by layer 3. Skin, fatty tissues, fibro-glandular tissues, cancerous tissues are represented by layer 4. In the three-dimensional view, layer 1 has 4 cells, layer 2 has 16 cells, layer 3 has 20 cells and layer 4 has 24 cells. The above 64 cell model is considered in the simulation. A two-dimensional view of the 38 cell model is shown in figure 6.6. It is used to

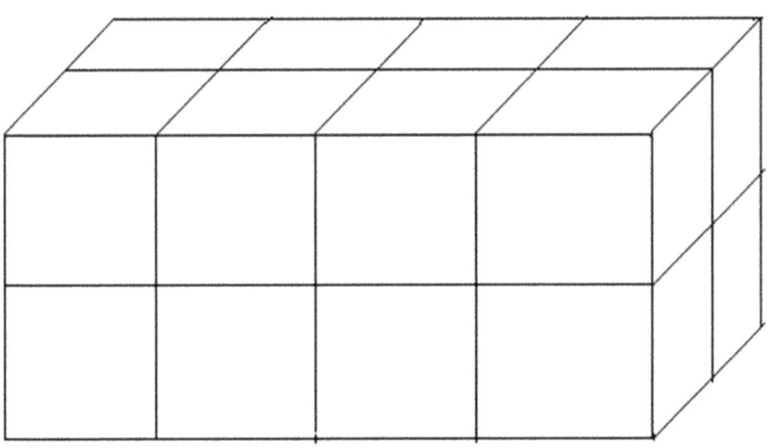

Figure 6.2. Simple human breast model. Source: [23].

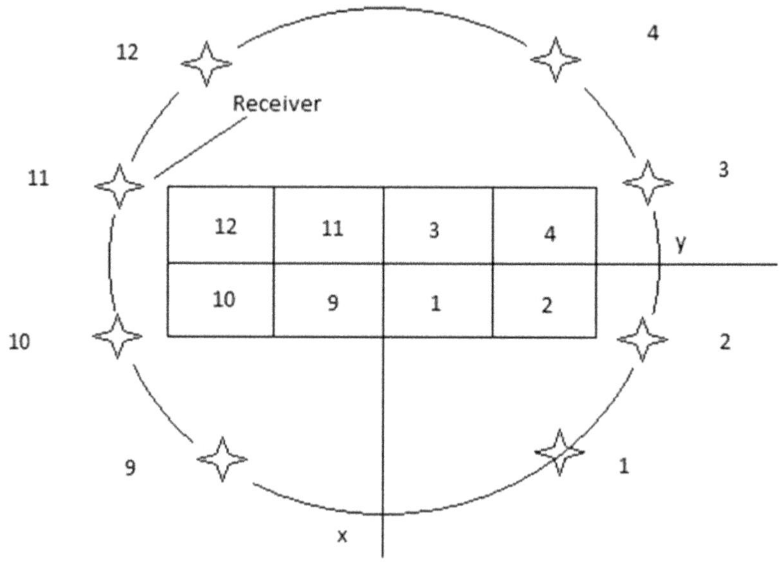

Figure 6.3. Top layer of simple breast model (bi-static system). Source: [23].

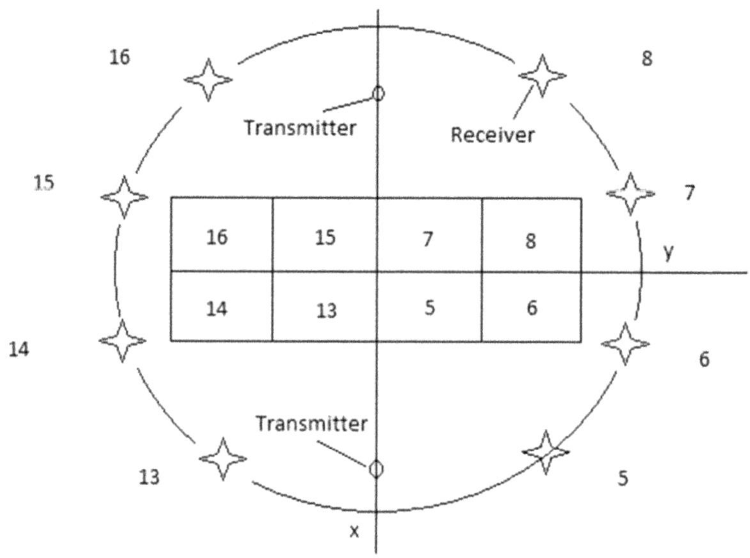

Figure 6.4. Bottom layer of simple breast model (bi-static system). Source: [23].

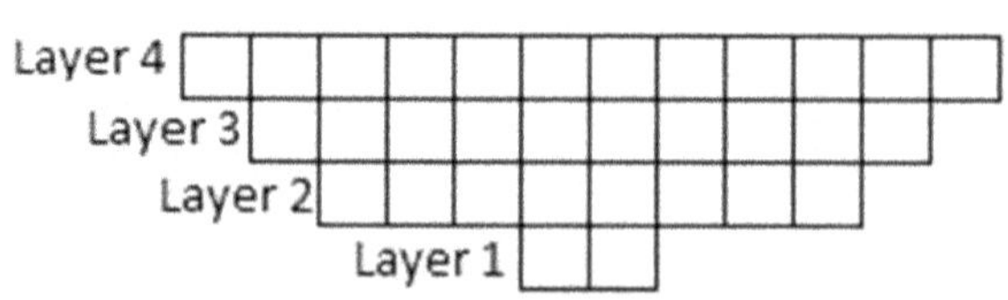

Figure 6.5. 2D view of 64 cell human breast model. Source: [23].

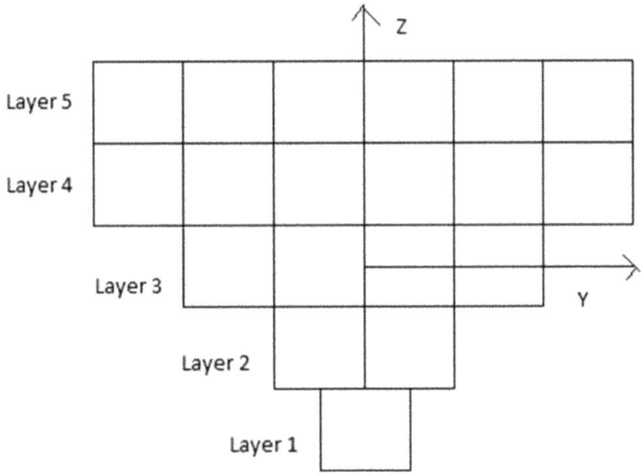

Figure 6.6. 2D view of 38 cell human breast model. Source: [23].

evaluate performance of the surrounding medium. It has one more layer as compared to the 64 cell model.

6.3.2 Symmetry exploitation using group theory

Matrix B_1 is calculated by solving the volume integral of Green's function. The structure of matrix B_1 is shown by using equation (6.43).

$$B_1 = \begin{bmatrix} b_{11} & b_{12} & \dots & b_{1n} \\ b_{21} & b_{22} & \dots & b_{2n} \\ \cdot & \cdot & \dots & \cdot \\ \cdot & \cdot & \dots & \cdot \\ b_{m1} & b_{m2} & \dots & b_{mn} \end{bmatrix} \tag{6.43}$$

In equation (6.43), m and n are number of receivers and cells, respectively. Each element of B_1 is also a 3×3 matrix.

$$b_{11} = \begin{bmatrix} b_{11}^{xx} & b_{11}^{xy} & b_{11}^{xz} \\ b_{11}^{yx} & b_{11}^{yy} & b_{11}^{yz} \\ b_{11}^{zx} & b_{11}^{zy} & b_{11}^{zz} \end{bmatrix} \tag{6.44}$$

b_{11} element of matrix B_1 is shown by equation (6.44). Each element of matrix B_1 is symmetric [5, 6]. This symmetry of measurement domain is exploited by using group theory. Basic group theory operators are shown by equations (6.45), (6.46) and (6.47).

$$R_1(x, y, z) = (-x, y, z) \tag{6.45}$$

$$R_2(x, y, z) = (x, -y, z) \tag{6.46}$$

$$R_3(x,\ y,\ z) = (x,\ y,\ -z) \tag{6.47}$$

The group formed by above operators is shown by equation (6.48).

$$G = \{I,\ R_1,\ R_2,\ R_3,\ R_1R_2,\ R_2R_3,\ R_3R_1,\ R_1R_2R_3\} \tag{6.48}$$

Octant and group multiplication tables are described in [5, 6]. Now, consider figures 6.3 and 6.4 for the next few lines. Receivers and cells numbered as 1, 2 have coordinates $(x,\ y,\ z)$, so they are represented by identity element of group. Receivers and cells numbered as 3, 4 have coordinates $(-x,\ y,\ z)$, so they are represented by R_1 element of group. Receivers and cells numbered as 5, 6 have coordinates $(x,\ y,\ -z)$, so they are represented by R_3 element of group. Receivers and cells numbered as 7, 8 have coordinates $(-x,\ y,\ -z)$, so they are represented by R_1R_3 element of group. Receivers and cells numbered as 9, 10 have coordinates $(x,\ -y,\ z)$, so they are represented by R_2 element of group. Receivers and cells numbered as 11, 12 have coordinates $(-x,\ -y,\ z)$, so they are represented by R_1R_2 element of group. Receivers and cells numbered as 13, 14 have coordinates $(x,\ -y,\ -z)$, so they are represented by R_2R_3 element of group. Receivers and cells numbered as 15, 16 have coordinates $(-x,\ -y,\ -z)$, so they are represented by $R_1R_2R_3$ element of the group. Equation (6.49) represents the transformation matrix [6].

$$V = \frac{1}{2\sqrt{2}}\begin{bmatrix} +I_s & +I_{s1} & +I_{s3} & -I_{s2} & +I_{s2} & -I_{s3} & -I_{s1} & -I_s \\ +I_s & +I_{s1} & -I_{s3} & +I_{s2} & +I_{s2} & -I_{s3} & +I_{s1} & +I_s \\ +I_s & -I_{s1} & +I_{s3} & +I_{s2} & +I_{s2} & +I_{s3} & -I_{s1} & +I_s \\ +I_s & -I_{s1} & -I_{s3} & -I_{s2} & +I_{s2} & +I_{s3} & +I_{s1} & -I_s \\ +I_s & +I_{s1} & +I_{s3} & -I_{s2} & -I_{s2} & +I_{s3} & +I_{s1} & +I_s \\ +I_s & +I_{s1} & -I_{s3} & +I_{s2} & -I_{s2} & +I_{s3} & -I_{s1} & -I_s \\ +I_s & -I_{s1} & +I_{s3} & +I_{s2} & -I_{s2} & -I_{s3} & +I_{s1} & -I_s \\ +I_s & -I_{s1} & -I_{s3} & -I_{s2} & -I_{s2} & -I_{s3} & -I_{s1} & +I_s \end{bmatrix} \tag{6.49}$$

Transformation matrix elements are given by equations (6.50), (6.51), (6.52) and (6.53).

$$I_s = \text{diag}(I_0,\ I_0,\ \ldots I_0) \tag{6.50}$$

$$I_{s1} = \text{diag}(I_1,\ I_1,\ \ldots I_1) \tag{6.51}$$

$$I_{s2} = \text{diag}(I_2,\ I_2,\ \ldots I_2) \tag{6.52}$$

$$I_{s3} = \text{diag}(I_3,\ I_3,\ \ldots I_3) \tag{6.53}$$

Now, matrices I_0, I_1, I_2 and I_3 are given by equations (6.54), (6.55), (6.56) and (6.57), respectively.

$$I_0 = \begin{bmatrix} 1 & 0 & 0 \\ 0 & 1 & 0 \\ 0 & 0 & 1 \end{bmatrix} \tag{6.54}$$

$$I_1 = \begin{bmatrix} -1 & 0 & 0 \\ 0 & 1 & 0 \\ 0 & 0 & 1 \end{bmatrix} \tag{6.55}$$

$$I_2 = \begin{bmatrix} 1 & 0 & 0 \\ 0 & -1 & 0 \\ 0 & 0 & 1 \end{bmatrix} \tag{6.56}$$

$$I_3 = \begin{bmatrix} 1 & 0 & 0 \\ 0 & 1 & 0 \\ 0 & 0 & -1 \end{bmatrix} \tag{6.57}$$

Matrices B_1, $J^{\mathrm{p}} = R^{\epsilon}E$, and E_{s} are block-diagonalized by using equations (6.58), (6.59) and (6.60), respectively.

$$B_{1\mathrm{b}} = VB_1V^T \tag{6.58}$$

$$J_{\mathrm{b}}^{\mathrm{p}} = VJ^{\mathrm{p}} \tag{6.59}$$

$$E_{\mathrm{b}}^{\mathrm{s}} = VE^{\mathrm{s}} \tag{6.60}$$

6.4 Inverse scattering problem formulation

The Levenberg–Marquardt method is used to solve the inverse scattering problem of microwave breast imaging [7–9]. Different methods are applied to solve the inverse scattering problem for microwave breast imaging in [10–14]. A model driven approach and stochastic optimization methods are described for microwave breast imaging in [15–17]. Matrix inversion is needed per iteration in the Levenberg–Marquardt method. The inverse scattering problem without group theory is solved by using equation (6.61).

$$[\Delta\epsilon] = (J_{\mathrm{a}}^T J_{\mathrm{a}} + \lambda \mathrm{diag}(J_{\mathrm{a}}^T J_{\mathrm{a}}))^{-1} J_{\mathrm{a}}^T (\vec{E}^{\mathrm{s}} - \widehat{\vec{E}}^{\mathrm{s}}) \tag{6.61}$$

In equation (6.61), J_{s} is Jacobian matrix. It is calculated by taking a partial derivative of the scattered electric field with respect to complex permittivity of each cell. $(\vec{E}^{\mathrm{s}} - \widehat{\vec{E}}^{\mathrm{s}})$ is the residual scattered electric field column vector. $[\Delta\epsilon]$ is change in complex permittivity. It is obtained at each iteration. λ is regularization parameter or damping factor. The inverse scattering problem with group theory is solved by using equation (6.62).

$$[\Delta\epsilon] = (J_{\mathrm{b}}^T J_{\mathrm{b}} + \lambda \mathrm{diag}(J_{\mathrm{b}}^T J_{\mathrm{b}}))^{-1} J_{\mathrm{b}}^T (\overrightarrow{E_{\mathrm{b}}^{\mathrm{s}}} - \widehat{\overrightarrow{E_{\mathrm{b}}}}^{\mathrm{s}}) \tag{6.62}$$

In equation (6.62), J_{b} is a Jacobian matrix. It is calculated by taking a partial derivative of block-diagonalized scattered electric field with respect to complex permittivity of each cell. $(\overrightarrow{E_{\mathrm{b}}^{\mathrm{s}}} - \widehat{\overrightarrow{E_{\mathrm{b}}}}^{\mathrm{s}})$ is residual block-diagonalized scattered electric field column vector.

6.5 Simulation parameters and noise consideration

Simulation parameters are given for the 64 cell model and saline is used as the surrounding medium. Frequency of 500 MHz is considered in simulation, which provides better penetration depth and enough resolution. Complex permittivity values of table 6.1 are used to calculate volume averaged complex permittivity for each cell [18]. Cell size and number of cells vary but volume remains constant during the whole simulation process. Radius of the receiver circle is 13 cm. In a bi-static system, a dipole antenna of 2 cm is used. Two transmitters are at 9 cm from the centre of the body. Size of receiver is the same as cell size. A scattered field at receivers' locations is obtained by solving the forward problem. Now, noise is added to it by using equation (6.63) and complex permittivity value of each cell is reconstructed by solving the inverse scattering problem.

$$\vec{E}^{s} = B\vec{E} + n \tag{6.63}$$

In equation (6.63), n is additive white Gaussian noise column vector. Root mean square error (RMSE) in complex permittivity is calculated by using equation (6.64).

$$\text{RMSE} = \sqrt{\frac{\sum_{i=1}^{K}(\epsilon_i - \widehat{\epsilon}_i)^2}{K}} \tag{6.64}$$

In equation (6.64), ϵ_i is an original permittivity value. $\widehat{\epsilon}_i$ is reconstructed permittivity value. K is total number of cells used in the model.

6.6 Results

Simulation time is calculated by inverting the matrix only once. Now, comparison of matrix inversion time is shown with and without group theory in table 6.2.

Table 6.2 gives a clear idea about effect of group theory on matrix inversion time. Matrix inversion time is reduced by applying group theory. A graph of RMSE in complex permittivity versus SNR is shown in figure 6.7. RMSE with group theory is higher than RMSE without group theory. A graph of overall simulation versus number of cells is shown in figure 6.8. Overall simulation time includes time to simulate all iterations with overhead time. Overall simulation time increases with

Table 6.1. Complex permittivity values for different breast tissues. Source: [23].

Biological tissues	Complex permittivity
Breast fat	$5.5 - j1.32$
Skin dry	$44.92 - j26.19$
Skin wet	$48.62 - j25.32$
Glandular tissues	$20 - j14.38$
Nipple	$45 - j25.16$
Blood vessels	$46.23 - j21.07$
Cancerous tissues	$65 - j32$

Table 6.2. Matrix inversion time in seconds. Source: [23].

Number of cells	Matrix inversion time	Matrix inversion time
	Without group theory	With group theory
64	0.102	0.087 2
512	0.896	0.62
1024	1.982	1.15

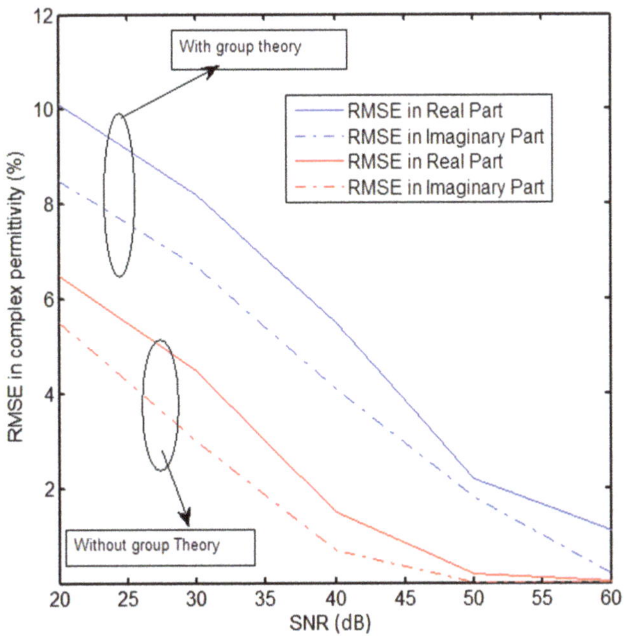

Figure 6.7. RMSE (%) in complex permittivity versus SNR (dB) (bi-static system). Source: [23].

number of cells. Overall simulation time with group theory is less than that without group theory. A graph of RMSE in complex permittivity versus SNR is shown in figure 6.9. It is clear that RMSE with group theory is higher than RMSE without group theory. Graph of RMSE in complex permittivity versus SNR is shown for a 38 cell model in figure 6.10. It is quite clear that saline is a better surrounding medium as compared to air [1].

6.7 Summary

Matrix formulation is described by using method of moment for microwave breast imaging. Symmetry is exploited in a microwave breast imaging system by using group theory. Overall simulation time is reduced considerably with group theory. By using group theory, approximately 30% to 35% computation time is reduced. The Levenberg–Marquardt method is implemented with and without group theory.

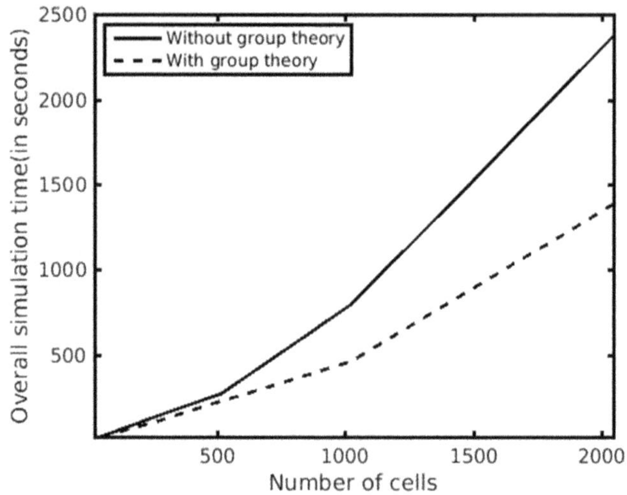

Figure 6.8. Overall simulation time versus number of cells. Source: [23].

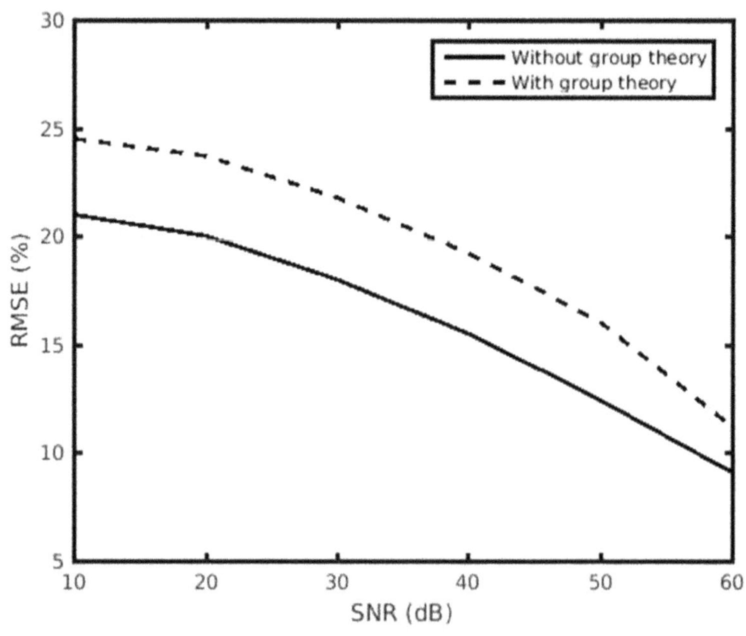

Figure 6.9. RMSE (%) in complex permittivity versus SNR (dB) for 1024 cells (mono-static system). Source: [23].

Matrix inversion with group theory is faster than without group theory because group theory converts matrices into block-diagonalized form. RMSE in complex permittivity is higher with group theory. This is considered as compensation to get computational efficiency. However, for SNR greater than 50 dB, RMSE in complex permittivity without group theory is approximately the same as RMSE in complex permittivity with group theory. Overall microwave image reconstruction time is

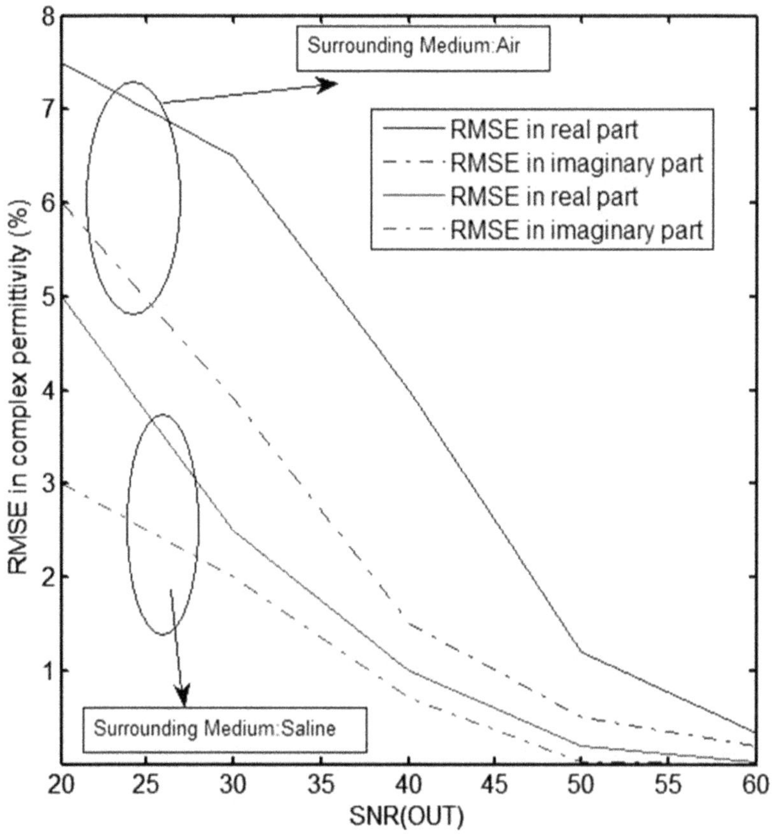

Figure 6.10. RMSE (%) in complex permittivity versus SNR (dB) for 38 cells (bi-static system). Source: [23].

reduced by exploiting symmetry using group theory. The performance of saline is better than air as surrounding medium because it provides better matching with human breasts than air. A multiple view (mono-static system) is better than a bi-static system because of redundant measurement data.

References

[1] Ghodgaonkar D K, Gandhi O P and Hagmann M J 1983 Estimation of complex permittivities of 3D inhomogeneous biological bodies *IEEE Trans. Microw. Theory Techn.* **31** 442–6

[2] Livesay D E and Chen K 1974 Electromagnetic fields induced inside arbitrarily shaped biological bodies *IEEE Trans. Microw. Theory Techn.* **22** 1273–80

[3] Hohmann G W 1975 Three dimensional induced polarization and electromagnetic modeling *Geophysics* **40** 305–24

[4] Harrington R F 1993 *Field Computation by Moment Methods* (Piscataway, NJ: IEEE Press) pp 1–79

[5] Cohoon D K 1980 Reduction of the cost of solving an Integral Equation arising in electromagnetic scattering through the use of group theory *IEEE Trans. Antennas Propag.* **28** 104–7

[6] Ghodgaonkar D K and Ismail R 2000 Exploiting symmetry in electromagnetic imaging problems by using group representation theory *Bull. Malaysian Math. Sci. Soc.* **23** 33–44

[7] Rubaek T, Kim O S and Meincke P 2009 Computational validation of a 3-D microwave imaging system for breast-cancer screening *IEEE Trans. Antennas Propag.* **57** 2105–15

[8] Zaeytijd J D, Franchois A, Eyraud C and Geffrin J 2007 Full-wave three-dimensional microwave imaging with a regularized Gauss–Newton method: theory and experiment *IEEE Trans. Antennas Wave Propag.* **55** 3279–92

[9] Park C S and Jeong B S 1999 Reconstruction of a high contrast and large object by using the hybrid algorithm combining a Levenberg–Marquardt algorithm and a genetic algorithm *IEEE Trans. Magn.* **35** 1582–5

[10] Rubaek T, Meaney P M, Meincke P and Paulsen K D 2007 Nonlinear microwave imaging for breast-cancer screening using Gauss–Newton's method and the CGLS inversion algorithm *IEEE Trans. Antennas Propag.* **55** 2320–31

[11] Fang Q, Meaney P M and Paulsen K D 2006 Singular value analysis of the Jacobian matrix in microwave image reconstruction *IEEE Trans. Antennas Propag.* **54** 2371–80

[12] Ney M M, Smith A M and Stuchly S S 1984 A solution of electromagnetic imaging using pseudoinverse transformation *IEEE Trans. Med. Imaging* **3** 155–62

[13] Pichot C, Jofre L, Peronnet G and Bolomey J 1985 Active microwave imaging of inhomogeneous bodies *IEEE Trans. Antennas Propag.* **33** 416–25

[14] Garnero L, Franchois A, Hugonin J, Pichot C and Joachimowicz N 1991 Microwave imaging complex permittivity reconstruction by simulated annealing *IEEE Trans. Microw. Theory Techn.* **39** 1801–7

[15] Belkebir K, Kleinman R E and Pichot C 1997 Microwave imaging location and shape reconstruction from multifrequency scattering data *IEEE Trans. Microw. Theory Techn.* **45** 469–76

[16] Caorsi S, Gragnani G L, Pastorino M and Rebagliati M 1996 A model driven approach to microwave diagnostics in biomedical applications *IEEE Trans. Microw. Theory Techn.* **44** 1910–20

[17] Pastorino M 2007 Stochastic Optimization methods applied to microwave imaging:a review *IEEE Trans. Antennas Propag.* **55** 538–48

[18] Andreuccetti D, Fossi R and Petrucci C 1997 An Internet resource for the calculation of the dielectric properties of body tissues in the frequency range 10 Hz–100 GHz (IFAC-CNR, Florence (Italy), 1997. Based on data published by C Gabriel et al in 1996) http://niremf.ifac.cnr.it/tissprop/

[19] Pozar D M 1989 *Microwave Engineering* (New York: Addison-Wesley) pp 547–93

[20] Dianat S A and Saber E S 2009 *Advanced Linear Algebra for Engineers with MATLAB* (Boca Raton, FL: CRC Press)

[21] Patel H N and Ghodgaonkar D K 2015 Computationally efficient microwave imaging of human breast model using group theory *IEEE MTT-S Int. Microwave and RF Conf. (Hyderabad, 10–12 December 2015)* pp 81–4

[22] Patel H N and Ghodgaonkar D K 2016 The effect of noise on complex permittivity reconstruction in mathematical breast model *IEEE Int. Conf. on Systems in Medicine and Biology (IIT Kharagpur, 4–7 January 2016)* pp 13–16

[23] Patel H N 2019 Microwave imaging for breast cancer detection using 3D level set based optimization, FDTD method and method of moments *PhD Dissertation* Dhirubhai Ambani Institute of Information and Communication Technology

Chapter 7

Finite difference time domain for microwave imaging

Finite difference time domain (FDTD) is used to solve Maxwell's equations on the discrete grid. The relation of the grid size and stability is given to avoid problems in simulation. Maxwell's equations are descritized by using the Yee grid approach with input waves. Equations are derived for solving the forward problem through the FDTD approach. Concfocal algorithm is described and evaluated by using the FDTD technique. Space–time beamforming for better microwave image reconstruction is shown in this chapter. Skin–breast artifact removal techniques are described with important approaches. Matched filter FDTD based time reversal is applied to solve the inverse scattering problem for breast cancer detection. The FDTD approach is applied in breast cancer detection through microwave image reconstruction.

7.1 Introduction to finite difference time domain

Finite difference time domain method was invented by Kane S Yee in 1966 [1]. He demonstrated an approximate solution of Maxwell's equations by using a discrete grid structure for the first time. Detailed derivations are included in a subsequent chapter. Finite difference approximations were used to calculate spatial and time domain derivatives. A Yee grid is shown in figure 7.1. figure 7.1 shows E_x, E_y, E_z, H_x, H_y and H_z components of electromagnetic fields. This Yee grid is useful in the calculation of spatial derivatives and curl of electromagnetic fields.

7.1.1 Grid size and stability

The one-cell spatial dimensions are just a fraction of a wavelength and equal in all directions $\Delta x = \Delta y = \Delta z$ [1]. Time domain dimension is equal to Δt. In Maxwell's equations, spatial dimensions are related to time domain dimension. The relationship

doi:10.1088/978-0-7503-2592-9ch7

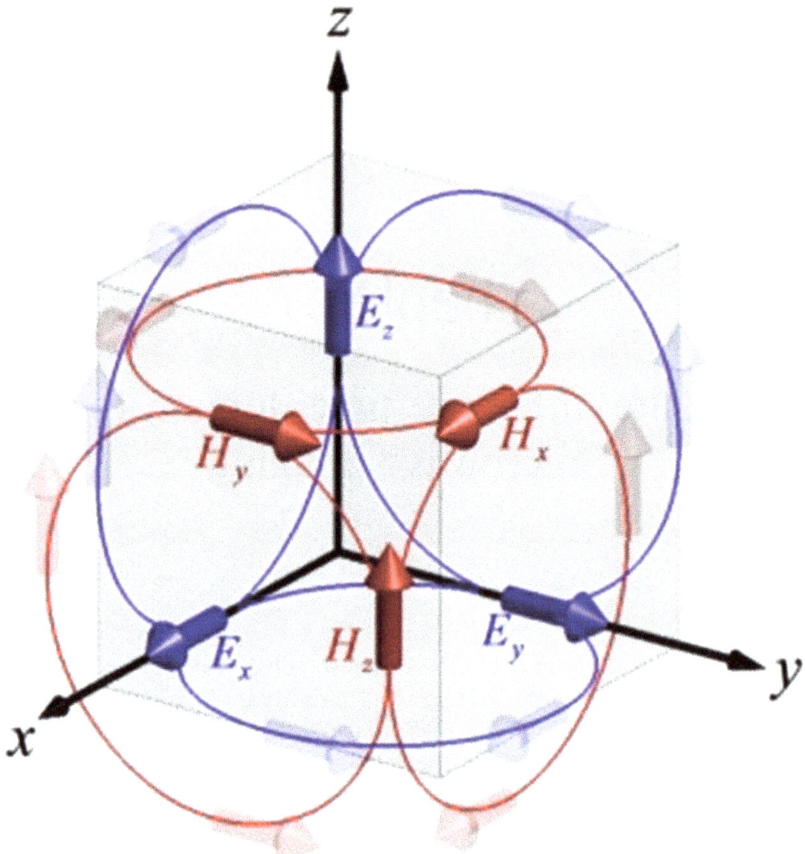

Figure 7.1. Yee grid for the approximate solutions of the Maxwell's equations. Reprinted with permission from Rumpf (2020) https://empossible.net/wp-content/uploads/2020/01/Lecture-Formulation-of-1D-FDTD.pdf.

between space increment and time increment must be satisfied for computational stability [1]. The stability criteria are shown by using equation (7.1) [1].

$$\sqrt{(\Delta x)^2 + (\Delta y)^2 + (\Delta z)^2} > c\Delta t \tag{7.1}$$

In equation (7.1), c is the velocity of light, If maximum light velocity is assumed to be $c_{\max}$ then stability criteria is given by equation (7.2).

$$\sqrt{(\Delta x)^2 + (\Delta y)^2 + (\Delta z)^2} > c_{\max}\,\Delta t \tag{7.2}$$

The above equations ensure that the wave does not travel faster than c or $c_{\max}$. Stability criteria must be followed for fruitful computations on the Yee grid.

7.1.2 Input wave for Yee grid computations

Incident plane wave is modeled as half a sine wave. The width of the sine wave is assumed as α units. The square grid has sides of length 4α in two dimensions. If only two components are assumed for incident wave then spatial dimensions are given by equation (7.3).

$$\Delta x = \Delta y = \frac{\alpha}{8} \tag{7.3}$$

Time domain dimension value is given by equation (7.4).

$$\Delta\tau = c\Delta t = \frac{1}{2}\Delta x = \frac{\alpha}{16} \tag{7.4}$$

The incident signal is delayed for practical computation on the Yee grid. The incident signal for the two-dimensional problem is given by equation (7.5).

$$E(x, y, t) = \sin\left(\frac{(x - 50\alpha + ct)\pi}{8\alpha}\right) \tag{7.5}$$

In equation (7.5), $0 \leqslant x - 50\alpha + ct \leqslant 8\alpha$. Magnetic field can be found by using the relation of impedance with electromagnetic fields in equation (7.6).

$$H(x, y, t) = \frac{1}{Z}E(x, y, t) \tag{7.6}$$

The above equations are used in the implementation of FDTD algorithm for electromagnetic problems. Sinusoidal steady state electromagnetic problems are solved by using FDTD for dielectric sphere, cylindrical metal cavity and missile-like cavity [2]. Total field and scattered field simulations are done by applying FDTD to Maxwell's equations on the Yee grid.

7.1.3 Two-dimensional FDTD analysis of microwave breast imaging

Microwave passive imaging imposes a complex radiometer design with lots of constraints including noise elimination. Microwave active imaging is emerging very fast to complement existing imaging techniques. Confocal imaging has long been used in optics. Now, confocal technique is used with microwave imaging for better diagnosis. In confocal imaging, illumination is focused on a particular body region and scattered signals are collected by refocusing them at the point of illumination origin [2]. Spatial resolution is better for transmitted and received signals in confocal microwave imaging. There are basic properties of breast tissues at microwave frequencies. Microwaves interact with biological tissues according to their water content. The significant contrast in dielectric or electric properties of malignant tumors and healthy breast tissues at microwave frequencies is crucial as compared to mammography and ultrasound imaging techniques. This results in higher scattering of microwave signals from tumor as compared to healthy breast tissues. The attenuation in normal breast tissues is less than 4 dB cm^{-1} up to 10 GHz. It is possible to detect breast tumors which are located about 5 cm beneath the skin. Confocal technique can suppress unwanted scattered signals from skin and veins. A chirp radar system is used in 3–10 GHz band which produces focused, pulsed and low power beam for breast cancer detection. Chirp radar signals propagate through the breast and these signals backscatter when a tumor is encountered in the breast. The backscattered signals are collected by the antenna which is located out of the breast focal point. A three-dimensional image of the tumor can be constructed by scanning the breast systematically. The spatial resolution depends on the size of the antenna aperture and the depth resolution depends on time-gating. Narrow impulse or FM chirp radar pulse illumination is used to achieve time-gating. The depth resolution and the clutter suppression are a function of the microwave signal processing software, application and equipment. The confocal microwave imaging detects different types of biological tissues based on their water content and it uses backscattered signals from the whole tumor. Microwave confocal imaging has the ability to complement x-ray based mammography in early stage breast tumor detection and other malignancy with high water content. Microwave is non-ionizing and it offers comfortable and pain-free breast imaging. The relative permittivity versus frequency graph is shown in figure 7.2 for tissues with low and high water content [2–6]. As shown in figure 7.2, tissues with low and high water content have different permittivity values for microwave frequencies. For tissues with different water content, a conductivity versus frequency graph is shown in figure 7.3 [2–6]. In the breast, the ratio of malignant tumor to healthy tissues conductivity values is about 6.4:1 and ratio of malignant tumor to healthy tissues permittivity values is about 3.8:1 [2, 7].

7.1.4 Healthy breast tissue dielectric properties

The relative permittivity and conductivity versus frequency for healthy breast tissues were measured around 1 GHz and 3 GHz [7, 8]. The biological tissues are not

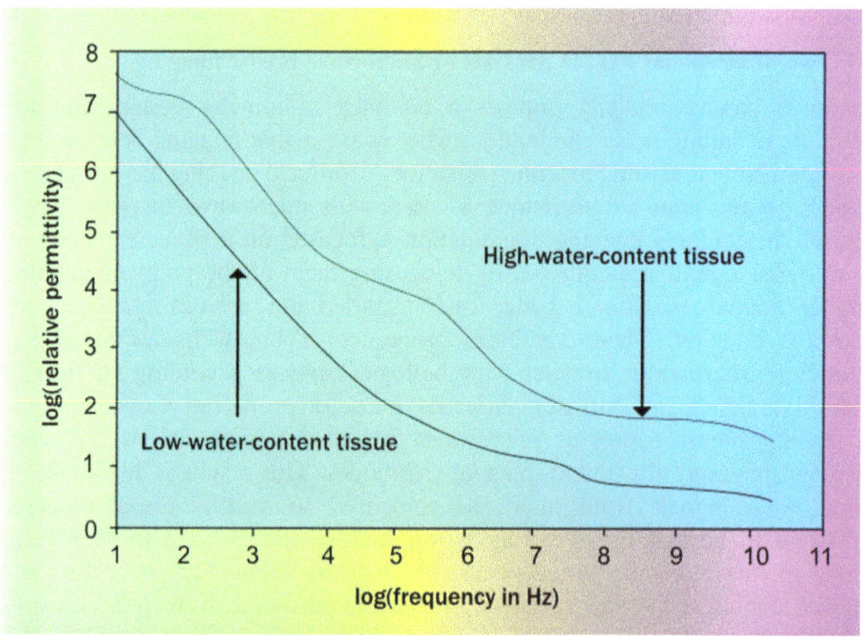

Figure 7.2. Relative permittivity versus frequency for tissues with different water contents. Copyright (1998) IEEE. Reprinted, with permission from [23].

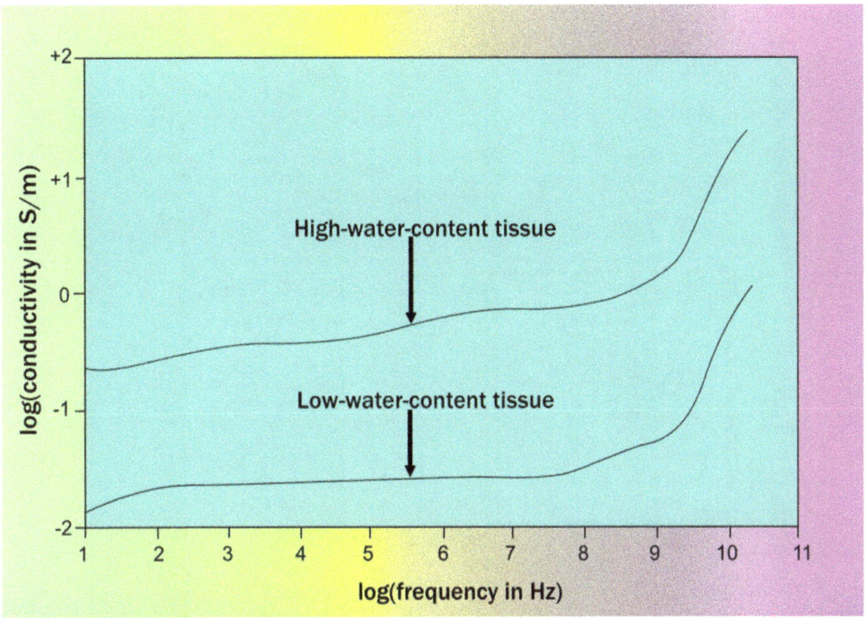

Figure 7.3. Conductivity versus frequency for tissues with different water contents. Copyright (1998) IEEE. Reprinted, with permission from [23].

polarized instantaneously due to external electromagnetic field. This effect was modeled by incorporating a Debye model in the calculation [7, 8].

$$\epsilon_r(f) = \epsilon_\infty - \frac{j\sigma}{2\pi f \epsilon_0} + \frac{\epsilon_s - \epsilon_\infty}{1 + j\dfrac{f}{f_p}} \tag{7.7}$$

In equation (7.7), f is the frequency in Hz, $\epsilon_0 = 8.854 \times 10^{-12}$ F m^{-1}, $\epsilon_s = 10$, $f_p = 2.5 \times 10^{10}$ Hz and $\sigma = 0.5$ S m^{-1}. A conductivity and permittivity versus frequency graph is shown in figure 7.4 for healthy breast tissues [2, 7–9]. Foster and Schwan have developed an empirical relationship between dielectric parameters and moisture content for microwave frequencies. The empirical model equations are given below [10].

$$\epsilon_r' = 1.71 f^{1.13} + \frac{\epsilon_s - 4}{1 + \left(\dfrac{f}{25}\right)^2} \tag{7.8}$$

$$\sigma = 1.35\sigma_{0.1} f^{0.13} + 0.002\,22 f^2 \left[\frac{\epsilon_r - 4}{1 + \left(\dfrac{f}{25}\right)^2}\right] \tag{7.9}$$

In equations (7.8) and (7.9), f is frequency in GHz, $\sigma_{0.1} = 0.05$ and $\epsilon_s = 8.5$ were calculated by using Foster and Schwan data. Figure 7.4 shows good agreement

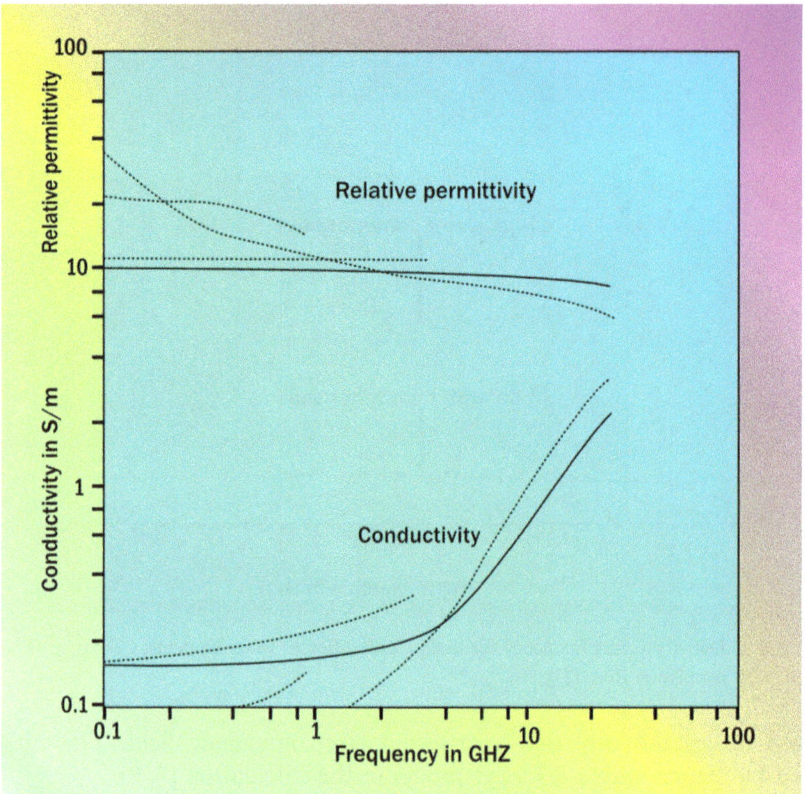

Figure 7.4. Relative permittivity and conductivity as a function of frequency for normal breast tissue as measured by Joines *et al* [7] (dashes) and by Chaudhary *et al* [8] (dash–dot) compared with Foster's and Schwan's Debye model (solid) and empirical model (dash–dot–dot) [9]. Copyright (1998) IEEE. Reprinted, with permission from [23].

between measured data and Debye model for permittivity and conductivity above 0.3 GHz. The empirical model given by equations (7.8) and (7.9) provide a better fit for permittivity than the Debye model. Two- dimensional FDTD and confocal microwave imaging system for breast cancer detection provides better results. The confocal technique and time-gating improve the backscatter detection of a malignant tumor by suppressing clutter due to heterogeneous breasts.

7.1.5 Design of antenna array

Video pulse RADAR is used to detect mines, pipes and natural resources buried inside the Earth's surface. Researchers want to use same type of RADAR to detect malignant tumors hidden inside biological tissues. It is difficult to detect small or weak scattering tissue structures due to reflections from the ends of impulse excited antennas. The resistively loaded bowtie antenna element for confocal microwave imaging is useful to overcome the above problem [11]. The structure of bowtie antenna is shown in figure 7.5 [11]. The side view of the antenna is also important to

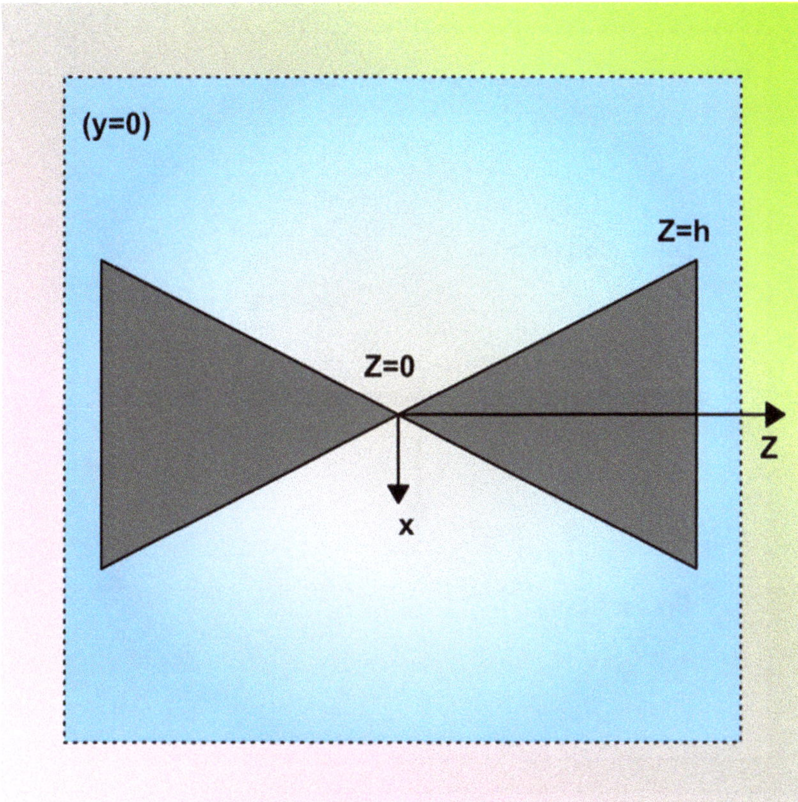

Figure 7.5. Structure of bowtie antenna. Copyright (1998) IEEE. Reprinted, with permission from [23].

understand the geometry of the system. Figure 7.6 shows a side view of the bowtie antenna [11]. Figure 7.6 shows the placement of antenna, lossy dielectric and breast tissues. The flare length of the antenna is about 4 cm with angle of 53° and it is placed at the surface of the breast. The skin layer of 1 mm is included in the proposed breast model. The material used to design the antenna has the following conductivity.

$$\sigma(z) = \sigma_0 \cdot \frac{1 - \dfrac{z}{h}}{1 + \left(\dfrac{\sigma_0}{\sigma_{1/2}} - 2\right) \cdot \left(\dfrac{z}{h}\right)} \text{ S m}^{-1} \tag{7.10}$$

In equation (7.10), $\frac{z}{h}$ is the normalized axial distance along the antenna, σ_0 depends on the metal chosen for antenna feed point design, $\sigma_{\frac{1}{2}}$ is chosen to suppress the reflected pulse. The large block of lossy dielectric is used to embed this antenna and this lossy dielectric provides matching with permittivity and conductivity of the normal breast tissues. The antenna is excited by the signal, as given in equation (7.11).

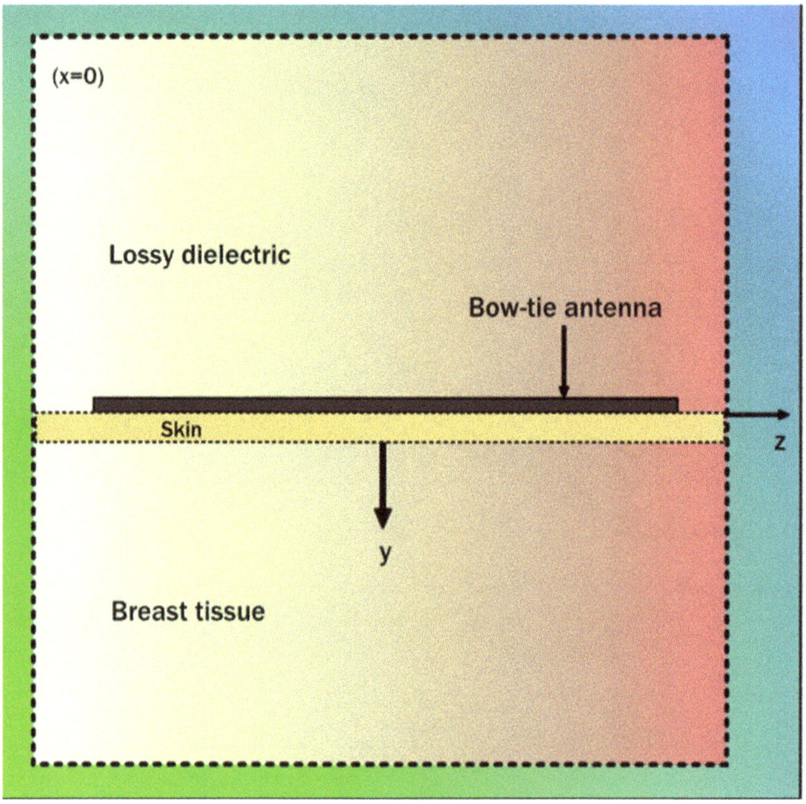

Figure 7.6. Side view of bowtie antenna. Copyright (1998) IEEE. Reprinted, with permission from [23].

$$V(t) = V_0 \sin[2\pi f(t - t_0)]e^{-\left[\frac{t-t_0}{\tau}\right]^2} \tag{7.11}$$

In equation (7.11), $f = 6\,\text{GHz}$, $\tau = 0.133$ ns and $t_0 = 4\tau$ [11]. This antenna array provides better breast tumor detection at an early stage. Large-scale 3D FDTD simulations of the breast cancer detection system provide promising results.

7.2 Microwave image formation using confocal technique

Signals are recorded using confocal technique, these signals have early and late time content. The early time content has incident wave, reflections from skin and antenna resonance. The late time signals have tumor backscatter waves and signals due to clutter. The goal of signal processing is to reduce the early time content and tumour backscatter response improvement. The image reconstruction steps are shown below [12].

1. **Calibration:** Calibration is the process to remove the incident signals and skin reflections from the recorded signals. It is assumed that the incident pulses and skin reflections are symmetric at all antenna locations. Patient orientation and image formation planes are shown in figure 7.7 for a planar system. The calibration signal is the average of the reflected returns at each antenna

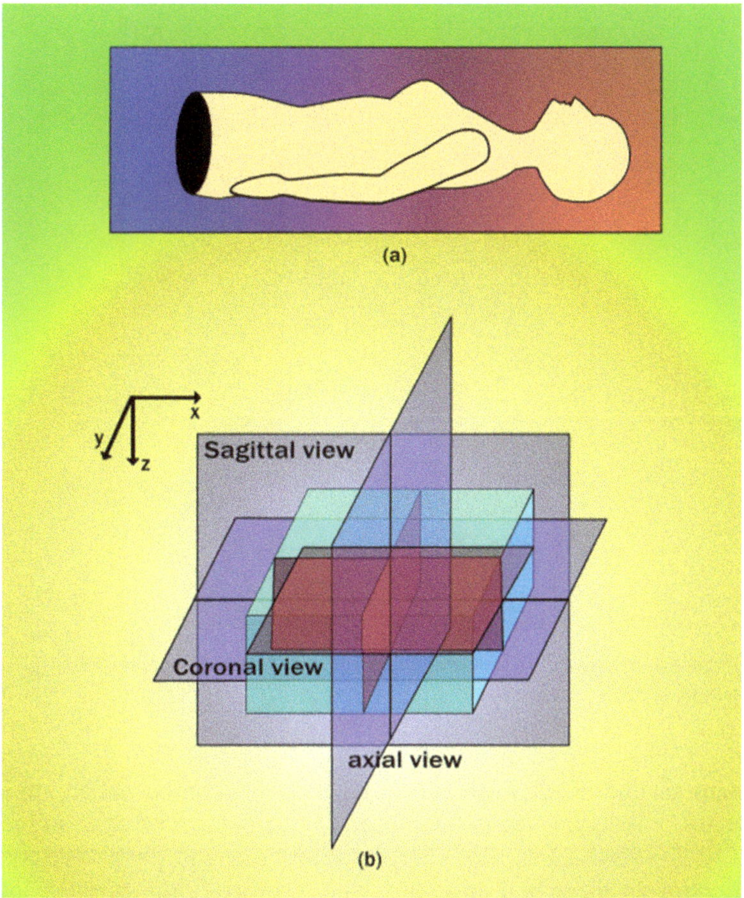

Figure 7.7. Planar system: (a) Patient orientation; (b) Image plane. Copyright (2002) IEEE. Reprinted, with permission from [12].

for the planar system. This calculated signal is subtracted from actual received signal at each antenna. Antennas are located at some distance from skin, so the incident wave and skin backscattering are seperated in time for a cylindrical system. Patient orientation and image formation planes are shown in figure 7.8 for a cylindrical system. Reflections or backscattered signals are recorded at each antenna without the breast model and these signals are subtracted from the actual response for each antenna. Skin reflections are dominant in the signals received at the antennas. Calibration reduces or removes unnecessary signals from the system.

2. **Integration:** The integration of the calibrated signals is the next important step [12]. The differentiated Gaussian pulse is used as an input signal which has zero crossing at its center point in time. The back scatter signal also has zero crossing at the center point, so there is maximum at the center point after integration of the calibrated signals.

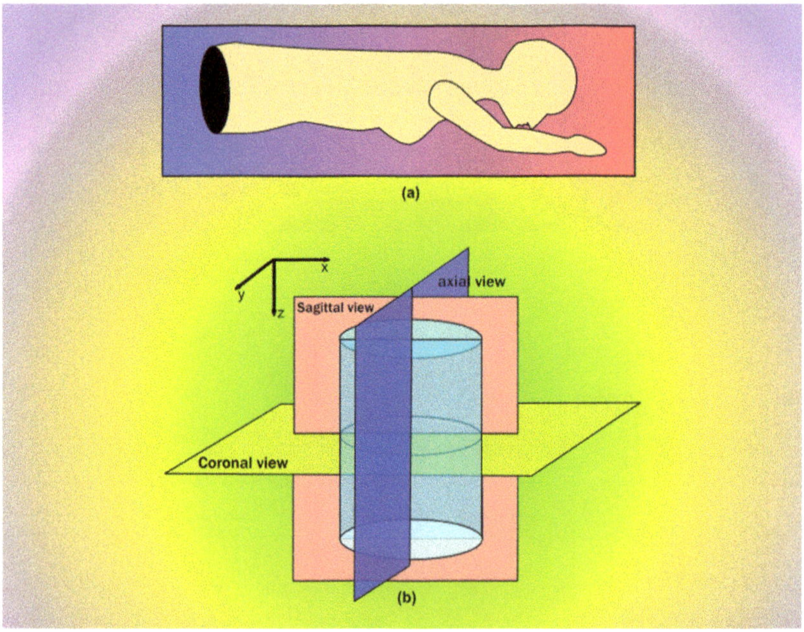

Figure 7.8. Cylindrical system: (a) Patient orientation; (b) Image plane. Copyright (2002) IEEE. Reprinted, with permission from [12].

3. **Compensation:** Radial spreading and path loss compensation are applied as the next important step in the process [12]. Spherical wave amplitude reduces due to radical spreading compensation, whereas path loss compensates reduction in the signal amplitude due to propagation through lossy breast tissues. Compensation factors of the planar system can be estimated by FDTD simulation of the system. Radial spreading compensation is calculated by using a $1/r$ model, where r is the distance of the antenna. Path loss is neglected for the cylindrical configuration. The propagation distance is recorded at each time step; processed signals are calculated then appropriate compensation factors are applied for planar and cylindrical systems [12].
4. **Image reconstruction:** The processed signals are artificially focused at a specific point in the breast. Distances are calculated from each antenna to the focal point then they are converted to time delays. The time delays are used to get the contribution of each processed signal component. All signal contributions are added to get the final sum. Square of this final sum is used to assign intensity value to pixel. The intensity values at a particular location are given by equation (7.12) [12].

$$I(\vec{r}) = \left(\sum_{n=1}^{N} B_n(\tau_n(\vec{r})) \right)^2 \tag{7.12}$$

In equation (7.12), B_n is the processed backscatter signal at the nth antenna located at $\vec{r}_n$ and $\tau_n(\vec{r}) = 2|\vec{r} - \vec{r}_n|/(v\Delta t)$ is the discrete time delay from the nth antenna to artificial focal point at location $\vec{r}$, v is the velocity of the signal propagation in the medium. Here medium is assumed to be homogeneous breast tissue medium. The focal point is scanned to new location in the 3D region of interest, and this process is repeated.

7.3 Space–time beamforming

Microwave imaging space–time (MIST) beamforming was proposed for detecting backscattered signals from small-size malignant tumors in [13]. This method has the ability to detect the presence and location of potential microwave scatterers such as malignant tumors in breast. Each antenna array element sequentially transmits low power ultrawideband (UWB) signals into the breast and records the backscattered energy. The UWB signals can be generated as a time domain impulse or by swept frequency input. Backscattered signals are spatially focused by a beamformer to identify clutter caused by the heterogeneous nature of breast tissues and noise. The spatial focus is achieved by applying time shift to received signals for alignment of the reflections at a particular potential location. Now, these time aligned signals are passed through a bank of finite impulse response filters for each antenna channel, addition is performed to generate output of the beamformer. A least square method is used to design weights of finite impulse response (FIR) filters, so the backscatter signals from potential locations have unit gain while eliminating frequency dependent propagation effects. The time-gating is used by beamformer to calculate backscatter energy from a potential location. If a malignant tumor is present at the potential location then it results in large energy. Proper change in time shifts, time-gating and FIR filter weights are done to scan different locations by the beamformer. Energy as a function of location provides backscattered signal strength as an image. The beamformer provides robustness with respect to the signal variations due to tumor properties such as shape and size. The estimate of backscattered waves from a particular location is obtained through beamformer for detailed tissue property analysis.

7.4 Removal of skin–breast artifact

N antenna elements are considered and the signal at the ith antenna is denoted as $b_i(t)$, and each received signal is sampled as $b_i[n]$. Backscatter signals have contributions from skin–breast interface, clutter due to breast heterogeneity, potential tumor lesions and noise. The backscatter due to skin–breast interface dominates other signals and it may exist beyond the time of backscatter from tumor lesions, so it is essential to remove skin–breast response for accurate tumor detection. Skin–breast backscatter signals are similar but they are not identical due to heterogeneity of the breast at different locations. If skin–breast backscatter signals are identical then they are eliminated by subtracting average backscatter signal from each channel. Figure 7.9 shows skin–breast backscatter in each channel is formed as a filtered combination of the signal in all other channels [13]. The skin–breast response in the first channel at the nth sample is estimated for $2J + 1$

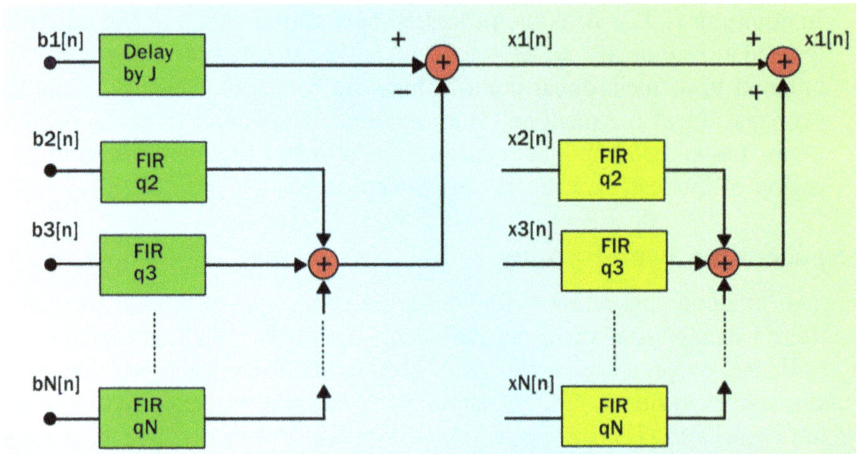

Figure 7.9. Skin–breast backscatter removal at first antenna. Copyright (2003) IEEE. Reprinted, with permission from [13].

successive samples centered on the nth sample in other $N-1$ channels. The $(2J+1) \times 1$ vector of time samples in the ith antenna channel is shown in equation (7.13).

$$b_i[n] = [b_i[n-j], \ldots, b_i[n], \ldots, b_i[n+J]^T], \ 2 \leqslant i \leqslant N. \tag{7.13}$$

Let $b_{2N}[n] = [b_2^T[n], \ldots, b_N^T[n]]^T$ be the combined data in channels 2 through N. q_i is the $(2J+1) \times 1$ vector of FIR filter coefficients in the ith channel and $q = [q_2^T, \ldots, q_N^T]^T$ is the combined FIR filter coefficients from channels 2 to N. The optimal filter coefficient vector is chosen to satisfy equation (7.14).

$$q = \text{argmin} \sum_{n=n_0}^{n_0+m-1} |b_1[n] - q^T b_{2N}[n]|^2 \tag{7.14}$$

The solution to the above equation is given in [13, 14].

$$q = R^{-1}p \tag{7.15}$$

$$R = \frac{1}{m} \sum_{n=n_0}^{n_0+m-1} b_{2N}[n] b_{2N}^T[n] \tag{7.16}$$

$$p = \frac{1}{m} \sum_{n=n_0}^{n_0+m-1} b_{2N}[n] b_1[n] \tag{7.17}$$

Sample covariance matrix R is formed due to high degree of similarity among skin–breast backscattering for N channels. R can be approximated as shown in equation (7.18) if it is ill-conditioned.

$$R_p = \sum_{i=1}^{p} \lambda_i u_i u_i^T \tag{7.18}$$

In equation (7.18), λ is the eigenvalue and u is the corresponding eigenvectors. The inverse of R is found by applying equation (7.19).

$$R_p^{-1} = \sum_{i=1}^{p} \frac{1}{\lambda_i} u_i u_i^T \tag{7.19}$$

Now, the skin–breast artifact is eliminated from the entire data set of the first channel by using equation (7.20).

$$x_1[n] = b_1[n] - Q^T b_{2N}[n] \tag{7.20}$$

The values of n_0 and m are chosen such that value of q is determined from a portion of the data in which residuals are negligible and condition of equation (7.21) is satisfied [13].

$$s_1[n] - Q^T s_{2N}[n] \approx 0 \tag{7.21}$$

Now, expanding values of $b_1[n]$ and $b_{2N}[n]$ in equation (7.20) [13].

$$\begin{aligned} x_1[n] &= s_1[n] - q^T s_{2N}[n] + d_1[n] - q^T d_{2N}[n] \\ &\approx d_1[n] - q^T d_{2N}[n] \end{aligned} \tag{7.22}$$

The residual signal is distorted by term $q^T s_{2N}[n]$, which is small due to average across N channels and $d_{2N}[n]$ do not add in phase. $d_{2N}[n]$ can be approximated by using $x_{2N}[n]$ as shown in equation (7.23) [13].

$$x_{2N}[n] = [x_2[n - J], \ldots, x_2[n + J], \ldots, x_N[n - J], \ldots, x_N[n + J]]^T \tag{7.23}$$

The final equation (7.24) represents data at first channel after removing skin–breast artifact [13].

$$\hat{x}_1[n] = x_1[n] + q^T x_{2N}[n] \tag{7.24}$$

The block diagram of microwave imaging based space–time beamforming is shown in figure 7.10 [13]. The microwave imaging space–time beamformer is applied to get an image of backscattered energy as a function of scan location r. The MIST generates a weighted combination of the time delayed versions of the backscattered signals for each scan location, as shown in figure 7.10 [13]. The final equation (7.25) can be derived with the help of [13].

$$w = (AA^T + \lambda I)^{-1} A f_d^T \tag{7.25}$$

A is the system matrix, f_d is the residual, w is the weight vector of filter. The above equation can be computed with the help of [13]. Microwave imaging space–time beamforming can detect milimeter sized breast tumors by reducing skin–breast artifact and noise. Experimental 3D MIST for multilayer breast phantom is proposed in [15] by modification 2D MIST.

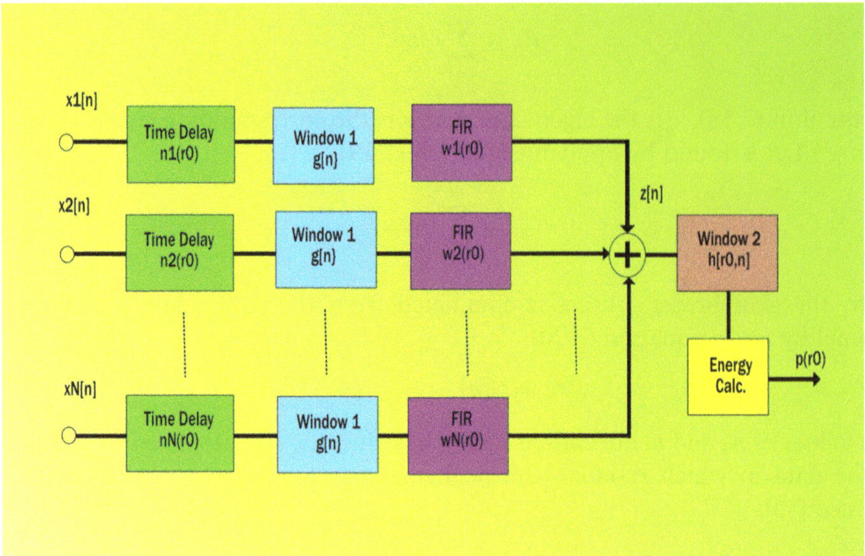

Figure 7.10. Microwave imaging based space–time beamforming. Copyright (2003) IEEE. Reprinted, with permission from [13].

7.5 FDTD based time reversal for microwave breast cancer detection

Finite difference time domain based time reversal eliminates wave attenuation so it is suitable for lossy and inhomogeneous breast medium [16]. Single UWB pulse excitation is used with the multiple receivers to detect 3 mm diameter tumors. The focusing is achieved even though background medium properties are not known *a priori*. Time reversed FDTD equations are easy to obtain through simple modifications in traditional FDTD equations [16, 17]. The following equalities hold for $t' = -t$.

$$\rho(t') = \rho(t) \tag{7.26}$$

$$E(t') = E(t) \tag{7.27}$$

$$B(t') = -B(t) \tag{7.28}$$

$$J(t') = -J(t) \tag{7.29}$$

The time evolution of the computational time reversal algorithm is represented as $t = T - n'\Delta t$, where T indicates time at which backpropagation begins. Transverse magnetic time reversal FDTD equations are given by (7.30), (7.31) and (7.32) [16].

$$\begin{aligned} E_x^{n'+\frac{1}{2}}(j, k) = E_x^{n'-\frac{1}{2}}(j, k) - \frac{\Delta t}{\epsilon \Delta}\Bigg[H_z^{n'}\left(\frac{j+1}{2}, k\right) - H_z^{n'}\left(\frac{j-1}{2}, k\right) \\ - H_y^{n'}\left(j, \frac{k+1}{2}\right) + H_y^{n'}\left(j, \frac{k-1}{2}\right)\Bigg] + \sigma\Delta E_x^{n'+\frac{1}{2}(j,k)} \end{aligned} \tag{7.30}$$

$$H_y^{n'+1}\left(j, \frac{k+1}{2}\right) = H_y^{n'}\left(j, \frac{k+1}{2}\right) + \frac{\Delta t}{\epsilon\Delta}\left[E_x^{n'+\frac{1}{2}}(j, k+1) - E_x^{n'+\frac{1}{2}}(j, k)\right] \quad (7.31)$$

$$H_z^{n'+1}\left(\frac{j+1}{2}, k\right) = H_z^{n'}\left(\frac{j+1}{2}, k\right) - \frac{\Delta t}{\epsilon\Delta}\left[E_x^{n'+\frac{1}{2}}(j+1, k) - E_x^{n'+\frac{1}{2}}(j, k)\right] \quad (7.32)$$

In the above equations, $\Delta x = \Delta y = \Delta$ is the spatial grid dimensions and Δt is the increment in time domain. The $(n' + 1/2)$ time step represents the next step in the back propagation. n' and Δt represent iteration step and temporal increment, respectively. Electric field distribution can be written as shown in equation (7.33).

$$E_x(r, t) = \phi(T - t)*K(r, t) \quad (7.33)$$

The above equation represents time convolution, K is given by equation (7.34).

$$K(r, t) = \frac{1}{4\pi r}\delta\left(t + \frac{|r|}{c}\right) - \frac{1}{4\pi r}\delta\left(t - \frac{|r|}{c}\right) \quad (7.34)$$

In the above equations, $\phi(t)$ is the excitation pulse or waveform, K is kernel distribution. Important aspects of computational time reversal are performed in time domain for breast cancer detection. It chooses the most optimal time instant when the wave focuses back to the scatterer which depends on location of the scatterer. In order to determine the optimal time instant for successful detection of target location, the inverse source problem is useful. In the time reversal process, the converging and diverging waves are used to achieve focusing for a very small time interval. The time reversal field reaches its peak value when focusing occurs at the optimal time instant. Whenever the signals are focused back to the source scatterer then it produces an image with a sharp peak at the target location. The entropy criteria is useful to find out optimal time instant and image. The FDTD time reversal (TR) technique is simple and effective for microwave breast imaging. Three-dimensional FDTD TR technique is shown for microwave breast imaging in [18].

7.5.1 Matched filter FDTD based time reversal

Matched filter FDTD based time reversal has the ability to detect backscattered signals from a tumor without any *a priori* information about skin layer and breast inhomogeneities. This proposed method is similar to the matched filter technique for land mine detection [20]. The information about characteristics of target response is needed to apply matched filter FDTD based TR. The input of the matched filter algorithm for the target signal at receiver i is shown in equation (7.35).

$$s_i(t) = ar_0(t - \tau_i) \quad (7.35)$$

In equation (7.35), $r_0(t)$ represents the early time backscattered field response, τ_i is the delay, a is the scaling factor. Tumor response estimation from the total field is similar to estimating the parameters a and τ_i in equation (7.35). These parameters depend on the location of the tumor with respect to receivers and its size.

These parameters are written as $\theta = (a, \tau_i)$. This random vector is estimated by maximizing the log-likelihood function of equation (7.36)[20, 21].

$$\ln f(\theta|x) = \ln f(x, \theta) - \ln f(x) \tag{7.36}$$

In the above equation $f(\theta|x)$ is the conditional or posterior probability density function, $f(x, \theta)$ is the joint probability density function, $f(x)$ is the marginal probability density function. Equation (7.36) is also known as the maximum *a posteriori* probability (MAP) estimate of θ [21]. The measured vector x is the total electric field at receiver i as shown by equation (7.37) [19].

$$y_i = y_i^0 + c \tag{7.37}$$

In the above equation, y_i^0 is a (deterministic) signal vector in time domain for the skin–breast contributions at the ith receiver. Skin thickness and breast tissue variations lead to change in y_i from reference signal y_i^0 and c is nonzero for such a case. The variations in skin thickness and breast tissues are random so variable c can be assumed as Gaussian random variable with zero mean and variance σ^2. The Gaussian distribution can be applied to variable y_i by using equation (7.38) [19].

$$f(x) = f(y_i) = \prod_{j=1}^{M} \frac{1}{\sqrt{2\pi\sigma^2}} e^{-[y_i(n) - y_i^0(n)]^2/2\sigma^2} \tag{7.38}$$

The total electric field follows normal distribution as shown by equation (7.38). The joint probability function $f(x, \theta)$ is given by equation (7.39).

$$f(x, \theta) = f(y_i, s_i) = \prod_{j=1}^{M} \frac{1}{\sqrt{2\pi\sigma^2}} e^{\,[y_i(n) - y_i^0(n) - s_i(n)]^2/2\sigma^2} \tag{7.39}$$

Now, log-likelihood ratio can be computed as shown in equation (7.40) [19].

$$L(y_i, s_i) = \frac{1}{2\sigma^2} \sum_{j=1}^{M} [y_i(n) - y_i^0(n)]^2 - [y_i(n) - y_i^0(n) - s_i(n)]^2 \tag{7.40}$$

The square can be expanded to get the final equation (7.41).

$$L(y_i, s_i) = \frac{1}{2\sigma^2} \sum_{j=1}^{M} 2s_i(n)[y_i(n) - y_i^0(n)] - s_i^2(n) \tag{7.41}$$

In the above equation, it is clear that $L(y_i)$ is a correlation operation where correlation between clutter free signal $y_i(n) - y_i^0(n) = d_i(n)$ and tumor signal $(s_i(n))$ is considered. The equivalent correlation equation can be given by (7.42).

$$C(\tau) = \int \frac{d_i(t) s_i(t + \tau)}{\sqrt{\langle d_i \rangle} \sqrt{\langle s_i \rangle}} \tag{7.42}$$

In equation (7.42), ⟨⟩ denotes average energy, $C(\tau)$ is invariant to the scaling factor a. The steps are shown below to estimate tumor-like target response [19].

1. Calculate residual as well as reference signal $d_i(n) = y_i(n) - y_i^0(n)$.
2. Calculate log-likelihood ratio by using equation (7.41) as a function of n_i
3. Find out value of a which maximizes the peak of step 2.
4. Now, use the available $s_i(n) = ar_0(n - n_i)$ as the estimate of the tumor.

The above four steps are used in the algorithm to estimate tumor-like response in the breast tissues. The performance of this method is better with the underlying assumption.

7.6 Summary

FDTD is described to solve Maxwell's equations on a discrete grid. Grid size and stability relation is explained with mathematical equations. The input wave for FDTD solution on a Yee grid and two-dimensional FDTD analysis for microwave imaging are discussed. The dielectric properties of healthy breast tissues are described for cancer detection. An overview of the antenna array design is given with an example from the literature. Confocal, space–time beamforming, removal of skin–breast methods and FDTD based time reversal for microwave imaging are given in this chapter. This chapter provides an overview of FDTD for breast cancer detection using microwave imaging to early stage researchers.

References

[1] Yee K 1966 Numerical solution of initial boundary value problems involving Maxwell's equations in isotropic media *IEEE Trans. Antennas Propag.* **14** 302–7

[2] Taflove A 1980 Application of the finite-difference time-domain method to sinusoidal steady-state electromagnetic-penetration problems *IEEE Trans. Electromagn. Compat.* **EMC-22** 191–202

[3] Gabriel C 1996 Compilation of the dielectric properties of body tissues at RF and microwave frequencies *Final technical rept. 15 Sep 93-14 Dec 94* 1996–0037 Radiofrequency Radiation Division, Brooks AFB, TX, USA

[4] Gabriel C, Gabriel S and Corthout E 1996 The dielectric properties of biological tissues: I. Literature survey *Phys. Med., Biol.* **41** 2231–49

[5] Gabriel S, Lau R W and Gabriel C 1996 The dielectric properties of biological tissues: II. Measurements on the frequency range 10 Hz to 20 GHz *Phys. Med., Biol.* **41** 2251–69

[6] Gabriel S, Lau R W and Gabriel C 1996 The dielectric properties of biological tissues: III. Parametric models for the dielectric spectrum of tissues *Phys. Med., Biol.* **41** 2271

[7] Joines W T, Dhenxing Y Z and Jirtle R L 1994 The measured electrical properties of normal and malignant human tissues from 50 to 900 MHz *Med. Phys.* **21** 547–50

[8] Chaudhary S S, Mishra R K, Swarup A and Thomas J M 1984 Dielectric properties of normal and malignant human breast tissues at radiowave and microwave frequencies *Indian J. Biochem., Biophys.* **21** 76–9

[9] Foster K R and Schepps J L 1981 Dielectric properties of tumor and normal tissue at radio through microwave frequency *J. Microwave Power* **16** 107–19

[10] Foster K R and Schwan H P 1989 Dielectric properties of tissues and biological materials: a critical review *Crit. Rev. Biomed. Eng.* **17** 25–104
[11] Hagness S C, Taflove A and Bridges J E 1999 Three-dimensional FDTD analysis of a pulsed microwaved confocal system for breast cancer detection: design of an antenna-array element *IEEE Trans. Antennas Propag.* **47** 783–91
[12] Fear E C, Li X, Hagness S C and Stuchly M A 2002 Confocal microwave imaging for breast cancer detection: localization of tumors in three dimensions *IEEE Trans. Biomed. Eng.* **49** 812–22
[13] Bond E J, Li X, Hagness S C and Van Veen B D 2003 Microwave imaging via spacetime beam-forming for early detection of breast cancer *IEEE Trans. Antennas Propag.* **51** 1690–705
[14] Haykin S 1996 *Adaptive Filter Theory* 3rd edn (Upper Saddle River, NJ: Prentice-Hall)
[15] Li X, Davis S K, Hagness S C, Van der Weide D W and Van Veen B D 2004 Microwave imaging via space-time beam-forming: experimental investigation of tumour detection in multilayer breast phantoms *IEEE Trans. Microw. Theory Techn.* **52** 1856–65
[16] Kosmas P and Rappaport C 2005 Time reversal with FDTD method for microwave breast cancer detection *IEEE Trans. Microw. Theory Techn.* **53** 2317–22
[17] Altman C and Suchy K 1991 *Reciprocity, Spatial Mapping and Time Reversal in Electromagnetics* (Amsterdam: Kluwer)
[18] Kosmas P and Rappaport C M 2006 FDTD-based time reversal for microwave breast cancer detection-localization in three dimensions *IEEE Trans. Microw. Theory Techn.* **54** 1921–7
[19] Kosmas P and Rappaport C 2006 A matched fllter FDTD-based time reversal approach for microwave breast cancer detection *IEEE Trans. Antennas Propag.* **54** 1257–64
[20] Linnehan R 2002 Mitigating ground clutter effects for mine detection with lightweight artificial dielectrics *M.S. Thesis* Northeastern University
[21] Scharf L L 1991 *Statistical Signal Processing* (New York: Addison-Wesley)
[22] Yin T and Ali F H 2015 Adaptive combining via correlation exploration for ultrawideband breast cancer imaging *IEEE Antennas Wirel. Propag. Lett.* **14** 587–90
[23] Hagness S C, Taflove A and Bridges J E 1998 Two-dimensional FDTD analysis of a pulsed microwave confocal system for breast cancer detection: fixed-focus and antenna-array sensors *IEEE Trans. Biomed. Eng.* **45** 1470–9

IOP Publishing

Breast Image Reconstruction and Cancer Detection
Using Microwave Imaging

Hardik N Patel, Deepak K Ghodgaonkar and Jasjit S Suri

Chapter 8

Review of machine learning based image reconstruction for different imaging modalities

Image reconstruction problem is formulated for inverse scattering effect of electromagnetic imaging. Traditional reconstruction techniques are described briefly. Machine learning approaches are discussed for different imaging modalities and applications. Machine learning approaches are described for computed tomography (CT), magnetic resonance imaging (MRI), positron emission tomography (PET), and photoacoustic imaging. Applications, computational power, algorithm, type of neural network and comparison with other approaches are discussed in this chapter. performance analysis is done for some selected machine learning methods.

8.1 Introduction

Over the past years, artificial intelligence has attracted researchers in almost all areas of science, technology and engineering. Image reconstruction and image analysis are two main pillars in the medical imaging process. In the image reconstruction stage, images are reconstructed from the tomographic measurements/raw data/features. In the image analysis stage, diagnostic features/readings are extracted from these reconstructed images. Applied machine learning research is evolving very fast in computer vision and image analysis. Computer vision and image analysis are used to extract features from the existing images (images to features). Tomographic reconstruction is applied to reconstruct images of internal structure from measurement data (features to images). Deep neural networks have amazing learning capability which attracted researchers to apply these methods in image reconstruction (imaging). Four types of different imaging modalities are considered in this review article. Inverse problems are solved in image reconstruction or imaging. In this review article, different deep neural networks are reviewed for inverse problems, computed tomography (CT), magnetic resonance imaging (MRI), positron emission

doi:10.1088/978-0-7503-2592-9ch8

tomography (PET) and photoacoustic imaging. Image reconstruction or inverse problems are solved in many applications like remote sensing, cancer detection, nondestructive testing, and medical imaging. The objective of this chapter is to provide a platform for new researchers so they can make a smooth transition.

8.1.1 Image reconstruction (inverse) problem formulation

Image reconstruction is basically an inverse problem. In any imaging modality, internal structure of objects or organs is unknown. Signals or waves are applied to objects or organs for their internal structure reconstruction. Incident signals or waves interact with internal structure of an object or an organ. Signals or waves received after this interaction are known as data. Based on these noise affected measurement data and known system matrix, internal structure of objects or organs is reconstructed. This type of problem can be formulated as given below.

$$Ax = \hat{b} \tag{8.1}$$

In the above equation, $\hat{b} = b + n$, where column vectors b and n are measured data and noise, respectively. A is the system's matrix, x is unknown. The problem of (8.1) is very challenging because of the nonlinear mapping function. In medical imaging, unknown x represents internal structure of an organ. Figure 8.1 explains about forward and inverse problems in medical imaging.

The patient would like to know about the diagnosis of a particular body part or organ. The first stage in figure 8.1 is data measurement using imaging setup and the patient's organ or body part. Data collection or measurement phase is generally known as the forward problem. After data collection, it is fed to a computer or embedded system (part of the imaging system) where a computational imaging algorithm reconstructs an image of the internal structure of the patient's body part or organ. This image reconstruction phase is known as the inverse problem.

8.2 Traditional image reconstruction techniques

There are many traditional techniques used to date for image reconstruction. Filtered back projection is the most widely used analytical technique in computed tomography based image reconstruction [89–91, 96]. A block diagram of filtered back projection is shown in figure 8.2. Associated noise of measurements is ignored by these methods and tries to reduce this artifact's effect by post-filtering operations [89–91].

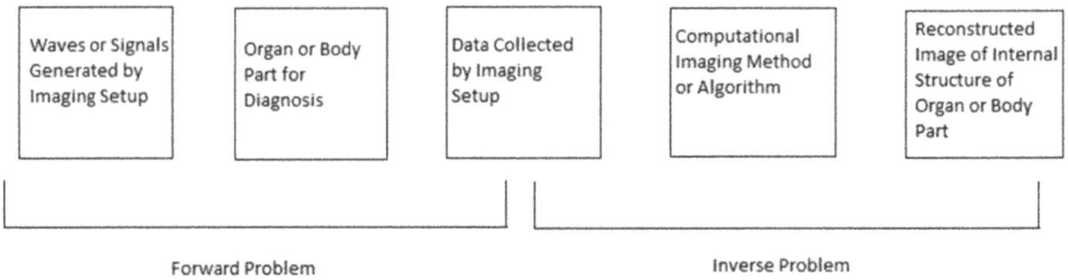

Figure 8.1. Block diagram of forward and inverse problems in medical imaging.

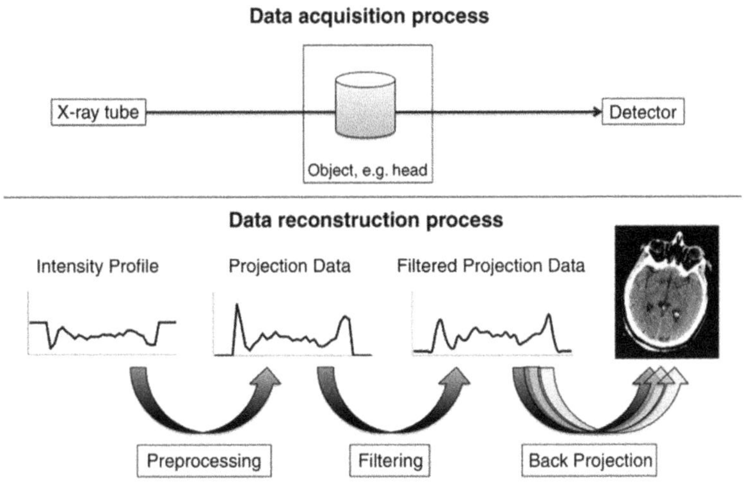

Figure 8.2. Forward backward projections [91]. Reprinted with permission from [4], copyright RSNA 2015.

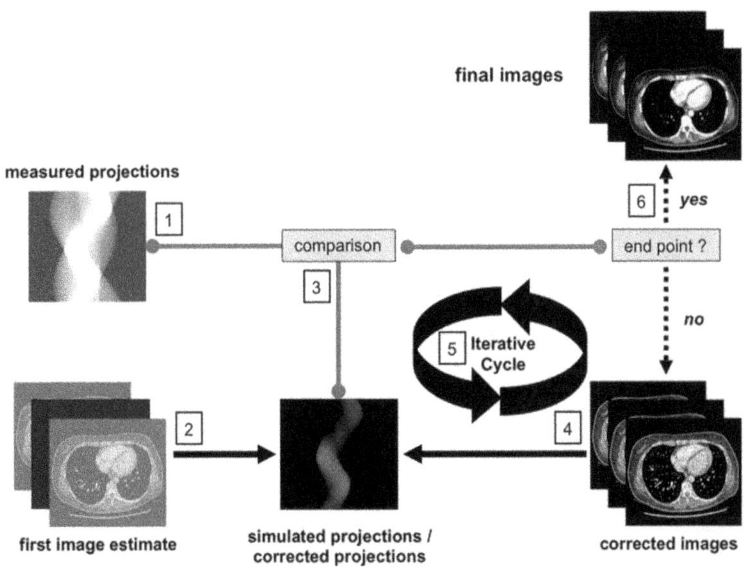

Figure 8.3. Iterative image reconstruction scheme [91]. Reprinted with permission from [4], copyright RSNA 2015.

Iterative reconstruction is also a commonly used technique in CT image reconstruction. The whole process of iterative reconstruction is shown in figure 8.3. As shown in figure 8.3, measured data (projections) is compared with reconstructed data (projections) at every iteration to get the best reconstructed image as a result. Algebraic reconstruction technique, simultaneous algebraic reconstruction technique, maximum likelihood expectation maximization and penalized likelihood are also used for CT image reconstruction [91]. In iterative technique, the forward problem is solved at each iteration to get a reconstructed image.

8.3 Machine learning techniques for image reconstruction

Machine learning is very popular and a fast growing field in all areas of science, technology and engineering. There are four types of machine learning techniques as given below.

- Supervised learning.
- Unsupervised learning.
- Semi-supervised learning.
- Reinforcement learning.

A labeled data set is required in supervised learning. The data set is divided into training, validation and test. Training data is used to train the machine learning model. Validation data is used to tune the parameters of the model. Test data is used to validate the model designed. On the other hand, unsupervised learning does not require a labeled data set. Clustering algorithm is an example of unsupervised learning. Semi-supervised learning uses both supervised and unsupervised learning algorithms. Reinforcement learning has an environment and agent. The agent may be a system or software, and environment depends on the problem.

A neural network is a part of machine learning techniques. Basically, the neural network has an input layer, hidden layers and output layers. If the neural network has more than two hidden layers then it is known as a deep neural network.

Input to a deep neural network is imaging data captured by a particular imaging technique. Output is a reconstructed image of the internal structure of a body organ or part. There are different types of neural networks. The most widely used neural networks are shown in this chapter. Convolutional neural network (CNN) is one of the most widely used neural networks in an image reconstruction problem. The general architecture of CNN is shown in figure 8.4. The architecture of a general adversarial neural network is shown in figure 8.5.

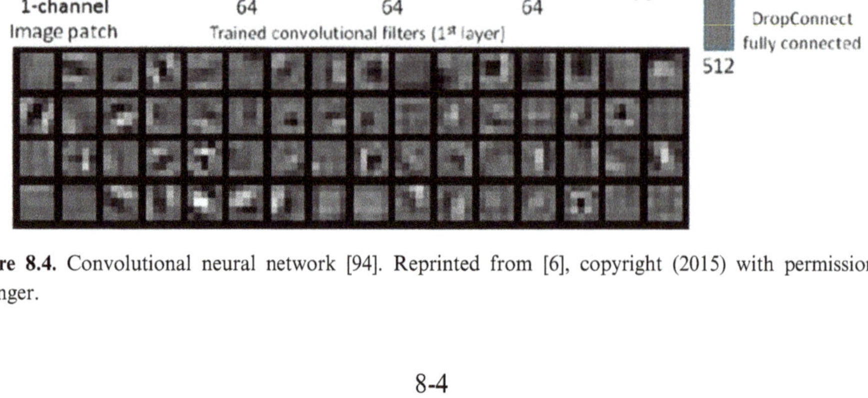

Figure 8.4. Convolutional neural network [94]. Reprinted from [6], copyright (2015) with permission of Springer.

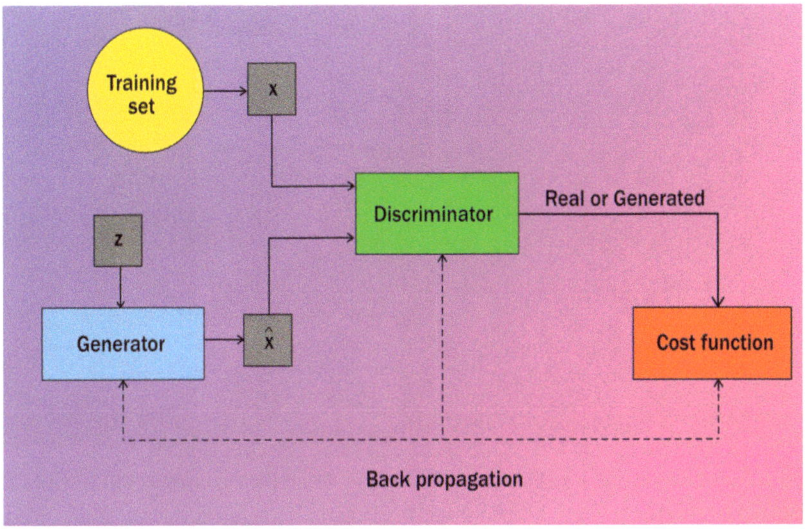

Figure 8.5. Generative adversarial network [95]. Copyright (2017) IEEE. Reprinted with permisssion from [7].

Now we consider the equation given below as a cost functional.

$$l_{\text{mse}} = ||g_\phi(y) - x||^2 \tag{8.2}$$

In equation (8.2), we find y such that the mean square error between measured and reconstructed data is minimal. The cost functional in predefined feature space is given as equation (8.3).

$$l_f = ||\psi(g_\phi(y)) - \psi(x)||^2 \tag{8.3}$$

Now equations (8.2)and (8.3) are implemented by figure 8.6.

8.3.1 Machine learning based solution of inverse problems

A deep autoregressive model is used in [90] to solve inverse computational imaging problems with deep pixel-level prior. Consider a natural image represented by $n \times n$ matrix I. The measurements are represented by matrix M and it can be written as $M = f(I)$. The aim of the inverse problem is to reconstruct original image I from the measurements M. Deep neural networks are generally used to learn inverse mapping $I = g(M)$, where g is a deep neural network and minimizing the reconstruction error on a set of training examples I_j, M_j. The autorgressive model is used to model the distribution of the natural images $p(I)$. Maximum *a posteriori* estimation is used to formulate the inverse problem in [90]. The estimated image $\hat{I}$ is written as equation (8.4).

$$\hat{I} = \log(p(I|M)) \tag{8.4}$$

The problem of reconstructing the original image I can be modeled as stochastic gradients using pixel dropout by equation (8.5).

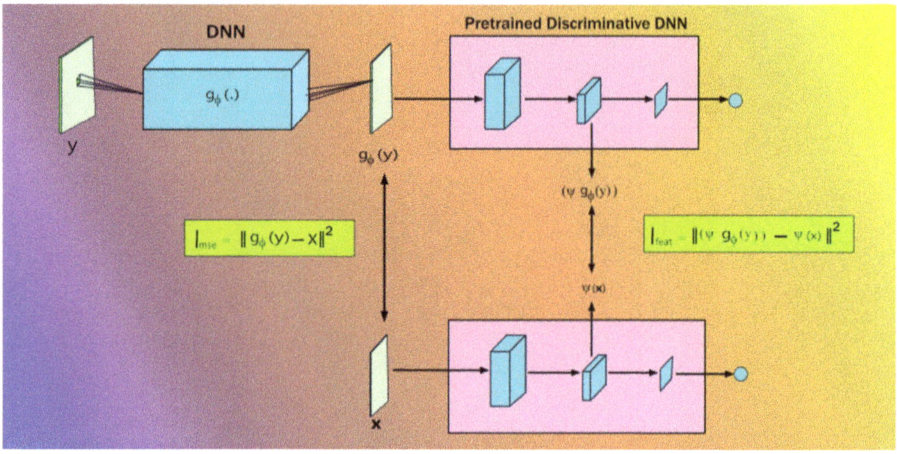

Figure 8.6. General deep learning architecture for inverse problems [94]. Copyright (2018) IEEE. Reprinted with permission from [14].

Table 8.1. Analysis of deep learning for inverse problems.

Problem type	Algorithm	NN type	Library and tools	Comparison
Inverse problems	Deep-pixel autoregressive prior [90]	CNN	MATLAB	TVAL3 and OneNet
	Deep convolutional framelets [91]	CNN	GTX 1080 Ti GPU, i7-7770 CPU, Python, Tensorflow	Red-net, U-net, FBP
	DCNN [92]	CNN	MatConvNet, Titan Black GPU	FBP, TV, U-net
	MoDL [93]	CNN	Python, Tensorflow, GPU	CG-ET-WS, SD-ET-WS

$$H_k = I_k + \alpha N \circ \nabla_x \log(p_\theta(I_k)) \tag{8.5}$$

In equation (8.5), N is a random binary mask with the percentage of zeros decided by the pixel dropout ratio. An inverse problem solution by deep convolutional framelets is proposed in [91]. An updated equation with deep convolutional framelet is given by equation (8.6).

$$f_{n+1} = \mu Dg + (I - \mu D)Q(f_n) \tag{8.6}$$

In equation (8.6), D is diagonal matrix, Q is deep convolutional framelet output. The above equation is solved by using a different deep neural network in [91]. Table 8.1 shows the analysis of deep learning for inverse problems.

U-Net has been modified to solve inverse problems in imaging [92]. A model based deep learning architecture is proposed in [93] for the solution of inverse problems. Regularized optimization equation for inverse problem is given by equation (8.7).

$$x = \arg min||Ax - b||_2^2 + \lambda||N_w(x)||^2 \quad (8.7)$$

In equation (8.7), first term and second terms are data consistency and regularization, respectively. There are many deep learning based algorithms which reconstruct images by using equation (8.8).

$$X_{\text{rec}} = \tau_w(A^H b) \quad (8.8)$$

In equation (8.8), τ_w is a learned CNN, the operator A^H transforms measurement data to the image domain. In order to apply proper inversion, a modified version of equation (8.8) is used as (8.9).

$$X_{\text{rec}} = \tau_w(A^H Ax) \quad (8.9)$$

The CNN is able to invert the normal operator $A^H A$ for the reconstruction of an image. The gradient of the cost function is calculated by using equation (8.10).

$$(\nabla_{z_{k-1}} C) = (A^H A + \lambda I)^{-1}(\nabla_{x_k} C) \quad (8.10)$$

In equation (8.10), $(\nabla_{z_{k-1}} C)$ is the gradient of cost function. The above equation is solved by conjugate gradient method.

8.3.2 Machine learning in computed tomography

Minimization is a large-scale optimization problem in imaging. This problem is generally solved by gradient descent or modified versions of it (quasi-Newton or Newton) with higher order derivatives. Regularization is included for ill-posed inverse problems in imaging. Many regularization schemes make the objective functional non-differentiable. Proximal approach is developed to deal with non-smooth objective functionals [89]. Table 8.2 shows the analysis of deep learning in CT. The proximal equivalent of the gradient descent method is given by equation (8.11).

$$f_{i+1} = \text{prox}_{\tau G}(f_i) \quad (8.11)$$

In equation (8.11), τ is the step size and the proximal operator is defined by equation (8.12).

$$\text{prox}_{\tau G}(f) = \arg min\left[G(f') + \frac{1}{2\tau}||f' - f||_X^2\right] \quad (8.12)$$

primal and dual variables are updated in alternating manner in the proximal primal-dual schemes. Primal-dual hybrid gradient (PDHG) is a well known algorithm and it is also known as the Chambolle–Pock algorithm [89]. Equation (8.13) shows the structure of the minimization problem for which PDHG algorithm is used.

$$\min[F(K(f)) + G(f)] \quad (8.13)$$

In equation (8.13), K: $X \to U$ is a nonlinear operator, U is a Hilbert space and F: $U \to R$ and G: $X \to R$ are functionals on the dual/primal spaces. Equation (8.14)

Table 8.2. Analysis of deep learning for CT.

Imaging modality	Algorithm	NN type	Library and tools	Comparison
	Learned primal-dual [89]	CNN	ODL, TensorFlow, GTX 1080 TI	FBP, TV, FBP+U-Net Denoising
	LEARN [90]	CNN	MATLAB, MatConvNet, Intel i7 6800K CPU and 64 GB RAM, GTX Titan Xp	PWLS, Gamma-Reg, FBP, FBP-ConvNet
	Deep learning method [91]	Neural network which learns mapping	Tensorflow, NVIDIA GTX 1080, an Intel Xeon E5-1630 v3 @ 3.70 GHz and 64 Gb RAM,	Parker, U-Net, wTV
	PWLS [92]	Machine learning	MATLAB	FBP, PWLS-Edge Preserving (EP), PWLS-DL (dictionary learning), PWLS-Square Transform
	CNN projected gradient descent [93]	CNN	MATLAB, Titan X GPU	FBP, FBP-Conv
	Statistical iterative reconstruction [94]	CNN-CBCT	COCO, GTX1080Ti	FDK, TV
	Deep reinforcement learning [95]	CNN	Python with TensorFlow, Intel Xeon 3.5 GHz CPU processor, Nvidia GPU	None
	Generative adversarial network with Wasserstein distance and perceptual loss [96]	GAN	Python with Tensorflow, NVIDIA Titan XP GPU	CNN, WGAN, GAN

Wavelet residual network [89]	CNN	MATLAB, MATConvNet, GTX 1080	FBP
DenseNet and deconvolution [90]	DD-Net	Tensorflow, Intel Core i5-7400 CPU and 16 GB RAM, Nvidia GPU	FBP, PWLS
Multi resolution framing U-Net [91]	CNN	MatConvNet toolbox MATLAB 2015a, GTX 1080 Ti, i7	FBP, U-Net, Dual frame U-Net
CNN based metal artifact reduction [92]	CNN	Matlab, MatConvNet, GeForce GTX 970 GPU	BHC, LI, NMAR
3-D convolutional encoder–decoder network [93]	Convolutional encoder–decoder	TensorFlow NVIDIA Titan Xp GPU	LDCT, RED-CNN, WGAN-VGG
Deep CNN [93]	CNN	MATLAB, MatConvNet	MBIR
CNN [94]	CNN	MATLAB 2015b, Intel i7 6700K CPU, 16 GB RAM and GTX 980 Ti	ASD-POCS, K-SVD, BM3D
Residual encoder–decoder CNN [95]	CNN	MATLAB 2015b on a PC (Intel i7 6700K CPU and 16 GB RAM), GTX 1080	TV-POCS, K-SVD, BM3D, KAIST-Net, CNN10
GAN [96]	GAN	Theano and Lasagne, NVIDIA Titan X GPU, 12 GB RAM	FBP
K-sparse autoencoder [89]	ANN	Tensorflow	TV-Prior, Dictionary-Prior

shows the total variation regularized computed tomography problem which is solved by PDHG.

$$\min||p(f) - g||_2^2 + \lambda||\nabla f||_1 \tag{8.14}$$

The proximal operator is replaced by learned proximal in the learned PDHG. Primal and dual spaces are extended to have some memory in learned primal-dual. It allows the neural network to learn about how to combine a previous update with the result of the operator evaluation. It updates learned proximal operators at each iteration [89]. Compressive sensing is used in tomographic reconstruction from sparse data or undersampled measurements. Regularization is used with iterative schemes to reconstruct images in sparse computed tomography. Learned experts' assessment based reconstruction network (LEARN) is used in [90] to determine different parameters of regularized iterative schemes. The network architecture is developed based on equation (8.15).

$$x^{t+1} = x^t - \left[\lambda^t A^T(Ax^t - y) + \sum_{k=1}^{K}(G_k^t)^T\gamma_k^t(G_k^t x^t)\right] \tag{8.15}$$

In equation (8.15), K is number of regularizers, G_k is transform matrix of convolutional operator for CT image x, γ is the derivative of the potential function. Neural network architecture corresponding to equation (8.15) is shown in figure 8.7 [90].

A cone beam back projection layer is proposed with a deep learning approach which can optimize correction steps in volume and projection domain [91].

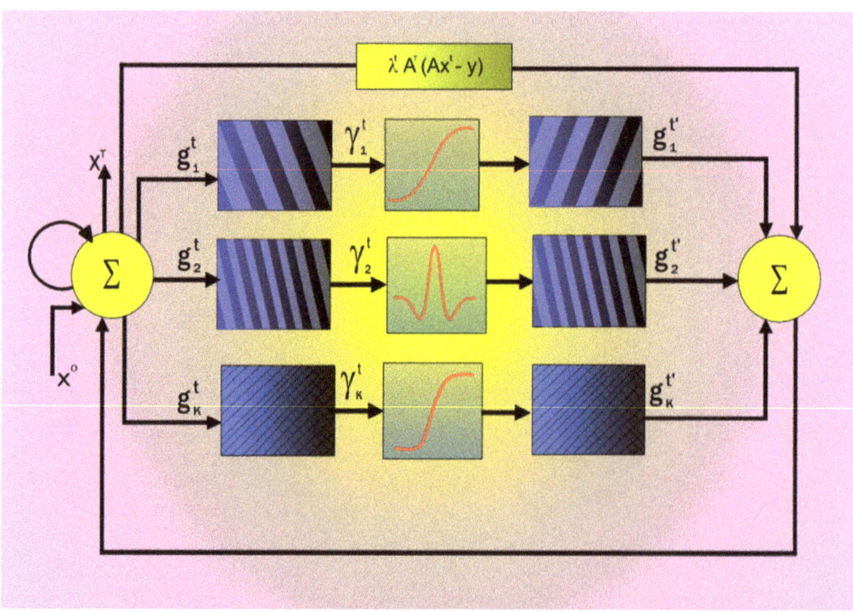

Figure 8.7. Neural network architecture corresponding to equation (8.15). Copyright (2018) IEEE. Reprinted with permisssion from [26].

It provides better performance than other analytical algorithms with almost the same computational complexity as other algorithms. Compensation of weights and apodization windows are learned automatically by the proposed neural network [91]. Penalized weighted least squares with regularization based on union of learned transforms (PWLS-ULTRA) is proposed for low dose 3D computed tomography image reconstruction in [92]. Image update and sparse coding-clustering are two important steps in the PWLS-ULTRA. It provides quality reconstruction as compared to filtered back projections (FBP) and PWLS. The CNN based projected gradient descent method is proposed for consistent CT image reconstruction in [93]. The loss function is given by equation (8.16).

$$J(\theta)\sum_{n=1}^{N}\sum_{q=1}^{Q}||x^{q} - \mathrm{CNN}_{\theta}(\widetilde{x^{q,\,n}})||_2^2 \tag{8.16}$$

Stochastic gradient descent is used up to T epochs for the optimization process. CNN is trained to reduce loss function of equation (8.16). The work of [93] is generic in nature so it can be used for different imaging modalities and inverse problems. Neural network based statistical iterative reconstruction is proposed for cone beam CT in [94]. Loss function used in [94] is given by equation (8.17).

$$L = \frac{1}{M}\sum_{k=1}^{M}||F(x_k;\,\theta) - (x_k - y_k)||_2^2 \tag{8.17}$$

In equation (8.17), F is the neural network operation, M is the batch size, x_k, y_k are the kth original image in the batch, respectively. Data deficiency and noise level are taken care of by the proposed neural network based method of [94]. The transfer learning approach is used to deal with data deficiency and the data-driven approach is used to learn potential regularization terms to deal with noise. Parameter tuning policy network (PTPN) is used with reinforcement learning approach for iterative CT reconstruction in [95]. PTPN training is done via deep reinforcement learning by using equation (8.18).

$$Q^{*}(s,\,a) = r + \gamma\max Q^{*}(s',\,a') \tag{8.18}$$

In equation (8.18), r is the reward achieved by the optimal action a based on the current state s. s' is the next state after taking action a. The function $Q^{*}(s,\,a)$ is parameterized by CNN, $Q(s,\,a) \approx Q(s,\,a;\,W)$, W can be found by minimizing the loss function $L(W) = [r + \gamma\max_{a'}Q(s',\,a';\,W) - Q(s,\,a;\,W)]^2$, which penalizes deviation from the equation (8.18). The loss function is given by equation (8.19) for target term $y = r + \gamma\max_{a'}Q(s',\,a';\,W')$.

$$L(W) = [y - Q(s,\,a;\,W)]^2 \tag{8.19}$$

The learning is implemented in stages with W' unchanged. W is updated to minimize the loss function. The gradient of loss function with respect to variable W is given by equation (8.20).

$$\frac{\partial L}{\partial W} = -[r + \gamma \max Q(s', a'; W') - Q(s, a: W)]\frac{\partial Q(s, a; W)}{\partial W} \tag{8.20}$$

The last term is computed by the back propagation approach in the neural network training process. W is updated as $W^{l+1} = W^l - \sigma\frac{\partial L}{\partial W}$, where σ and l are learning rate and index of iteration, respectively. PTPN is trained by using the neural network architecture shown in figure 8.8 [95].

Low dose CT image denoising is proposed by using generative adversarial network (GAN) with Wasserstein distance and perceptual loss [96]. Wasserstein distance based GAN (WGAN) solves equation (8.21) as a minmax optimization problem to get both G and D.

$$\text{minmax} L_{\text{WGAN}}(D, G) = -\mathbb{E}_x[D(x)] + \mathbb{E}_z[D(z)] + \lambda \mathbb{E}_{\hat{x}}[(||\nabla_{\hat{x}}||_2 - 1)^2] \tag{8.21}$$

In equation (8.21), Wasserstein distance estimation is performed by the first two terms, the last term is the gradient penalty for the regularization of the network. A deep convolutional framelet based wavelet residual network is proposed for denoising of low dose CT images [89]. DenseNet and deconvolution are proposed together for a sparse view CT reconstruction in [90]. The DD-Net network architecture of [90] is shown in figure 8.9.

The above network consists of 45 layers including four densed blocks, eight deconvolution layers, five convolution layers, batch normalization, rectified linear unit (ReLU) qand pooling operators. A very good image reconstruction is achieved by using DenseNet and deconvolution in [90]. U-Net is proposed in [91] through deep convolutional framelets for the sparse view CT. The architectures of different U-Net variants are shown in figure 8.10 [91].

The proposed variants are better than conventional U-Nets for the sparse view CT application. CNN is proposed for metal artifact reduction (MAR) for x-ray based CT [92]. The cost function of equation (8.22) is minimized in the CNN training.

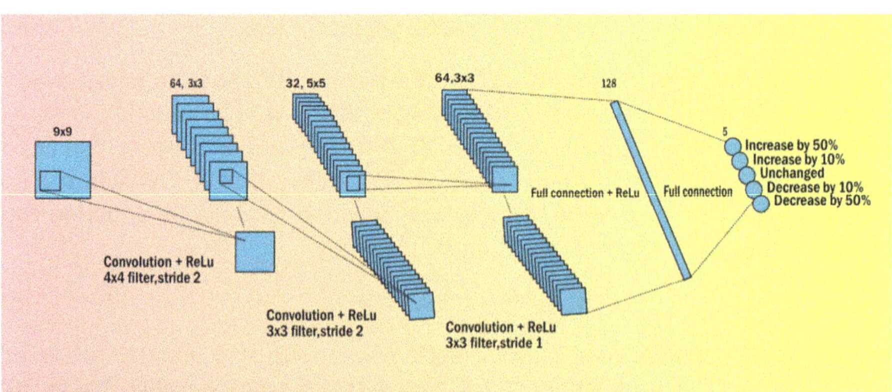

Figure 8.8. Neural network architecture for training of PTPN. Copyright (2018) IEEE. Reprinted with permisssion from [31].

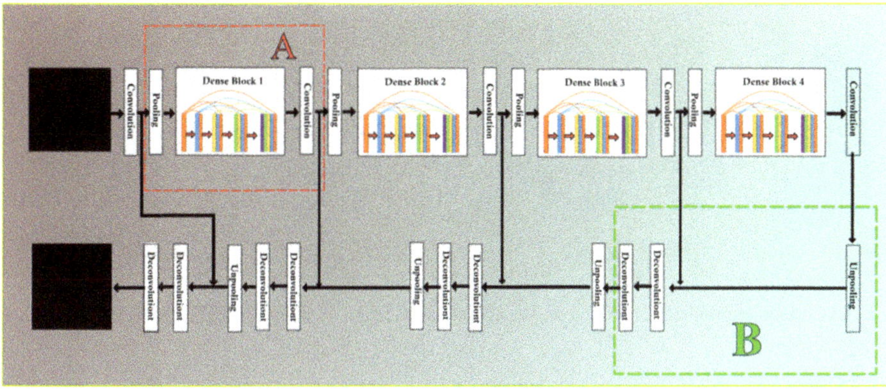

Figure 8.9. Network architecture of the DD-Net. Copyright (2018) IEEE. Reprinted with permisssion from [34].

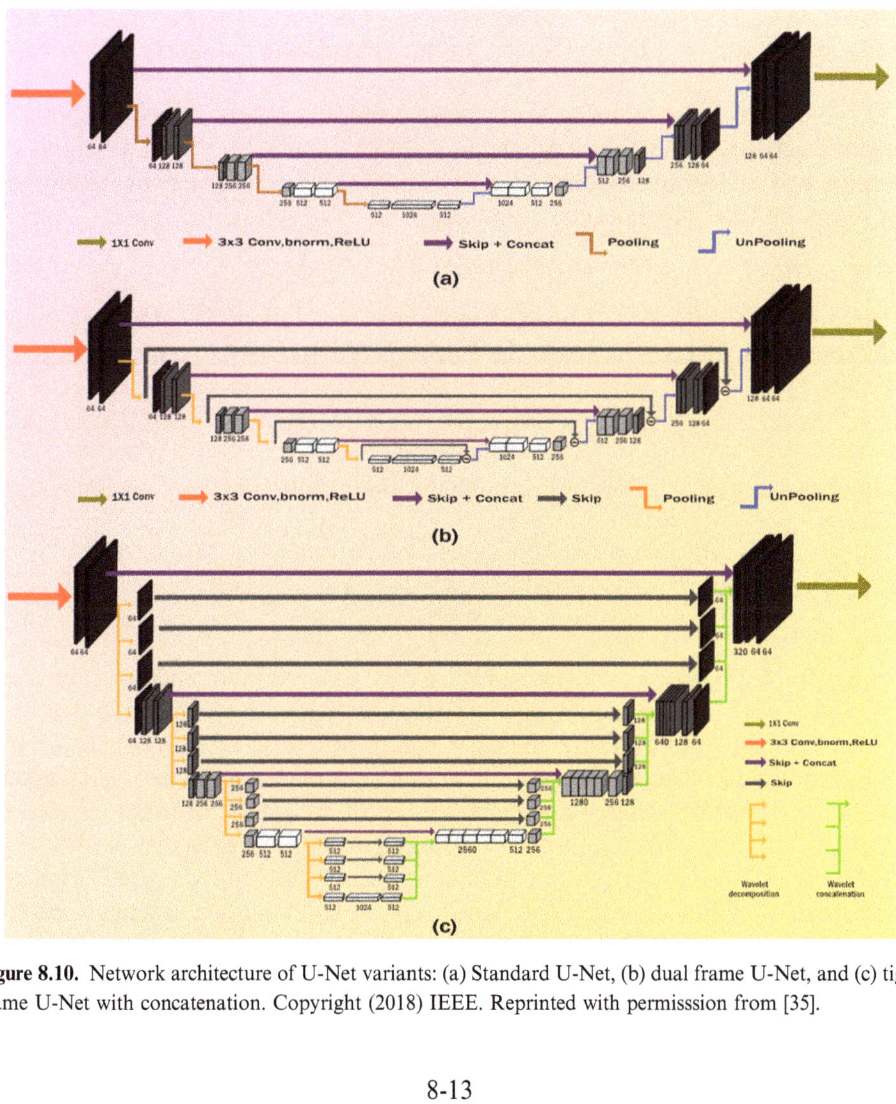

Figure 8.10. Network architecture of U-Net variants: (a) Standard U-Net, (b) dual frame U-Net, and (c) tight frame U-Net with concatenation. Copyright (2018) IEEE. Reprinted with permisssion from [35].

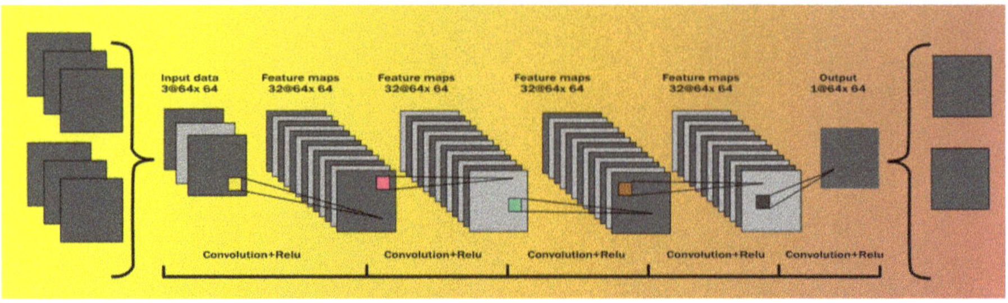

Figure 8.11. Architecture of CNN for metal artifact reduction. Copyright (2018) IEEE. Reprinted with permisssion from [36].

$$H = \arg\min \frac{1}{R}\sum_{r=1}^{R} ||H(u_r) - v_r||_F^2 \tag{8.22}$$

In equation (8.22), (u_r, v_r) is the training sample pair, H is the function to be determined, $||\cdot||_f$ is the Forbenius norm. The CNN workflow is shown in figure 8.11.

There are five convolution layers between input and output layers of CNN. The nonlinear activation function is defined as $\mathrm{ReLU}(x) = \max(0, x)$ and it is applied to the output of each convolutional layer. The output after applying convolution and ReLU can be formulated as equation (8.23).

$$c_l(u) = \mathrm{ReLU}(W_l{*}C_{l-1}(u) + b_l) \tag{8.23}$$

In equation (8.23), $l = 1, \ldots, L - 1$, * indicates convolution, W_l and b_l are weigths and biases in the lth layer, respectively. Equation (8.24) is used to represent output at last layer.

$$C_L(u) = W_L{*}C_{L-1}(u) + b_L \tag{8.24}$$

The parameter estimation is done through the minimization of loss function given by (8.25).

$$\mathrm{Loss}(U, V, \Theta) = \frac{1}{R}\sum_{r=1}^{R} ||C_L(u_r) - v_r||_F^2 \tag{8.25}$$

In equation (8.25), $U = u_1, \ldots, u_R$ and $V = v_1, \ldots, v_R$ are input and target datasets, respectively. 3D convolutional encoder–decoder network is designed by using transfer learning from a 2D trained network for low dose CT reconstruction [93]. 3D convolutional encoder–decoder denoising approach has better performance. Low dose CT based detection and classification of metastatic liver lesions used the results of 2016 low dose CT grand challenge [94–96]. 4D extended cardiac torso (XCAT) phantom is designed and simulated by using PET, SPECT and CT imaging modalities [89, 90]. A statistical method is proposed for image reconstruction in multislice helical CT [91]. The advantages are faster acquisition and wide organ coverage for routine clinical diagnostics. Dictionary learning based image reconstruction is proposed in [92] for low dose CT. Now considering K and N to be integers and R the real space, a dictionary is represented by a matrix $D \in R^{N\times K}$ whose column $d_k \in R^{N\times 1}$ (where k is varying from 1 to K) is an N dimensional vector, which is known as an atom. Generally, the dictionary is either redundant or over-complete, that is $N \ll K$. An image patch of size $\sqrt{N} \times \sqrt{N}$ pixels can be expressed as an N dimensional vector $x \in R^{N\times 1}$. Now, a patch x is either exactly or approximately represented as a sparse liner combination of the atoms in the dictionary D as shown by equation (8.26).

$$||x - D\alpha||_2^2 \leqslant \epsilon \tag{8.26}$$

In equation (8.26), $\epsilon \geqslant 0$ is a small error and the representation vector $\alpha \in R^{k\times 1}$, $||\alpha||_0 \ll N \ll K$ with $||.||_0$ being the l_0-norm. The dictionary redundancy means the number of atoms is larger than the length of an atom. The optimization problem of equation (8.27) is solved to get sparse representation $\alpha \in RK$ of an image patch $x \in RN \times 1$ with respect to a given dictionary $D \in RN \times K$. $\min||\alpha||_0$ such that

$$||x - D\alpha||_2^2 \leqslant \epsilon \tag{8.27}$$

Equation (8.27) is rewritten in unconstrained form as equation (8.28).

$$\min||x - D\alpha||_2^2 + v||\alpha||_0 \tag{8.28}$$

In equation (8.28), v is the Lagrange multiplier. Equations (8.27) and (8.27) directly are NP-hard, so an approximate alternative strategy is desirable. There are several approaches available, such as matching pursuit and orthogonal matching pursuit algorithms. The l_0 norm can be replaced by l_1 norm to make the problem convex. Consider a training set of S patches, the dictionary learning is used to get a dictionary that makes each patch in the training set sparsely represented by the atoms in this dictionary. Patch set matrix $X \in R^{N\times S}$ with a patch $X_s \in R^{N\times 1}$ is a column vector of X, and the sparse representation vector as a matrix $\alpha \in R^{K\times S}$ with the representation $\alpha_s \in R^{K\times 1}$ a column vector of $\alpha \in R^{K\times S}$. Now the dictionary learning is to solve the problem shown by equation (8.29).

$$\min \sum_{s=1}^{S}(||x_s - D\alpha_s||_2^2 + v_s||\alpha_s||_0) \tag{8.29}$$

Image denoising is done through dictionary learning technique. Let a vector $z \in R^{M\times 1}$ represent a noise image of $H \times W$ pixels and a vector $x \in R^{M\times 1}$ denote its corresponding filtered version, $M = H \times W$. A set of small overlapping patches are extracted from the image. The size of patches has $H - \sqrt{N} + 1 \times W - \sqrt{N} + 1$ with a sliding distance of one pixel. Now, the denoising procedure is to minimize the objective function by using equation (8.30).

$$\min||x - z||_2^2 + \lambda\sum_{s=1}^{S}(||E_s x - D\alpha_s||_2^2 + v_s||\alpha_s||_0) \tag{8.30}$$

8.3.3 Physics of low dose x-ray CT

The statistics of x-ray based measurements are mostly represented by a Poisson distribution as equation (8.31).

$$I_i \sim \text{Poisson}(b_i e^{-[Ax]_i} + r_i) \tag{8.31}$$

In equation (8.31), $i = 1, \ldots, N_m$, A is a system matrix of projection operator, x is a vector of attenuation coefficients, N_m is the number of measurements, N_v is the number of image voxels, b_i is x-ray source intensity of the ith ray, r_i is the background scattering and noise. The sinogram data is expressed as equation (8.32).

$$y_i \sim N\left([Ax]_i, \frac{\bar{I}_i}{(\bar{I}_i - r_i)^2}\right) \tag{8.32}$$

In equation (8.32), $\bar{I}_i = E[I_i]$. Beam hardening can be produced by the polychromatic x-ray in actual practice. The linearity of projection data and attenuation coefficients is not a valid assumption due to rare detection of low energy x-ray photons by detectors. There are photon starvation artifacts due to heavy attenuation and absorption of x-ray photons in bones. Machine learning applications are given in table 8.3 for magnetic resonance imaging (MRI), positron emission tomography (PET) and photoacoustic imaging.

8.4 Performance analysis of proposed approaches

The learned primal-dual algorithm of [89] is a general framework for solution of inverse problems that combines model based reconstruction with deep learning. This learned iterative reconstruction scheme uses CNNs in both the reconstruction and data space, and these are connected by the forward operator and its adjoint. Proximal operators are replaced by parametric operators and these parametric operators are derived by using training data. The performance of learned primal-dual is good irrespective of quality of data (table 8.4). Learned Experts' Assessment-based Reconstruction Network (LEARN) is a novel approach to tune regularization parameters from training data [90].

The overall performance of LEARN is good in artifact reduction, feature preservation, and computational speed with 50 neural network layers. This model was directly motivated by the numerical scheme for solving the optimization problem based on physical, mathematical and application-relevant knowledge. Hence, the resultant neural network architecture, the LEARN network in this study, was well motivated in the first place, and then optimized via training and testing using machine learning techniques. This setup offers us unique insights into how the LEARN network achieves its excellent performance. Unlike most deep learning approaches for reconstruction, the new layer of [91] permits joint optimization of correction steps in volume and projection domain. The FBP algorithm is converted into parallel-beam geometry during neural network implementation [91]. In this approach, projection domain weights are learned from the image domain using this new layer. By training, these algorithms can adapt to cases for which no

Table 8.3. Analysis of deep learning for MRI, PET, photoacoustic imaging.

Imaging modality	Algorithm	NN type	Library and tools	Comparison
MRI	Convolutional RNN [90]	RNN	Theano and Lasagne	k-t FOCUSS, k-t SLR, 3D CNN
	GAN [91]	GAN	Tensorflow, Tensorpack	DeepADMM, DeepCascade,
	Deep De-Aliasing Generative Adversarial Networks [92]	GAN	Python wrapper (TensorLayer) TensorFlow3	TV, SIDWT, RecPF, DLMRI, PANO
	Greedy Mask selection [93]	NN	MATLAB's Parallel Computing Toolbox, 256 CPUs, For the NN decoder, 40 GPU nodes, Python	TV, BP, BM3D and NN decoders
	MLP [93]	NN	Caffe, Intel Quad Core i7-3770 3.4 GHz and NVIDIA Geforce GTX TITAN-x	C-based pLORAKS, S-based pLORAKS
	CNN [94]	CNN	MatConvNet, MATLAB 2015a, GTX 1080 Ti Intel i7	TV and PR-FOCUSS
	Deep ADMM-Net [95]	NN	Intel core i7-4790k CPU	TV, RecPF, SIDWT, PANO, BM3D
	Cascade CNN [89]	CNN	GeForce GTX 1080, Theano	DLTG, kt-SLR, L+S
	Deep Residual Learning Network [90]	CNN	MATLAB, MATConvNet, GTX 1080, I7-4770 CPU	Complex-net
PET	Deep Learning Prior and Local Linear Fitting [93]	CNN	MATLAB (2016a) using MEX and CUDA, GPU frameworks in MATLAB, Caffe	Gaussian, TV, DnCNN, NLM
	Artificial Neural Network Enhanced Bayesian [94]	NN Bayesian	Caffe	MAP, MLP
Photoacoustic	CNN [90]	CNN	ntel Core i5-6600k CPU with 32 GB of RAM, Nvidia GTX Titan X	—
	Deep gradient descent [91]	CNN	MATLAB, Python, Titan Xp GPU	DGD, U-Net, TV

Table 8.4. Performance analysis of proposed approaches.

Approach	NN type	Optimizer	Performance metric	Best case
Learned primal-dual [89]	CNN	Adam	SSIM	0.989
Learn [90]	CNN	Projected Gradient Descent	SSIM	0.986
Deep learning [91]	CNN	Adam	SSIM	0.795
PWLS-ULTRA [92]	–	–	SSIM	0.981
Projected gradient descent [93]	CNN	Gradient Descent	SSIM	0.332
Statistical iterative CBCT [94]	CNN	ADAM	SSIM	1.0
Deep reinforcement learning [95]	Reinforcement Learning	ADMM	relative Error	4.22
GAN-WD [96]	GAN	ADAM	SSIM	0.809 0
Deep convolutional framelet [89]	CNN	SGD	SSIM	0.899
DenseNet and deconvolution [90]	CNN	Adam	RMSE and SSIM	0.000 67 and 0.93
Framing U-Net [91]	CNN	ADMM	SSIM	0.899
CNN [92]	CNN	ADMM	SSIM	0.977
Convolutional encoder–decoder [93]	CNN, GAN	Adam	SSIM	0.919
Deep CNN using directional wavelets [93]	CNN	Iterative	NRMSE	0.016
CNN [94]	CNN	SGD	NRMSE	0.016
RED-CNN [95]	CNN	Adam	SSIM	0.975 4
Convolutional RNN [90]	RNN	Adam	SSIM	0.985
GAN with cyclic loss [91]	GAN	Adam	NRMSE	0.05
DAGAN [92]	GAN	Adam	SSIM	0.04
Learning framework [93]	–	Greedy	NMSE	0.806
MLP [93]	Deep NN	–	nRMSE	0.04
Domain adaption [94]	CNN	SGD	NMSE	0.018 6
Deep ADMM-Net [95]	CNN	ADMM	NMSE	0.037 9
Deep cascade CNN [89]	CNN	Adam	MSE	0.000 8
Deep residual [90]	CNN	–	SSIM	0.914
DnCNN [93]	CNN	ADMM	NRMSE	0.26
ANN enhanced Bayesian [94]	ANN	MAP, ML	NMSE	0.03
CNN [90]	CNN	–	AUC	0.989 0
Model based [91]	CNN	DGD	SSIM	0.945

analytical closed-form solution is known. Penalized weighted least square with ultra regularization is proposed for low dose CT problems in [92]. The union of square transforms is pre-learned from numerous image patches extracted from a data set of CT images or volumes. The proposed PWLS-based cost function is optimized by alternating between a CT image reconstruction step, and a sparse coding and clustering step. The proposed approach of [92] achieves better image quality and speed as compared to learned over-complete synthesis dictionaries. A new image reconstruction approach of [93] replaces the projector in a projected gradient descent (PGD) with a CNN. Unlike existing iterative image reconstruction algorithms, these CNN based approaches usually lack a feedback mechanism to enforce that the reconstructed image is consistent with the measurements. A relaxed version of PGD has been proposed in [93] wherein gradient descent enforces measurement consistency,while a CNN recursively projects the solution closer to the space of desired reconstruction images. The proposed framework is generic and can be used to solve a variety of inverse problems including super resolution, deconvolution, accelerated MRI, etc. This can bring more robustness and reliability to the current deep-learning-based techniques. A deep reinforcement learning based PTPN is shown in figure 8.8 [94]. PTPN performs better than manual tuning of parameters during image reconstruction problems.

8.5 Summary

Machine learning based image reconstruction methods are described for inverse problems, CT, MRI, PET, photoacoustic imaging techniques. Algorithm, neural network type, library and tools and comparison for all machine learning methods are discussed. The performance is analysed and compared for selected machine learning methods.

References

[1] http://bighttp://www.epfl.ch/demo/jtomography/

[2] Oliveira *et al* Comparison among tomographic reconstruction algorithms with a limited data *Int. Nuclear Atlantic Conf.-INAC 2011* **2011**

[3] Geyer L L, Schoepf U J, Meinel F G, Nance J W Jr, Bastarrika G, Leipsic J A, Paul N S, Rengo M, Laghi A and De Cecco C N 2015 State of the art: iterative CT reconstruction techniques *Radiology* **276** 339–57

[4] https://skymind.ai/wiki/deep-reinforcement-learning

[5] https://ieee-tmi.org/images/slides/slide30.jpg

[6] Roth *et al* 2015 Detection of sclerotic spine metastases via random aggregation of deep convolutional neural network classifications *Recent Advances in Computational Methods and Clinical Applications for Spine Imaging* (Cham: Springer) pp 3–12

[7] Ponti *et al* 2017 30 Everything you wanted to know about deep learning for computer vision but were afraid to ask *2017 30th SIBGRAPI Conf. on Graphics, Patterns and Images Tutorials (SIBGRAPI-T)* (Piscataway, NJ: IEEE) pp 17–41

[8] Lin H W, Tegmark M and Rolnick D 2017 Why does deep and cheap learning work so well? *J. Statist. Phys.* **168** 1223–47

[9] LeCun Y, Bengio Y and Hinton G 2015 Deep learning *Nature* **521** 436–44

[10] Wang G, Kalra M and Orton C G 2017 Machine learning will transform radiology significantly within the next 5 years *Med. Phys.* **44** 2041–4

[11] Wang G, Ye J C, Mueller K and Fessler J A 2018 Image reconstruction is a new frontier of machine learning *IEEE Trans. Med. Imaging* **37** 1289–96

[12] Latif J, Xiao C, Imran A and Tu S 2019 Medical imaging using machine learning and deep learning algorithms: a review *2019 2nd Int. Conf. on Computing, Mathematics and Engineering Technologies (iCoMET)* (Piscataway, NJ: IEEE) pp 1–5
[13] Anwar S M, Majid M, Qayyum A, Awais M, Alnowami M and Khan M K 2018 Medical image analysis using convolutional neural networks: a review *J. Med. Syst.* **42** 226
[14] Lucas A, Iliadis M, Molina R and Katsaggelos A K 2018 Using deep neural networks for inverse problems in imaging: beyond analytical methods *IEEE Signal Process Mag* **35** 20–36
[15] McCann M T, Jin K H and Unser M 2017 Convolutional neural networks for inverse problems in imaging: A review *IEEE Signal Process Mag* **34** 85–95
[16] Wang G 2016 A perspective on deep imaging *IEEE Access* **4** 8914–24
[17] Greenspan H, van Ginneken B and Summers R M 2016 Guest editorial deep learning in medical imaging: overview and future promise of an exciting new technique *IEEE Trans. Med. Imaging* **35** 1153–9
[18] Dave A, Vadathya A K, Subramanyam R, Baburajan R and Mitra K 2019 Solving inverse computational imaging problems using deep pixel-level prior *IEEE Trans. Comput. Imaging* **5** 37–51
[19] Ye J C, Han Y and Cha E 2018 Deep convolutional framelets: a general deep learning framework for inverse problems *SIAM J. Imag. Sci.* **11** 991–1048
[20] Jin K H, McCann M T, Froustey E and Unser M 2017 Deep convolutional neural network for inverse problems in imaging *IEEE Trans. Image Process.* **26** 4509–22
[21] Aggarwal H K, Mani M P and Jacob M 2017 *MoDL: Model based deep learning architecture for inverse problems. [Online].* Available: 1712.02862
[22] Zhao C, Zhang J, Wang R and Gao W 2018 CREAM: CNN-REgularized ADMM framework for compressive-sensed image reconstruction *IEEE Access* **6** 76838–53
[23] Qiao Z, Liang D, Tang S and Halpern H 2019 Optimization-based image reconstruction from fast-scanned, noisy projections in EPR imaging *IEEE Access* **7** 19590–601
[24] He J, Yang Y, Wang Y, Zeng D, Bian Z, Zhang H, Sun J, Xu Z and Ma J 2019 Optimizing a parameterized plug-and-play ADMM for iterative low-dose CT reconstruction *IEEE Trans. Med. Imaging* **38** 371–82
[25] Adler J and Öktem O 2018 Learned primal-dual reconstruction *IEEE Trans. Med. Imaging* **37** 1322–32
[26] Chen H *et al* 2018 LEARN: learned experts assessment-based reconstruction network for sparse-data CT *IEEE Trans. Med. Imaging* **37** 1333–47
[27] Würfl T *et al* 2018 Deep learning computed tomography: learning projection-domain weights from image domain in limited angle problems *IEEE Trans. Med. Imaging* **37** 1454–63
[28] Zheng X, Ravishankar S, Long Y and Fessler J A 2018 PWLS-ULTRA: an efficient clustering and learning-based approach for low-dose 3D CT image reconstruction *IEEE Trans. Med. Imaging* **37** 1498–510
[29] Gupta H, Jin K H, Nguyen H Q, McCann M T and Unser M 2018 CNN based projected gradient descent for consistent image reconstruction *IEEE Trans. Med. Imaging* **37** 1440–53
[30] Chen B, Xiang K, Gong Z, Wang J and Tan S 2018 Statistical iterative CBCT reconstruction based on neural network *IEEE Trans. Med. Imaging* **37** 1511–21
[31] Shen C, Gonzalez Y, Chen L, Jiang S B and Jia X 2018 Intelligent parameter tuning in optimization-based iterative CT reconstruction via deep reinforcement learning *IEEE Trans. Med. Imaging* **37** 1430–9

[32] Yang Q *et al* 2018 Low dose CT image denoising using a generative adversarial network with Wasserstein distance and perceptual loss *IEEE Trans. Med. Imaging* **37** 1348–57
[33] Kang E, Chang W, Yoo J and Ye J C 2018 Deep convolutional framelet denosing for low-dose CT via wavelet residual network *IEEE Trans. Med. Imaging* **37** 1358–69
[34] Zhang Z, Liang X, Dong X, Xie Y and Cao G 2018 A sparse-view CT reconstruction method based on combination of DenseNet and deconvolution *IEEE Trans. Med. Imaging* **37** 1407–17
[35] Han Y and Ye J C 2018 Framing U-Net via deep convolutional framelets: application to sparse-view CT *IEEE Trans. Med. Imaging* **37** 1418–29
[36] Zhang Y and Yu H 2018 Convolutional neural network based metal artifact reduction in x-ray computed tomography *IEEE Trans. Med. Imaging* **37** 1370–81
[37] Shan H *et al* 2018 3D convolutional encoder–decoder network for low-dose CT via transfer learning from a 2D trained network *IEEE Trans. Med. Imaging* **37** 1522–34
[38] McCollough C H *et al* 2017 Low-dose CT for the detection and classification of metastatic liver lesions: results of the 2016 low dose CT grand challenge *Med. Phys.* **44** e339–52
[39] Yu L, Shiung M, Jondal D and McCollough C H 2012 Development and validation of a practical lower-dose-simulation tool for optimizing computed tomography scan protocols *J. Comput. Assisted Tomogr* **36** 477–87
[40] McCollough C H *et al* 2012 Achieving routine submillisievert CT scanning: Report from the summit on management of radiation dose in CT *Radiology* **264** 567–80
[41] Segars W P, Mahesh M, Beck T J, Frey E C and Tsui B M W 2008 Realistic CT simulation using the 4D XCAT phantom *Med. Phys.* **35** 3800–8
[42] Segars W P, Sturgeon G, Mendonca S, Grimes J and Tsui B M W 2010 4D XCAT phantom for multimodality imaging research *Med. Phys.* **37** 4902–15
[43] Thibault J-B, Sauer K D, Bouman C A and Hsieh J 2007 A three-dimensional statistical approach to improved image quality for multislice helical CT *Med. Phys.* **34** 4526–44
[44] Xu Q, Yu H, Mou X, Zhang L, Hsieh J and Wang G 2012 Low-dose x-ray CT reconstruction via dictionary learning *IEEE Trans. Med. Imaging* **31** 1682–97
[45] Kang E, Min J and Ye J C 2017 A deep convolutional neural network using directional wavelets for low-dose x-ray CT reconstruction *Med. Phys.* **44** e360–75
[46] Chen H *et al* 2017 Low-dose CT via convolutional neural network *Biomed. Opt. Exp.* **8** 679–94
[47] Chen H *et al* 2017 Low-dose CT with a residual encoder–decoder convolutional neural network *IEEE Trans. Image Process.* **36** 2524–35
[48] Wolterink J M, Leiner T, Viergever M A and Išgum I 2017 Generative adversarial networks for noise reduction in low-dose CT *IEEE Trans. Med. Imaging* **36** 2536–45
[49] Wu D, Kim K, El Fakhri G and Li Q 2017 Iterative low-dose CT reconstruction with priors trained by artificial neural network *IEEE Trans. Med. Imaging* **36** 2479–86
[50] Qin C, Schlemper J, Caballero J, Price A N, Hajnal J V and Rueckert D 2019 Convolutional recurrent neural networks for dynamic MR image reconstruction *IEEE Trans. Med. Imaging* **38** 280–90
[51] Quan T M, Nguyen-Duc T and Jeong W-K 2018 Compressed sensing MRI reconstruction using a generative adversarial network with a cyclic loss *IEEE Trans. Med. Imaging* **37** 1488–97
[52] Yang G *et al* 2018 DAGAN: Deep de-aliasing generative adversarial networks for fast compressed sensing MRI reconstruction *IEEE Trans. Med. Imaging* **37** 1310–21
[53] Gözcü B, Mahabadi R K, Li Y-H, Ilcak E, Cukur T, Scarlett J and Cevher V 2018 Learning-based compressive MR *IEEE Trans. Med. Imaging* **37** 1394–406

[54] Lustig M, Donoho D and Pauly J M 2007 Sparse MRI: the application of compressed sensing for rapid MR imaging *Mag. Res. Med.* **58** 1182–95

[55] Ravishankar S and Bresler Y 2011 MR image reconstruction from highly undersampled k-space data by dictionary learning *IEEE Trans. Med. Imaging* **30** 1028–41

[56] Ravishankar S and Bresler Y 2015 Efficient blind compressed sensing using sparsifying transforms with convergence guarantees and application to magnetic resonance imaging *SIAM J. Imag. Sci.* **8** 2519–57

[57] Jin K H, Lee D and Ye J C 2016 A general framework for compressed sensing and parallel MRI using annihilating filter based low-rank Hankel matrix *IEEE Trans. Comput. Imag* **2** 480–95

[58] Lee D, Jin K H, Kim E Y, Park S-H and Ye J C 2016 Acceleration of MR parameter mapping using annihilating filter-based low rank Hankel matrix (ALOHA) *Magn. Reson. Med.* **76** 1848–64

[59] Jin K H, Um J-Y, Lee D, Lee J, Park S-H and Ye J C 2017 MRI artifact correction using sparse+low-rank decomposition of annihilating filter-based Hankel matrix *Magn. Reson. Med.* **78** 327–40

[60] Hammernik K *et al* 2017 Learning a variational network for reconstruction of accelerated MRI data *Magn. Reson. Med.* **79** 3055–71

[61] Kwon K, Kim D and Park H 2017 A parallel MR imaging method using multilayer perceptron *Med. Phys.* **44** 6209–24

[62] Han Y, Yoo J, Kim H H, Shin H J, Sung K and Ye J C 2018 Deep learning with domain adaptation for accelerated projection-reconstruction MR *Magn. Reson. Med.* **80** 1189–205

[63] Yang Y, Sun J, Li H and Xu Z 2016 Deep ADMM-net for compressive sensing MRI *Proc. Adv. Neural Inf. Process. Syst.*

[64] Wang S *et al* 2016 Accelerating magnetic resonance imaging via deep learning *Proc. IEEE 13th Int. Sympos. Biomed. Imag. (ISBI)* 514–7

[65] Schlemper J, Caballero J, Hajnal J V, Price A N and Rueckert D 2017 A deep cascade of convolutional neural networks for dynamic MR image reconstruction *IEEE Trans. Med. Imaging* **37** 491–503

[66] Lee D, Yoo J, Tak S and Ye J 2018 Deep residual learning for accelerated MRI using magnitude and phase networks *IEEE Trans. Biomed. Eng.* **65** 1985–95

[67] Lee D, Yoo J and Ye J C 2017 Deep residual learning for compressed sensing MRI *Proc. IEEE 14th Int. Sympos. Biomed. Imag. (ISBI)* 15–8

[68] Daubechies I, Han B, Ron A and Shen Z 2003 Framelets: MRA-based constructions of wavelet frames *Appl. Comput. Harmon. Anal.* **14** 1–46

[69] Kim K *et al* 2018 Penalized PET reconstruction using deep learning prior and local linear fitting *IEEE Trans. Med. Imaging* **37** 1478–87

[70] Yang B, Ying L and Tang J 2018 Artificial neural network enhanced Bayesian PET image reconstruction *IEEE Trans. Med. Imaging* **37** 1297–309

[71] Ahn S *et al* 2015 Quantitative comparison of OSEM and penalized likelihood image reconstruction using relative difference penalties for clinical PET *Phys. Med. Biol.* **60** 5733–52

[72] Nuyts J, Beque D, Dupont P and Mortelmans L 2002 A concave prior penalizing relative differences for maximum-a-posteriori reconstruction in emission tomography *IEEE Trans. Nucl. Sci.* **49** 56–60

[73] Gong K *et al* 2017 Iterative PET image reconstruction using convolutional neural network representation *IEEE Trans. Med. Imaging* **38** 675–85

[74] Allman D, Reiter A and Bell M A L 2018 Photoacoustic source detection and reflection artifact removal enabled by deep learning *IEEE Trans. Med. Imaging* **37** 1464–77
[75] Hauptmann A *et al* 2018 Model based learning for accelerated, limited-view 3D photoacoustic tomography *IEEE Trans. Med. Imaging* **37** 1382–93
[76] Collins D L *et al* 1998 Design and construction of a realistic digital brain phantom *IEEE Trans. Med. Imag.* **17** 463–8
[77] Kalra M, Wang G and Orton C G 2017 Radiomics in lung cancer: Its time is here *Med. Phys.* **45** 997–1000
[78] Ravishankar S and Bresler Y 2013 Learning sparsifying transforms *IEEE Trans. Signal Process* **61** 1072–86
[79] Wohlberg B 2016 Efficient algorithms for convolutional sparse representations *IEEE Trans. Image Process.* **25** 301–15
[80] Chun I Y and Fessler J A 2018 Convolutional dictionary learning: acceleration and convergence *IEEE Trans. Image Process.* **27** 1697–712
[81] Gregor K and LeCun Y 2010 Learning fast approximations of sparse coding *Proc. Int. Conf. Mach. Learn.* 399–406
[82] Tishby N and Zaslavsky N 2015 Deep learning and the information bottleneck principle *Proc. IEEE Inf. Theory Workshop (ITW)* 1–5
[83] Ge R, Lee J D and Ma T 2017 Learning one-hidden-layer neural networks with landscape design arXiv:1711.00501
[84] Du S S and Lee J D 2018 On the power of over-parametrization in neural networks with quadratic activation arXiv:1803.01206
[85] Du S S, Lee J D, Tian Y, Póczos B and Singh A 2017 Gradient descent learns one-hidden-layer CNN: Don't be afraid of spurious local minima arXiv:1712.00779
[86] Jin K H and Ye J C 2015 Annihilating filter-based low-rank Hankel matrix approach for image in painting *IEEE Trans. Image Process.* **24** 3498–511
[87] Lee J, Jin K H and Ye J C 2016 Reference-free single-pass EPI Nyquist ghost correction using annihilating filter-based low rank Hankel matrix (ALOHA) *Magn. Reson. Med.* **76** 1775–89
[88] Chen Y, Chi Y, Fan J and Ma C 2019 Gradient descent with random initialization: Fast global convergence for nonconvex phase retrieval *Math. Prog.* **176** 5–37
[89] Sun J, Qu Q and Wright J 2016 A geometric analysis of phase retrieval *Proc. IEEE Int. Symp. Inf. Theory (ISIT)* 2379–83
[90] Sun J, Qu Q and Wright J 2015 When are nonconvex problems not scary? arXiv:1510.06096
[91] Zhu B, Liu J Z, Cauley S F, Rosen B R and Rosen M S 2018 Image reconstruction by domain-transform manifold learning *Nature* **555** 487–92
[92] Yoon Y H, Khan S, Huh J and Ye J C 2017 *Deep learning in RF sub-sampled B-mode ultrasound imaging* arXiv:1712.06096
[93] Wu D, Kim K, Dong B and Li Q 2017 *End-to-end abnormality detection in medical imaging* arXiv:1711.02074
[94] Deng J, Dong W, Socher R, Li L-J, Li K and Fei-Fei L 2009 ImageNet: A large-scale hierarchical image database *Proc. IEEE Conf. Comput. Vis. Pattern Recognit. (CVPR)*
[95] Feng R, Rundle D and Wang G 2018 Neural-networks-based photon-counting data correction: Pulse pileup effect arXiv:1804.10980
[96] Goodfellow I, Bengio Y, Courville A and Bengio Y 2016 *Deep Learning* (Cambridge, MA: MIT Press)

Hardik N Patel, Deepak K Ghodgaonkar and Jasjit S Suri

Chapter 9

Review of machine learning based image reconstruction for microwave breast imaging

Machine learning based image reconstruction approaches by microwave imaging are described in this chapter. Current challenges in the microwave diagnostic systems are discussed. Steps are discussed for the solution of microwave imaging problems with the current challenges. Data collection through microwave scanning and possible machine learning features are shown for breast cancer detection. Data processing steps are shown for microwave breast imaging. Diagnosis through different machine learning models is described in this chapter. Variational Bayesian inversion is described for microwave breast imaging and cancer detection. Deep neural networks based inverse scattering problem formulation is shown for microwave breast imaging.

9.1 Motivation

Significant academic research and commercial development have been done in microwave breast imaging during recent years. There are different microwave breast imaging studies which have proposed clinical trials [1–7]. The main target of microwave breast imaging is to detect tumors in human breasts by using different image reconstruction algorithms [8–12]. There is no huge advantage of continuous mammography screening in terms of long term survival according to [13, 14]. There are articles about automation in the breast diagnosis system to integrate signal or image pre-processing, segmentation and diagnosis by using machine learning [15, 16]. The systems of [15, 16] can help clinicians to diagnose breast cancer by identifying features in a signal or image which may not be observed through visual inspection. Machine learning based diagnosis systems can play a key role in the establishment of microwave breast imaging as an early stage breast cancer screening method. There are benign and malignant types of breast cancers with different

doi:10.1088/978-0-7503-2592-9ch9

dielectric properties, so microwave breast imaging can distinguish between malignant and benign tumors [2, 17–21]. Further investigations are required for the characterisation of microcalcifications, benign and malignant tissues in the microwave range. The shape and characterisation of tumors are widely recognised features for their malignancy [22–25]. Benign tumours are approximately elliptical and generally have well circumscribed margins and malignant tumors have irregular shapes and are surrounded by a radiating pattern of spikes [22–26]. It is already shown how microwave backscattered signals change due to presence of tumors in the breast [27–38]. Study shows that machine learning algorithms can learn from the backscattered signal pattern by using a simple data set. Machine learning is not still used in clinical breast diagnosis based on microwave imaging.

9.2 Machine learning in microwave imaging

A patient may sit or lie down on the microwave breast imaging prototype system while the breasts are illuminated by low power microwave signals. These incident signals are scattered back due to breast tissues and recorded on the system. Diagnosis of the type of tumor depends on the tumor signature retrieval through backscattered signal examination. Feature extraction methods were proposed with different classifiers to diagnose breast tumours [29–32]. Classification of breast tumour by using RADAR target signatures is proposed in [29, 30]. When breasts are illuminated by ultrawideband (UWB) pulse, significant scattering waves are generated from the strong scatterers like tumors present in the breast. These backscattered signals are used to reconstruct a UWB image of the breasts, where high scattering regions suggest the possible presence of the tumor. Signal analysis and classification are done by following the steps below.

- The recorded backscattered signals are downsampled by a factor of 16.
- Principal component analysis (PCA) is applied to each recorded scattered signal.
- Dimensionality reduction is applied.
- Classification is done by using linear and quadratic discriminant approaches.

The performance of quadratic discriminant classifier is better than the linear one. Support vector machine (SVM) based classification of early stage breast cancer is proposed based on UWB RADAR target signatures [31, 32]. The comparison of PCA, independent component analysis (ICA) and discrete wavelet transform (DWT) is done by using three classification approaches: linear discriminant analysis (LDA), quadratic discriminant analysis (QDA) and SVM [33]. The breast is modelled with tumors of different size, shape and location by using finite difference time domain (FDTD) and machine learning [29–32]. Evolved topology spiking neural network (SNN) with evolutionary algorithms is proposed as an accurate and robust UWB breast cancer classifier which can determine an optimal number of neurons, and interneuron connections [33, 34]. The SNNs are more closely related to biological neural networks as compared to artificial neural networks (ANNs) such as multi-layer perceptrons. Unlike ANN, SNNs use transient pulses for communication and computations which makes them computationally powerful. Natural evolution can be modeled by genetic algorithm (GA) through a set of computational operators. GA is a parallel and population based search approach which encodes each solution into a data structure known as a genome. High fitness solutions are computed through natural evolution of GA. Mutation is used to explore the solution search space, whereas crossover is used to get good solution building blocks.

The neuro evolution through augmenting topologies (NEAT) algorithm algorithm is used to work with SNN. NEAT algorithm creates networks of optimal size and these networks contain only neurons and connections. Self-organising maps are used to track the development of tumors from benign stage to different levels of malignancy, and this approach is able to distinguish between different shapes of tumors [35]. The tumor phantoms are developed with various sizes and shapes to immerse in the breast phantoms [36, 37]. Tumor diagnosis is combined with the microwave breast imaging system in [38]. Flow of the proposed microwave breast imaging and diagnosis system is shown in figure 9.1.

As shown in figure 9.1, the first step is numerical modeling of breast phantom, the second step is FDTD simulations, the third step is image reconstruction, the fourth step is identification of tumour response, and the fifth step is diagnosis of breast tumor (either benign or malignant). A gradient based time domain microwave tomography algorithm was used to reconstruct a microwave image of the breasts [38]. In this algorithm, the error between measured and estimated electromagnetic signals is minimized for the target. The least square problem is given by equation (9.1).

$$F(\epsilon_r, \sigma) = \int_0^T \sum_{m=1}^{M} \sum_{n=1}^{N} W(t) |E_{m,n}^{m}(t) - E_{m,n}^{e}(\epsilon_r, \sigma, t)|^2 dt \tag{9.1}$$

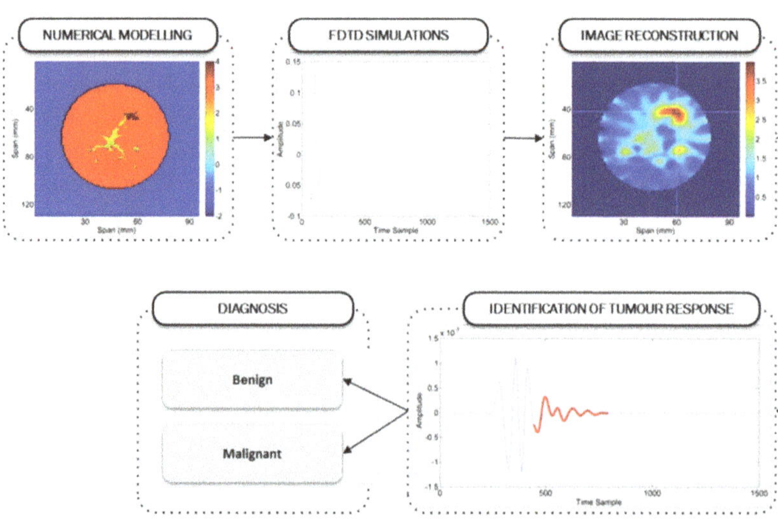

Figure 9.1. Flow of the proposed microwave breast imaging and diagnosis system. Source: [38].

The proposed system of figure 9.1 has better accuracy, sensitivity and specificity than the systems without post-processing. Now consider SVM based approach for microwave breast imaging [39–43].

$$E_{\text{tr}|\text{rs}} = (E_{\text{tr}|\text{rs}}^{\text{Re},x}, E_{\text{tr}|\text{rs}}^{\text{Im},x}, E_{\text{tr}|\text{rs}}^{\text{Re},y}, E_{\text{tr}|\text{rs}}^{\text{Im},y}, E_{\text{tr}|\text{rs}}^{\text{Re},z}, E_{\text{tr}|\text{rs}}^{\text{Im},z})^T \quad (9.2)$$

Consider the column vector representing electric field intensity as equation (9.2). Now consider figure 9.2 to understand the setup.

Now consider the breast tissue as a 3D lattice of classification cells. The number of cells is represented by N_x, N_y, N_z along three spatial axis. Each cell is either healthy ($X_{ijk} = -1$) or tumor cell $X_{ijk} = 1$, which gives the classification problem function as shown in equation (9.3).

$$F: \Gamma_E \rightarrow [X_{ijk}, i = 1 \ldots N_x, j = 1 \ldots N_y, k = 1 \ldots N_z] \quad (9.3)$$

In equation (9.3), $\Gamma_E = [E_{\text{tr}|\text{rs},\text{tr}=1\ldots T,\text{rs}=1\ldots R}]$. In order to solve the above problem by using single SVM classifier, it is converted into equation (9.4).

$$F: [\Gamma_E, i, j, k] \rightarrow X_{ijk} \quad (9.4)$$

A set of samples is formed as input–output pair to apply SVM which is known as the training set. Now, SVM classifier output is mapped to posterior probabilities for presence of the tumor provided that the received electric field is known.

$$PX_{ijk} = 1|\Gamma_E, i, j, k \quad (9.5)$$

In equation (9.5), PX_{ijk} is probability indicating presence of the tumor in the breast tissue cell. The hyperplane is used by SVM to classify a cell either as a healthy or tumor cell.

$$w^T\Gamma + b = 0 \quad (9.6)$$

Equation (9.6) is used to determine the class of each cell in breast tissue. The cost-sensitive ensemble classifier is proposed to detect breast cancer by using microwaves on phantoms and patients [44–46]. The performance of ensemble selection approach is better than with other ensemble classifiers. Empirical mode decomposition (EMD) and PCA based feature extraction is proposed with ensemble selection classifier in [47].

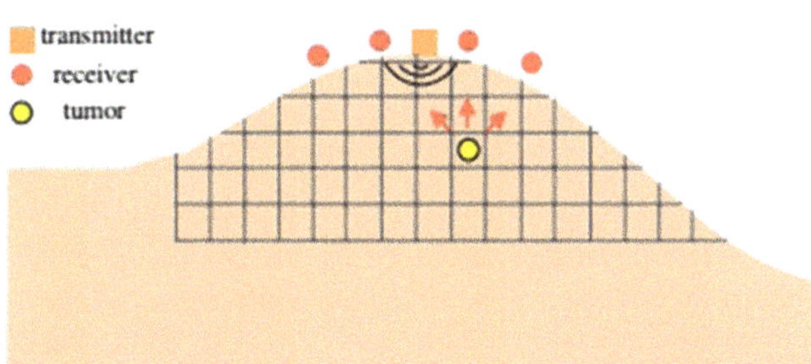

Figure 9.2. Transmitter and receiver setup. Reprinted from [67], copyright (2006), with permission from Elsevier.

9.2.1 Current challenges in microwave breast diagnosis systems

The breast cancer diagnosis studies reviewed above show that the tumor signature is affected by its shape. Now, machine learning is useful to develop a model which works on backscattered signals and learn to distinguish between malignant and benign tumours. Feature extraction and machine learning approaches to detect breast tumours are reviewed in this section. Clinically realistic data is quite complex to handle. Malignant and benign tumours are present in a variety of shapes, sizes and spiculations, which can easily change the backsctttered signals received at a specific antenna. The shape and size of breast changes from person to person with different distributions of fatty and glandular tissues. This diversity leads to diverse backscattered signals which further makes the design and development of a single platform for diagnosis a very complex task. There is difficulty in the tumor signature retrieval from the backscattered signals due to presence of a skin layer, which also varies from person to person. The magnitude of backscattered signals from skin is higher than that of tumor signature. High density of glandular tissues may be detected as a breast tumor, which results in a false positive. Tumors can occur at different locations inside the breast, so sometimes it is very difficult to detect them. Tumors of different sizes and shapes are located at different distances from a particular transmit–receive antenna pair. Even the various angles between transmit and receive antennas can affect the phase of the tumor signature. A number of strategies have been proposed which can remove large reflections due to skin layer and they also decrease the glandular tissue influence on the backscatter signals [49, 50]. Signal pre-processing by using windowing can time align and highlight the tumor response [38]. Time and frequency representations of the data could further capture the essence of the tumor signature while reducing the background noise [47, 48]. Some of the studies have used backscattered signals cpatured with the most informative transmit–receive antenna pairs for the tumor classification [33, 40, 42, 44–46]. There is no thorough investigation about antenna topology and optimal use of the information from each channel in the literature. There is a set of challenges present in converting microwave breast diagnosis systems to experimental and clinical evaluation due to several factors like patient position and movement, intra-patient menstrual cycle variations, hormonal changes, breast size, shape and composition variations.

9.2.2 Challenges in the development of robust machine learning classification models

A machine learning algorithm trained with particular training dataset should be adaptive to the new unseen data sets. As a common practice, the model is generally trained on the subset of data and tested on the unseen subset of data. The training set should be large to minimize variance in the model training. However, the performance evaluation proposed in the literature is not meaningful on the unseen data set which results into some degree of error. This can easily lead to over-optimistic performance reports. Overfitting of the machine learning model in the training and model selections phases and contamination of the information across the data set result in poor model validation. Cross-validation is a good strategy to prevent overfitting of the model during taining phase and it is widely used for the model selection. However, it has been shown that the cross- validation during the model selection can generate non generalisable and over-optimistic performance. This effect is often known as the selection bias [51, 52]. The type of pre-processing and feature based algorithms applied to the original data set should be considered for a machine learning based system. The feature extraction from the original data set is crucial to diagnostic performance. However, feature based algorithms and pre-processing are important in the contamination of the information between training and test sets. Contamination prevention method should be applied to training and test sets. Many of the challenges discussed above have not yet been explicitly solved for microwave breast systems through machine learning based diagnosis algorithms in the literature. Careful and consistent methods for model validation and performance evaluation should be adopted as best practice. Ultimately, it is meaningless to have the best machine learning models without proper evaluation strategy, which could make microwave breast diagnosis systems useless.

9.3 Flow of the machine learning based microwave breast imaging for cancer diagnosis

The flow of the machine learning based microwave breast imaging is given below for cancer diagnosis [55].

1. Data collection through microwave scanning
    - Design breast phantoms with tumors.
    - Choose antennas for multistatic system.
    - FDTD simulation.
2. Data processing
    - Apply tumor windowing only.
    - Apply feature extraction only.
    - Apply tumor windowing followed by feature extraction.
3. Machine learning based automatic diagnosis
    - Apply classification model.
    - Apply antenna grouping.
    - Final decision either benign or malignant.

Stage 1 is about data collection through breast tumor models, multistatic system and FDTD simulation. Stage 2 offers several options like tumor windowing (TW) or feature extraction (FE) or TW followed by FE. TW is used to select signal segments of interest, combined with feature extraction. Stage 3 is about diagnosis through classification, antenna grouping and final decision. 'Some channels might be more useful to improve diagnostic performance' is explored as a concept. Stage 3 algorithms are targeted to understanding the following points.

- Whether the angular distance between receiver and transmitter antennas determines its predictive power.
- Whether there is a relationship between tumor-channel distance and diagnosis performance.
- How to use each channel information with machine learning best practice.

9.3.1 Data collection through microwave scanning

Numerical data set was created by using breast pahtoms with tumours and FDTD electromagnetic simulation. The method is widely used in microwave breast imaging to model microwaves propagation and scattering within the breasts [53]. The tumor models are developed by using the algorithms proposed in [54]. A total of 72 tumors have been generated with average sizes ranging from 6 mm to 20 mm diameter. Benign tumors are created by using a smooth border, whereas spiculated borders are used for a malignant tumor [54]. Five different positions like four quadrant and centre locations are used to place the tumors in breasts. Data collection has been done by forming channels between transmitter and receiver antennas as shown in figure 9.3 [55].

The multistatic microwave measurement system is modeled with a concentric ring of twelve equally spaced Hertzian dipole antennas around the breast. Each antenna is modeled as an electric current source and the whole antenna system is immersed in the coupling medium with dielectric properties similar to fatty tissues. The FDTD simulation is performed using differentiated Gaussian pulse with the centre frequency of 6 GHz. The spatial resolution of the system is 1 mm and the sampling frequency is 600 GHz. The reference simulation is performed to remove antenna effects in the backscattered signals due to full breast phantom with tumors. In figure 9.3, antennas are represented as black diamonds surrounding the breast. A coronal view of one breast slice is shown including a malignant tumor in the glandular tissues. The paths from one transmitting antenna to the tumor and from tumor to the receiving antenna is shown by using dash and dot–dash lines,

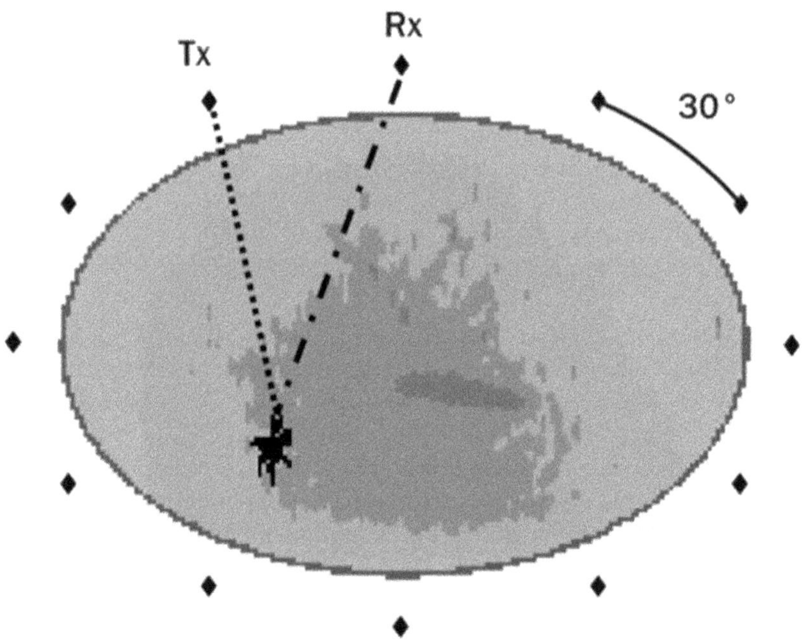

Figure 9.3. Data acquisition setup by using channels formed by transmitter and reciver antennas. Reprinted with permission from [55].

respectively. One microwave breast scan is composed of backscattered signals collected from 78 channels. A total of 1080 microwave scans are performed (3 breast models are combined with 72 tumour models at 5 different positions within the breast). A data set containing 84 240 backscattered signals is used in this work.

9.3.2 Data processing

This portion represents the processing methods used to prepare the data for the classification. Two methods, namely tumor windowing and feature extraction, are used to process the backscattered signals. The tumor location detection is a very important first step in the tumor windowing process. The round trip propagation delay between tumor and each channel is calculated based on the average propagation speed inside the heterogeneous breast model. The estimated tumor signature is then windowed from the backscattered signal. The approximate window length can be derived either empirically or analytically. The ideal length of window may be considered as 2.5 times the pulse width for the full tumor signature or response extraction. The propagation delay depends greatly on the average dielectric properties of each breast tissue. Reflections produced from tumors propagating through different paths are hard to align. The peak energy in each backscattered signal is detected in each backscattered signal and the time alignment is achieved in tumor response. Now downsampling is applied to get 30 GHz frequency for each windowed tumor response. The window length of the tumor signatures have 60 time samples after downsampling. The reflections from skin layer and a clutter from glandular tissues are eliminated after implementing tumor windowing. Signals collected from different channels are time aligned due to this. The tumor response is isolated as a result of TW and this tumor signature is given to the classification algorithm. Artifact removal is applied prior to windowing because it can compensate for the antenna effects. If only TW is applied then the windowed time domain signatures are treated as independent observations and they are given to the classification model as an input. Feature extraction is used to retrieve meaningful information embedded in a signal and it is also helpful in the dimensionality reduction of the problem compared to original data. Benign tumors result in a signal that tends to preserve the original structure of Gaussian peak, whereas malignant tumors result in more irregular signals due to heavy reflections from the tumor. Features targeted in this work are related to signal structure and frequency content for the diagnosis. The feature extraction proposed in this work depends on the different time and frequency peak analysis of the original data. Each group of features is calculated for the signal captured by each channel during each scan. No calculations are done across the data set and between tumor response, which prevents data contamination issues, so extraction of features is done independently on each observation.

Benign and malignant tumor signatures are shown in figure 9.4 [55]. Signals are captured under an ideal scenario to highlight the potential differences between benign and malignant tumor signatures. The captured signals are time aligned and windowed. The backscattered signal from a benign tumor has little distortion and the original Gaussian structure is preserved, as shown in figure 9.4(a), whereas

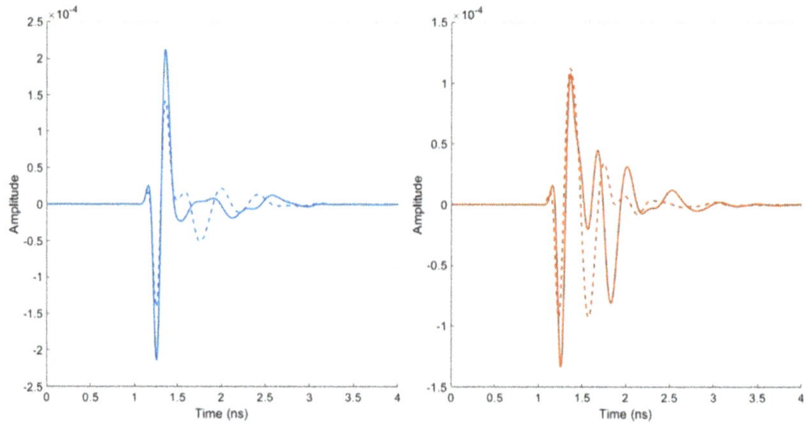

Figure 9.4. Benign tumour signature versus malignant tumour signature: (a) benign tumour response (b) malignant tumour response. Reprinted with permission from [55].

backscattered signal from a malignant tumor has a higher level of distortion, as shown figure 9.4(b). If features to be extracted from the signal are 30 then they are divided into four subgroups as shown in table 9.1 [55]. If feature extraction is applied directly to original backscattered signal then it is known as FE. If the feature extraction is applied after tumor windowing has been used on backscattered signal then it is known as TW+FE.

9.3.3 Diagnosis

First and second stages of the machine learning based diagnosis of microwave breast imaging are covered. Now, the third stage is about classification, antenna grouping and final decision. Random forest algorithm is used to classify the backscattered signals into malignant or benign [61]. Random forest is an ensemble method which works by generating many classification trees [62] and giving the class that is the mode of the classes of all individual trees. Each tree has been grown by a randomly sampled subset of features and observations from the entire data set. There is no correlation among randomly generated trees which results in low bias and low variance. Random forest provides generalisable models which do not overfit, and are fast and easy to understand [61]. One third of the observations of the original data set are left as out-of-bag (oob) during the training phase. The oob observations are used to evaluate performance error. This provides the generalisation ability of this model. The importance of each feature can also be determined by the random forests. The hyperparameters like number of trees, number of features, leaf size can be tuned by Bayesian optimisation. All channels contain information about a tumor but this information varies according to channel and location of tumor with respect to antennas in a channel and the relative distance between transmit and receive antennas in a channel. The channel angle, which is the angular distance between transmit and receive antennas in a channel, is also important. The variance in the tumor signatures

Table 9.1. List of 30 features divided in four subgroups.

Time domain features (calculated from the windowed signals)
1. Amplitudes of maximum positive peak
2. Amplitudes of maximum negative peak
3. Locations of maximum positive peak
4. Locations of maximum negative peak
5. Variance
6. Root mean squared error
7. Number of positive peaks
8. Number of negative peaks
9. Mean amplitudes of positive peaks
10. Mean amplitudes of negative peaks
11. Mean full width half maximum of the positive peaks
12. Mean full width half maximum of the negative peaks
13. Mean separation between positive peaks
14. Mean separation between negative peaks
15. Number of zero crossings
16. Integral of the signal
17. Integral of the absolute value of the signal
18. Positive percentage area of the signal
19. Negative percentage area of the signal
Autocorrelation features [56, 57]
20. Mean value of the autocorrelation sequence
21. Number of peaks in the autocorrelation sequence
22. Mean amplitudes of the peaks
23. Mean FWHM of the peak
24. Mean separation between peaks
Power spectral density features-estimate the PSD of signal using Welch's method [58]
25. Mean value of the Welch estimate
Power spectral density features-estimate the PSD of signal using periodogram method [59, 60]
26. Mean value of the periodogram estimate
27. Number of peaks in the periodogram
28. Mean amplitude of the peak
29. Mean FWHM of the peaks
30. Mean seperation between the peaks

in different channels can impact the performance of the classifier. This channel variance is proportional to the variance between signatures of benign and malignant tumours. In order to analyze the significance of intra-channel variance, three types of classification models are designed which utilize different channel angles in the classification algorithm. Three types of models are shown in figure 9.5 [55].

Equal angles (EA) models are used to classify signals only from a single channel angle. Equal angle combined (EAC) models are used to produce final diagnosis by combining predictions from different EA models at different channel angles. Multiple angles (MA) models classify signals collected by channels where the

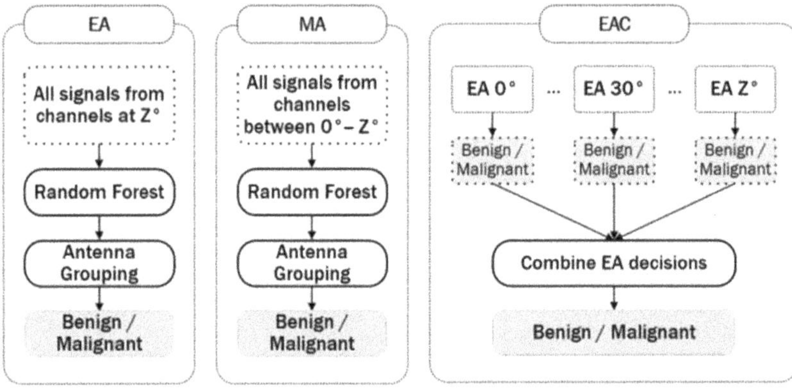

Figure 9.5. Three types of classification models implemented: EA (equal angles), MA (multiple angles) and EAC (equal angles combined). Reprinted with permission from [55].

transmit and receive antennas are separated by different angles. Performance evaluation of these three classification models can identify an optimal antenna pair topology in terms of channel angle which can result in improved diagnostic performance. The assumed architecture has one ring of 12 antennas equally distributed around the breast. Let X be the angle between the transmit and receive antennas in a channel, $X \in [0.180°]$ and X increases by steps of 30°. EA classification models have information from channels with an equal angle between transmit and receive antennas. Seven EA models have been built to evaluate the diagnostic performance of channels with equal angles. MA models have information from channels with different angles between transmit and receive antennas. Six MA models have been used in the work for the diagnostic performance evaluation. EAC models use all possible EA models to combine predictions of all. Comparison of EA, MA and EAC models are shown in table 9.2. The signal is then known as TW+FE.

As shown in table 9.2, different classification models are used to evaluate diagnosis performance for each of them. It is important to know how backscattered signals or features extracted from backscattered signals are used in the decision-making (diagnosis) process. Each scan has signatures collected from 78 different channels for independent classification. In a realistic clinical diagnostic scenario, a diagnosis is given based on the full scan. The process of final diagnosis is not discussed in existing literature or diagnostic results are reported based on the results from the independent channels. In order to explain final diagnosis, an antenna grouping algorithm is developed by which the independent channel predictions are grouped. Signals with low quality information about a tumor can result in incorrect predictions about malignancy. The antenna grouping algorithm has the ability to filter incorrect predictions from lower quality channels. Channels closer to the tumor generate more useful information for the diagnosis. The antenna grouping algorithm provides multiple views of the same tumor through different channel angles. The ranked antenna grouping considers W number of channels ordered by proximity to the tumor. W is increased in steps to perform antenna grouping. Cross-validation

Table 9.2. Comparison of EA, MA and EAC classification models.

Classification model number	EA	MA	EAC
1	0°	–	–
2	30°	0°–30°	0°–30°
3	60°	0°–60°	0°–60°
4	90°	0°–90°	0°–90°
5	120°	0°–120°	0°–120°
6	150°	0°–150°	0°–150°
7	180°	0°–180°	0°–180°

has been performed to evaluate diagnostic performance and mitigate sources of contamination during optimization of the classification model. The nested cross-validation is shown in figure 9.6 [55].

The entire dataset is divided into k stratified folds, containing equal representation from each class. $k = 5$ has been chosen in the study of [55]. For each outer fold the model is trained and hyperparameters are optimized. An unbiased estimate is provided by random forest as an oob error. The average of k fold is used as an indication of diagnostic performance.

9.4 Variational Bayesian inversion for microwave breast imaging

Microwave breast imaging is a nonlinear inverse scattering problem and it can be solved by Bayesian estimation framework. The breast is assumed to be composed of compact regions made of a restricted number of different homogeneous materials. Gauss–Markov–Potts distribution is used to define *a priori* knowledge. First joint posterior is defined for all unknowns, now variational Bayesian approximation is used compute the estimator and reconstruct the conductivity and permittivity profiles. This approximation has best separable probability law to approximate the true posterior distribution in the Kullback–Leibler sense. This results in an implicit parametric optimization scheme which is solved iteratively. The formulation is based on an integral equation of the electric field obtained by applying Green's function to the Helmholtz wave equations. The forward model consists of two coupled integral equations. The first equation is the observation type Fredholm first kind integral equation which relates the scattered field measurements to Huygens type sources induced within the breasts by incident waves. The second equation relates the total electric field inside the breasts to the induced sources. The forward problem is solved by using method of moments with pulse basis function and point matching which partition test domain D into N_D small elementary pixels with constant field inside each of them. Now consider contrast function X defined in D and null outside of the domain, such that $X(r) = (k^2(r) - k_1^2)/k_0^2$, where k_0 and k_1 are the propagation constants of free space and background medium, respectively. The Huygens type sources $w(r)$ are then defined as $w(r) = X(r)E(r)$, where $E(r)$ is the total field inside breasts.

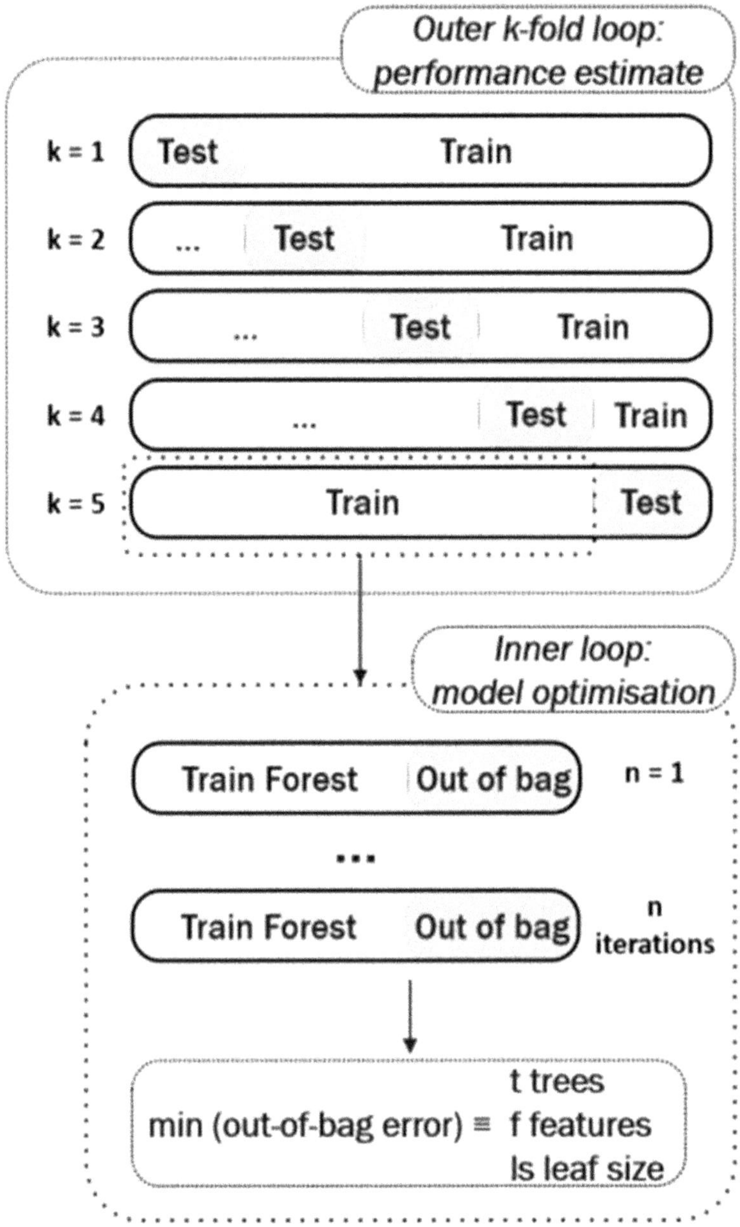

Figure 9.6. Nested cross-validation method. Reprinted with permission from [55].

$$y = G^0 w + \epsilon \tag{9.7}$$

$$w = XE^{\text{inc}} + XG^c w + \zeta \tag{9.8}$$

In equation (9.7), y is the vector of scattered electric field $y(r)$ at the measurement points r ($r \in S$), G^0 is the integral of Green's function, w is a vector with values of

$w(r')$ at the centers r' of the pixels, ϵ is the model error with Gaussian distribution. In equation (9.8), X is the diagonal matrix, G^c is the integral of the Green's function, ζ is the measurement error with Gaussian distribution. Equation (9.8) is solved first to compute induced sources w, where the contrast X, the incident field E^{inc} are kown. Equation (9.7) is solved to get scattered electric field vector y [64]. The inverse problem is solved to retrieve the unknown contrast X, or the relative permittivity ϵ_r and conductivity σ, from the known scattered electric field y and incident field E^{inc}. The conditional *a priori* probability law is shown by equation (9.9) [64].

$$p(\omega|X, v_\zeta) \propto \exp\left[-\frac{1}{2v_\zeta}||w - XE_{\text{inc}} - XG^C w||_D^2\right] \tag{9.9}$$

Now, scattered electric field equation (9.7) gives the conditional *a priori* probability law as shown by equation (9.10) [64].

$$p(y|w, v_\epsilon) \propto \exp\left[-\frac{1}{2v_\epsilon}||y - G^0 w||_S^2\right] \tag{9.10}$$

Now, introduce the *a priori* information for the solution of ill-posed inverse scattering problem. The reconstructed object is formed of a restricted number K homogeneous materials distributed in the compact regions. The compactness is represented by a hidden variable $z(r)$ associated with each pixel r for different regions. The classification label $z(r)$ of a pixel r is related to its neighbours by the Potts–Markov equation (9.11) [64].

$$p(z|\lambda) = \frac{1}{T(\lambda)} \exp\left[\lambda \sum_{r \in D} \sum_{r' \in v_r} \delta(z(r) - z(r'))\right] \tag{9.11}$$

In equation (9.11), λ is the Potts parameter that determines the correlation between neighbours, $T(\lambda)$ is a normalization factor and v_r is a neighbourhood of r which contains the four nearest pixels. It may be noted that the value of λ represents *a priori* behaviour of the hidden field. The homogeneous area depends on the value of λ in the final image. The critical value of lambda is represented by equation (9.12).

$$\lambda_c = \log(1 + \sqrt{K}) \tag{9.12}$$

The number of homogeneous areas remain low whereas small details of high contrast are very well preserved using the above equation. The breast consists of a finite number of different tissues which can be expressed by equation (9.13) [64].

$$p(x(r)|z(r) = k) = N(m_k, v_k) \tag{9.13}$$

In equation (9.13), $k = 1 \ldots K$. The above equation indicates that all the pixels with the same label represent the same tissue with contrast as Gaussian law with mean value m_k and a variance v_k. Now, two *a priori* models can be formulated on the basis of mean and variance estimation. According to the first model known as independent Gaussian mixture (IGM), the interaction between pixels is represented only by hidden field $z(r)$ while the contrast of the pixels is conditionally independent.

In IGM model, mean (m_k) and variance (v_k) depend only on the class k. The second model known as Gauss–Markov mixture (GMM) ensures the correlation between pixels of the same class through Markov field and it considers independent pixels of the other classes to preserve contours. This can be achieved by setting *a priori* mean of pixel contrast to the mean of its same class nearest neighbours. Now all the components are there to find the equation of the joint posterior law of the unknowns (X, w, z, ψ), where ψ is the set of hyperparameters of the model. The posterior probability is calculated by using the Bayes equation of (9.14).

$$\begin{aligned} p(X, w, z, \psi|y) &\propto p(y|w, v_\epsilon)p(w|X, v_\zeta)p(X|z, m, v)p(z|\lambda) \\ &\times p(m_k|\mu_0, \tau_0)p(v_k|\eta_0, \phi_0)p(v_\epsilon|\eta_\epsilon, \phi_\epsilon)p(v_\zeta|\eta_\zeta, \phi_\zeta) \end{aligned} \tag{9.14}$$

In equation (9.14), $p(y|w, v_\epsilon)p(w|X, v_\zeta)p(X|z, m, v)$ and $p(z|\lambda)$ are derived from equations (9.9), (9.10), (9.11) and (9.13), respectively. Gaussian and inverse gamma distibutions are assigned to means and variances by using the below equations [64].

$$\begin{aligned} p(m_k|\mu_0, \tau_0) &= N(\mu_0, \tau_0) \\ p(v_k|\eta_0, \phi_0) &= IG(\eta_0, \phi_0) \\ p(v_\epsilon|\eta_\epsilon, \phi_\epsilon) &= IG(\eta_\epsilon, \phi_\epsilon) \\ p(v_\zeta|\eta_\zeta, \phi_\zeta) &= IG(\eta_\zeta, \phi_\zeta) \end{aligned} \tag{9.15}$$

In equation (9.15), μ_0, η_0, ϕ_0, η_ϵ, ϕ_ϵ, η_ζ and ϕ_ζ are meta hyperparameters, N and IG represent normal and inverse gamma distributions, respectively. Now, variational Bayesian is used as an approximation for the posterior distribution represented by equation (9.15). A free-form separable law $q(u) = \prod_j q(x_j)$, with $u = X, w, z, \psi$, minimizes the Kullback–Leibler divergence $KL(q||p) = \int q \ln(q/p)$. The separable law can be defined by equation (9.16) [64].

$$q(u) = q(v_\epsilon)q(v_zeta)\prod_{i=1}^{N_D} q(x_i)q(w_i)q(z_i)\prod_{k=1}^{K} q(m_k)q(v_k) \tag{9.16}$$

Now, we search for the optimal form of q that minimizes the Kullback divergence. This results in the following parametric distributions.

$$\begin{aligned} q(w) &= N(\tilde{m}_w, \tilde{V}_w) \\ q(X) &= N(\tilde{m}_X, \tilde{V}_X) \\ q(z) &= \prod_r \tilde{\zeta_k(r)} \\ q(m_k) &= N(\hat{\mu}_k) \\ q(v_k) &= IG(\tilde{\eta}_k, \tilde{\phi}_k) \\ q(v_\epsilon) &= IG(\tilde{n}_\epsilon, \tilde{\phi}_\epsilon) \\ q(v_\zeta) &= IG(\tilde{\eta}_\zeta, \tilde{\phi}_\zeta) \end{aligned} \tag{9.17}$$

In equation (9.17), tilded variables are mutually dependent and iteratively computed. The probability of a hidden field of a pixel is computed from probabilities of its neighbours in the approximating law $\prod_r \tilde{\zeta_k}(r)$ [64]. Variational Bayesian approach results in the quality reconstruction of image in the inverse scattering problems.

9.5 Deep neural networks for microwave breast imaging

Quantitative and super-resolution are two main characteristics of nonlinear electromagnetic (EM) inverse scattering imaging technique. In this type of technique, more realistic interactions between internal structure of object and EM waves are considered as compared to conventional tomography. Intrinsic strong nonlinearity, ill-posedness and heavy computation costs are the main challenges in EM inverse scattering technique. The first step is to find the relationship between iterative method and deep neural networks (DNNs) for nonlinear EM inverse scattering. As a result, a novel DNN based approach is developed for nonlinear EM inverse problems (DeepNIS) [65]. Cascade of the multi-layer complex valued residual convolutional neural network (CNN) has been proposed as a DeePNIS in [65]. Three layers of DeepNIS are shown in figure 9.7 [65]. 2D MIMO configuration is used for measurement configuration. The object of interest is placed in the investigation domain D_{inv}. The object is illuminated by the TM-polarized incident waves $E_{\text{inc}}^{(n)}$, $n = 1, 2, \ldots, N$, where N is the total number of transmitters. The scattered electric field at the location r_m is given by equation (9.18).

$$E_{\text{sca}}(r_m) = k_0^2 \int_{D_{\text{inv}}} G(r_m, r')X(r')E_t(r')\mathrm{d}r' \tag{9.18}$$

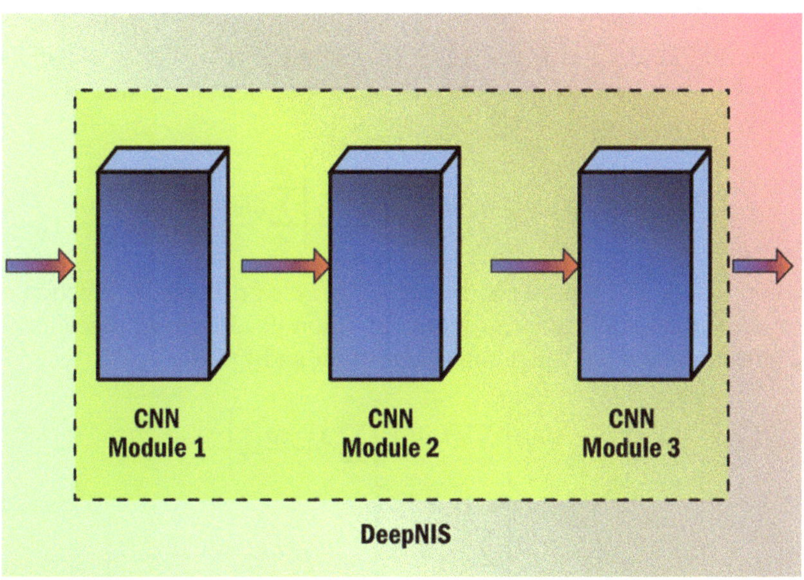

Figure 9.7. Three modules of CNN as DeepNIS. Copyright (2018) IEEE. Reprinted with permission from [65].

Now, scattered electric field is replaced by difference of total electric field and incident electric field.

$$E_t(r) - E_{inc}(r) = k_0^2 \int_{D_{inv}} G(r_m, r')X(r')E_t(r')dr' \tag{9.19}$$

In the above equations $r = (x, y)$ and $r' = (x', y')$ denote observation and source points, respectively, E_t total electric field, $G(r, r') = \frac{i}{4}H_0^{(1)}(k_0|r - r'|)$ represents the 2D Green's function in free space, $H_0^{(1)}$ is the first kind zeroth order Hankel function. The contrast function is defined as $X = k^2/k_0^2 - 1$, where k and k_0 are the wave numbers of the probed sample and background medium, respectively. The whole investigation domain is discretized in pixels such that the total electric field and contrast function can be assumed uniform in each pixel. As a result, the non linear EM inverse scattering problem is converted into the following coupled equations (9.20) and (9.21).

$$E_{sca} = G_d \cdot E \cdot X \tag{9.20}$$

$$E - E_{inc} = G_s \cdot E \cdot X \tag{9.21}$$

In equations (9.20) and (9.21), G_d, G_s are the integration of Green's function, E is total electric field and X is the contrast function. In general, iterative stratagies are used to solve the above equations. The contrast function is updated iteratively by using equation (9.22) [65].

$$X_{(k+1)} = \arg\min\left[\sum_n ||\delta E_{sca} - J_k\delta X||_2^2 + R(X)\right] \tag{9.22}$$

In equation (9.22), $\delta E_{sca} = E_{sca} - \delta E_{sca}(X_k)$ and $\delta X = X - X_k$, J_k is the Jacobian matrix at kth iteration. Now proximal approximation technique is applied to equation (9.22) to get equation (9.23).

$$X_{(k+1)} = D^H S\left(D_{X(k)} + D\left[\sum_n (J_k)^H J_k\right]\sum_n (J_k)^H \delta E_{sca}\right) \tag{9.23}$$

In equation (9.23), $S(\cdot)$ represents the element-wise soft threshold function and the subscript H denotes conjugate transpose. Equation (9.23) is rearranged as (9.24) to make conncetion between the iterative algorithm and DNN.

$$\begin{aligned} D_{X(k+1)} &= S\left(D_{X(k)} + D\left[\sum_n (J_k)^H J_k\right]\sum_n A_{(k)}\delta E_{sca}\right) \\ &= S\left(D_{X(k)} + D\left[\sum_n (J_k)^H J_k\right]\sum_n A_{(k)}(E_{sca} - G_d E_t X_k)\right) \\ &= S(P_{(k)}X_{(k)} + b_{(k)}) \end{aligned} \tag{9.24}$$

In equation (9.24), $P_{(k)} = D_{x_{(k)}} - D\left[\sum_n (J_k)^H J_k\right] \sum_n A_{(k)} G_d E_t$ and $b_{(k)} = D\left[\sum_n (J_k)^H J_k\right] \sum_n A_{(k)} E_{sca}$. In the deep learning terminology $P_{(k)}$ and $b_{(k)}$ are weight matrix and bias, respectively.

9.6 Summary

Machine learning based image reconstruction by using microwave imaging is described with current challenges in the diagnosis as well as in the development of robust machine learning classification models. Data collection methods are discussed for microwave breast imaging system. Both data processing and diagnosis are proposed with the help of literature. Variational Bayesian inversion and deep neural networks are discussed for microwave breast imaging. There is no standard scanning and machine learning based diagnosis process for microwave breast imaging. Most of the machine learning models are just implemented on a computer. Machine learning or AI based diagnosis, monitoring and treatment are not integrated as a system. An AI based system has been proposed for diagnosis, monitoring and treatment in the next chapters.

References

[1] Meaney P, Fanning M, Li D, Poplack S P and Paulsen K 2000 A clinical prototype for active microwave imaging of the breast, IEEE Trans. Microw *Theory Tech* **48** 1841–53

[2] Poplack S P, Tosteson T D, Wells W A, Pogue B W, Meaney P M, Hartov A, Kogel C A, Soho S K, Gibson J J and Paulsen K D 2007 Electromagnetic breast imaging: results of a pilot study in women with abnormal mammograms *Radiology* **243** 350–9

[3] Fear E C, Bourqui J, Curtis C, Mew D, Docktor B and Romano C 2013 Microwave breast imaging with a monostatic radar-based system: a study of application to patients, IEEE Trans. Microw *Theory Tech* **61** 2119–28

[4] Porter E, Coates M and Popović M 2016 An early clinical study of time-domain microwave radar for breast health monitoring *IEEE Trans. Biomed. Eng.* **63** 530–9

[5] Preece A W, Craddock I J, Shere M, Jones L and Winton H L 2016 MARIA M4: Clinical evaluation of a prototype ultrawideband radar scanner for breast cancer detection *J. Med. Imaging* **3** 033502

[6] Bannister P 2016 A novel microwave radar breast imaging system in a symptomatic breast clinic *Proc. BSBR Breast Imaging Research Network Workshop (Manchester, UK)*

[7] Fasoula A, Anwar S, Toutain Y and Duchesne L 2017 Microwave vision: from RF safety to medical imaging *Proc. 11th European Conf. on Antennas and Propagation (EuCAP) (Paris)* 2746–50

[8] Fear E C, Hagness S C, Meaney P M, Okoniewski M and Stuchly M A 2002 Enhancing breast tumor detection with near-field imaging *IEEE Microw. Mag.* **3** 48–56

[9] Nikolova N K and Webster J G 2014 Microwave biomedical imaging *Wiley Encyclopedia of Electrical and Electronics Engineering* (Hoboken, NJ: Wiley)

[10] Conceição R C, Mohr J J and O'Halloran M 2016 *An Introduction to Microwave Imaging for Breast Cancer Detection* (Basel: Springer)

[11] Bolomey J C, Lakhtakia A and Furse C M (ed) 2018 Crossed viewpoints on microwave-based imaging for medical diagnosis: from genesis to earliest clinical outcomes *The World of Applied Electromagnetics* (Cham: Springer) pp 369–414

[12] O'Loughlin D, O'Halloran M J, Moloney B M, Glavin M, Jones E and Elahi M A 2018 Microwave breast imaging: clinical advances and remaining challenges *IEEE Trans. Biomed. Eng.* **65** 2580–90

[13] Gøtzsche P C and Nielsen M 2011 Screening for breast cancer with mammography *Cochrane Database Syst. Rev.* **6** CD001877

[14] Biller-Andorno N and Jüni P 2014 Abolishing mammography screening programs? A view from the Swiss Medical Board *N. Engl. J. Med.* **370** 1965–7

[15] Suri J S and Rangayyan R M 2006 *Recent Advances in Breast Imaging, Mammography, and Computer-Aided Diagnosis of Breast Cancer* vol 15 (Bellingham, WA: SPIE)

[16] Jinshan T, Rangayyan R M, Jun X, El Naqa I and Yongyi Y 2009 Computer-aided detection and diagnosis of breast cancer with mammography: recent advances *IEEE Trans. Inf. Technol. Biomed.* **13** 236–51

[17] Olson S L, Fam B W, Winter P F, Scholz F J, Lee A K and Gordon S E 1988 Breast calcifications: analysis of imaging properties *Radiology* **169** 329–32

[18] Fondrinier E, Lorimier G, Guerin-Boblet V, Bertrand A F, Mayras C and Dauver N 2002 Breast microcalcifications: multivariate analysis of radiologic and clinical factors for carcinoma *World J. Surg.* **26** 290–6

[19] Buchbinder S S, Leichter I S, Lederman R B, Novak B, Bamberger P N, Coopersmith H and Fields S I 2002 Can the size of microcalcifications predict malignancy of clusters at mammography? *Acad. Radiol.* **9** 18–25

[20] Cox R F and Morgan M P 2013 Microcalcifications in breast cancer: lessons from physiological mineralization *Bone* **53** 437–50

[21] Ridley N, Iriarte A, Tsui L, Bore C, Shere M, Lyburn I and Bannister P 2017 Automatic labelling of lesions using radiofrequency feature discrimination *Proc. European Congress of Radiology (Vienna, Austria, 1–5 March 2017)*

[22] Stavros A T, Thickman D, Rapp C L, Dennis M A, Parker S H and Sisney G A 1995 Solid breast nodules: use of sonography to distinguish between benign and malignant lesions *Radiology* **196** 123–34

[23] Rangayyan R M, El-Faramawy N M, Desautels J E L and Alim O A 1997 Measures of acutance and shape for classification of breast tumors *IEEE Trans. Med. Imaging.* **16** 799–810

[24] Rahbar G, Sie A C, Hansen G C, Prince J S, Melany M L, Reynolds H E, Jackson V P, Sayre J W and Bassett L W 1999 Benign versus malignant solid breast masses: US differentiation *Radiology* **213** 889–94

[25] D'Orsi C, Sickles E, Mendelson E and Morris E 2013 ACR *BI-RADS® Atlas, Breast Imaging Reporting and Data System* American College of Radiology, Reston, VA

[26] Dorland W A N 2012 *Dorland's Illustrated Medical Dictionary* 32nd edn (Philadelphia, PA: Saunders/Elsevier)

[27] Chen Y, Gunawan E, Low K S, Wang S C, Soh C B and Putti T C 2008 Effect of lesion morphology on microwave signature in 2-D ultra-wideband breast imaging *IEEE Trans. Biomed. Eng.* **55** 2011–21

[28] Davis S, Van Veen B D, Hagness S C and Kelcz F 2008 Breast tumor characterization based on ultrawideband microwave backscatter *IEEE Trans. Biomed. Eng.* **55** 237–46

[29] Conceição R, O'Halloran M, Byrne D, Jones E and Glavin M 2010 Tumor classification using radar target signatures *Proc. Progress in Research and Electromagnetics Sympos.* vol 1 *(Cambridge, MA, 5–8 July 2010)* pp 346–9

[30] Conceição R C, O'Halloran M, Jones E and Glavin M 2010 Investigation of classifiers for early-stage breast cancer based on radar target signatures *Prog. Electromagn. Res.* **105** 295–311

[31] Conceição R C, O'Halloran M, Glavin M and Jones E 2010 Support vector machines for the classification of early-stage breast cancer based on radar target signatures *Prog. Electromagn. Res. B* **23** 311–27

[32] Conceição R C, O'Halloran M, Glavin M and Jones E 2011 Evaluation of features and classifiers for classification of early-stage breast cancer *J. Electromagn. Waves Appl* **25** 1–14

[33] O'Halloran M, McGinley B, Conceição R C, Morgan F, Jones E and Glavin M 2011 Spiking neural networks for breast cancer classification in a dielectrically heterogeneous breast *Prog. Electromagn. Res.* **113** 413–28

[34] O'Halloran M, Cawley S, McGinley B, Conceição R C, Morgan F, Jones E and Glavin M 2011 Evolving spiking neural network topologies for breast cancer classification in a dielectrically heterogeneous breast *Prog. Electromagn. Res. Lett.* **25** 153–62

[35] Jones M, Byrne D, McGinley B, Morgan F, Glavin M, Jones E, Conceição R C and O'Halloran M 2013 Classification and monitoring of early stage breast cancer using ultra wideband radar *Proc. 8th Int. Conf. on Systems (ICONS) (Seville, 27 January–1 February 2013)* pp 46–51

[36] Conceição R C, Medeiros H, O'Halloran M, Rodriguez-Herrera D, Flores-Tapia D and Pistorius S 2013 Initial classification of breast tumour phantoms using a UWB radar prototype *Proc. Int. Conf. on Electromagnetics in Advanced Applications (ICEAA) (Torino, Italy, 9–13 September 2013)* pp 720–3

[37] Conceição R C, Medeiros H, O'Halloran M, Rodriguez-Herrera D, Flores-Tapia D and Pistorius S 2014 SVM-based classification of breast tumour phantoms using a UWB radar prototype system *Proc. 31st URSI General Assembly and Scientific Symp. (URSI-GASS) (Beijing, China, 16–23 August 2014)* pp 1–4

[38] Oliveira B L, Shahzad A, O'Halloran M, Conceição R C, Glavin M and Jones E 2015 Combined breast microwave imaging and diagnosis system *Proc. Progress in Electromagnetics Research Sympos.* vol 1 *(Prague, Czech Republic, 6–9 July 2015)* pp 274–8

[39] Kerhet A, Raffetto M, Boni A and Massa A 2006 A SVM-based approach to microwave breast cancer detection *Eng. Appl. Artif. Intell.* **19** 807–18

[40] Byrne D, O'Halloran M, Jones E and Glavin M 2011 Support vector machine-based ultrawideband breast cancer detection system *J. Electromagn. Waves Appl.* **25** 1807–16

[41] Byrne D, O'Halloran M, Glavin M and Jones E 2011 Breast cancer detection based on differential ultrawideband microwave radar *Prog. Electromagn. Res.* **20** 231–42

[42] Santorelli A, Porter E, Kirshin E, Liu Y J and Popovic M 2014 Investigation of classifiers for tumor detection with an experimental time-domain breast screening system *Prog. Electromagn. Res.* **144** 45–57

[43] Conceição R C, Byrne D, Noble J A and Craddock I J 2016 Initial study for the investigation of breast tumour response with classification algorithms using a microwave radar prototype *Proc. 10th European Conf. on Antennas and Propagation (EuCAP) (Davos, Switzerland, 10–15 April 2016)* pp 1–2

[44] Li Y, Santorelli A, Laforest O and Coates M 2015 Cost-sensitive ensemble classifiers for microwave breast cancer detection *Proc. IEEE Int. Conf. on Acoustics, Speech and Signal Processing (ICASSP) (Brisbane, QLD, Australia, 19–24 April 2015)* pp 952–6

[45] Li Y, Santorelli A and Coates M 2016 Comparison of microwave breast cancer detection results with breast phantom data and clinical trial data: varying the number of antennas *Proc. 10th European Conf. on Antennas and Propagation (EuCAP) (Davos, Switzerland, 10–15 April 2016)* pp 1–5
[46] Li Y, Porter E, Santorelli A, Popović M and Coates M 2017 Microwave breast cancer detection via cost-sensitive ensemble classifiers: phantom and patient investigation *Biomed. Signal Process. Control* **31** 366–76
[47] Song H, Li Y, Coates M and Men A 2017 Microwave breast cancer detection using empirical mode decomposition features arXiv:1702.07608
[48] Song H, Li Y and Men A 2018 Microwave breast cancer detection using time-frequency representations *Med. Biol. Eng. Comput.* **56** 571–82
[49] Elahi M A, Shahzad A, Glavin M, Jones E and O'Halloran M 2014 Hybrid artifact removal for confocal microwave breast imaging *IEEE Antennas Wirel. Propag. Lett.* **13** 149–52
[50] Elahi M A, Glavin M, Jones E and O'Halloran M 2017 Adaptive artifact removal for selective multistatic microwave breast imaging signals *Biomed. Signal Process. Control* **34** 93–100
[51] Ambroise C and McLachlan G J 2002 Selection bias in gene extraction on the basis of microarray gene-expression data *Proc. Natl. Acad. Sci. USA* **99** 6562–6
[52] Cawley G C and Talbot N L C 2010 On over-fitting in model selection and subsequent selection bias in performance evaluation *J. Mach. Learn. Res.* **11** 2079–107
[53] O'Halloran M, Conceição R C, Byrne D, Glavin M and Jones E 2009 FDTD modeling of the breast: a review *Prog. Electromagn. Res.* B **18** 1–24
[54] Oliveira B L, O'Halloran M, Conceição R C, Glavin M and Jones E 2016 Development of clinically informed 3-D tumor models for microwave imaging applications *IEEE Antennas Wirel. Propag. Lett.* **15** 520–3
[55] Oliveira B L, Godinho D, O'Halloran M, Glavin M, Jones E and Conceição R C 2018 Diagnosing breast cancer with microwave technology: remaining challenges and potential solutions with machine learning *Diagnostics* **8** 36
[56] Buck J R, Daniel M M and Singer A 2002 *Computer Explorations in Signals and Systems Using MATLAB* (Upper Saddle River, NJ: Prentice-Hall)
[57] Stoica P and Moses R L 2005 *Spectral Analysis of Signals* (Upper Saddle River, NJ: Pearson Prentice-Hall)
[58] Welch P 1967 The use of fast Fourier transform for the estimation of power spectra: a method based on time averaging over short, modified periodograms *IEEE Trans. Audio Electroacoust.* **15** 70–3
[59] Auger F and Flandrin P 1995 Improving the readability of time-frequency and time-scale representations by the reassignment method *IEEE Trans. Signal Process.* **43** 1068–89
[60] Fulop S A and Fitz K 2006 Algorithms for computing the time-corrected instantaneous frequency (reassigned) spectrogram, with applications *J. Acoust. Soc. Am.* **119** 360–71
[61] Reiman L 2001 Random forests *Mach. Learn.* **45** 5–32
[62] Breiman L, Friedman J H, Olshen R A and Stone C J 1984 *Classification and Regression Trees* (Boca Raton, FL: Chapman & Hall)
[63] Spackman K A 1989 Signal detection theory: valuable tools for evaluating inductive learning *Proc. 6th Int. Workshop on Machine Learning* (San Francisco, CA: Morgan Kaufmann) pp 160–3

[64] Gharsalli L, Ayasso H, Duchêne B and Mohammad-Djafari A 2014 Variational Bayesian inversion for microwave breast imaging *Comput. Assisted Methods Eng. Sci.* **21** 199–210
[65] Li L, Wang L G, Teixeira F L, Liu C, Nehorai A and Cui T J 2018 DeepNIS: deep neural network for nonlinear electromagnetic inverse scattering *IEEE Trans. Antennas Propag.* **67** 1819–25
[66] Yao H M, Wei E I and Jiang L 2019 Two-step enhanced deep learning approach for electromagnetic inverse scattering problems *IEEE Antennas Wirel. Propag. Lett.* **18** 2254–8
[67] Kerhet A *et al* 2006 A SVM-based approach to microwave breast cancer detection *Eng. Appl. Artif. Intell.* **19** 807818

Hardik N Patel, Deepak K Ghodgaonkar and Jasjit S Suri

Chapter 10

Microwave image reconstruction methods

Microwave image reconstruction methods are described in this chapter. The Levenberg–Marquardt based inverse problem solution is described with regularization. The Gauss–Newton method is discussed in detail for microwave image reconstruction with least squares and Broyden–Fletcher–Goldfarb–Shannon (BFGS) quasi-Newton method. The Born iterative method is formulated for microwave breast imaging. An overview of the stochastic optimization method (genetic algorithm) is described for microwave breast imaging.

Microwave imaging has many applications like remote sensing, medical imaging, nondestructive testing, concealed weapon detection and through-wall imaging. All the above applications rely on the solution of the inverse problem. There are different methods and algorithms used for microwave breast imaging.

10.1 Levenberg–Marquardt method

Levenberg–Marquardt method is basically a combination of the methods proposed in [1, 2]. Microwave imaging based complex permittivity reconstruction is proposed in [3] by using the Levenberg–Marquardt method. An arbitrary cylindrical object is surrounded by a homogeneous medium and it is excited by transverse magnetic (TM) harmonic excitation [3]. The cylinder is oriented in the z direction and its cross-section in the xy plane. Water is considered as a surrounding medium. The permittivity at a point $r(x, y)$ of the cross-section is given by equation (10.1).

$$\epsilon(r) = \epsilon'(r) + i\epsilon''(r) \tag{10.1}$$

In equation (10.1), ϵ' is the relative dielectric permittivity and ϵ'' is proportional to the conductivity σ. The contrast function $c(r)$ with respect to the known surrounding medium complex permittivity ϵ_{sur} is given by equation (10.2).

doi:10.1088/978-0-7503-2592-9ch10

$$c(r) = \begin{matrix} \epsilon(r) - \epsilon_{\text{sur}}, r \in S \\ 0, \qquad\qquad r \notin S' \end{matrix} \tag{10.2}$$

$k(r) = k'(r) + ik''(r)$ is complex wave propagation with $k = k_0\sqrt{\epsilon}$, where $k_0 = \omega\sqrt{\epsilon_0\mu_0}$ is the propagation constant in vacuum. Incident, total and scattered electric fields are denoted by $E^i(r)$, $E(r)$, and $E^s(r)$, respectively. The first geometry has receivers equally spaced on the line which is a model for the planar microwave camera [4]. The second geometry has receivers equally spaced on the circle and it is considered as the model for a circular microwave scanner [5]. Incident wave illumination is different for linear and circular imaging domain geometries. Plane wave propagation is perpendicular to the line containing receivers for linear geometry. A cylindrical wave is considered for the circular geometry. The circular geometry produces better reconstructions than a linear one. The total and scatter electric fields are related by equation (10.3), which is known as the electric field integral equation (EFIE).

$$E_l(r) = E_l^{\text{i}}(r) + \int\int k_0^2 c(r')E_l(r')G(r, r')\text{d}r' \tag{10.3}$$

In equation (10.3), $l = 1\ldots L$, G is the free space Green's function $G(r, r') = (i/4)H_0^{(1)}(k_{\text{sur}}|r - r'|)$. The scattered electric field at receivers is calculated by equation (10.4).

$$E_l^{\text{s}}(s_{lm}) = \int\int k_0^2 c(r')E_l(r')G(s_{lm}, r')\text{d}r' \tag{10.4}$$

In equation (10.4), s_{lm} is the receiver locations, $l = 1\ldots L$ and $m = 1\ldots M$. Equations (10.3) and (10.4) are known as a forward scattering problem when the contrast c of object, incident field E_l^{i} in S and surrounding medium complex permittivity ϵ_{sur} are given and the scattered electric field E^{s} is unknown. When contrast is unknown then it is known as an inverse scattering problem. Equation (10.4) is nonlinear and the problem is ill-posed. This type of nonexistence can be solved with redefining the solution as the minimization of cost functional. Non-uniqueness is present in equation (10.4) due to nonlinearity and limited data set. The cost functional may result in local minima. The least square cost function and solution of equation (10.4) are sensitive to the errors and noise in the data so it is necessary to include some form of regularization. In Levenberg–Marquardt method cost functional is minimized by using least square approach. Prior information and bounds on complex permittivity, proper values of cell size and regularization parameter play an important role in the stability of the solution.

10.1.1 Forward problem

The forward problem is solved during each iteration of the Levenberg–Marquardt method so accuracy is very important in the solution of the forward problem. Discretization of equation (10.3) is done by applying method of moments with pulse basis functions and point matching [6]. The contrast and total electric field are both discretized by using the same pulse basis functions. Maximum cell size is restricted to $\lambda/5$ as proposed by [7], and contrast profile is assumed to be constant over one cell. Equations (10.3) and (10.4) can be converted into matrix form by applying method of moments and linear algebra.

$$[I - G^{\mathrm{r}}C]E_l = E_l^{\mathrm{i}} \tag{10.5}$$

Equation (10.5) represents the matrix form of equation (10.3) after applying discretization to it. The scattered electric field equation (10.4) can be converted into the matrix form of equation (10.6).

$$E_l^{\mathrm{s}} = G_l^{\mathrm{s}} E_l c \tag{10.6}$$

In equations (10.5) and (10.6) c, E_l, E_l^{i}, E_l^{s} are column vectors.

$$c = \begin{bmatrix} c_1 \\ \vdots \\ C_N \end{bmatrix} \tag{10.7}$$

$$E_l = \begin{bmatrix} E_{1,i} \\ \vdots \\ E_{l,N} \end{bmatrix} \tag{10.8}$$

$$E_l^{\mathrm{i}} = \begin{bmatrix} E_l^{\mathrm{i}}(r_1) \\ \vdots \\ E_l^{\mathrm{i}}(r_N) \end{bmatrix} \tag{10.9}$$

$$E_l^{\mathrm{s}} = \begin{bmatrix} E_l^{\mathrm{s}}(s_{l1}) \\ \vdots \\ E_l^{\mathrm{s}}(s_{lm}) \end{bmatrix} \tag{10.10}$$

In the above equations, G^{r} and G_l^{s} are matrices of the integrated Green's functions with $N \times N$ and $M \times N$ dimensions, respectively, and C and E_l are the diagonal matrices. The Green's functions matrix is independent of the view for circular geometry, therefore $G_l^{\mathrm{s}} = G^{\mathrm{s}}$. The electric field ($e_l$) is obtained by computing $[I - G^{\mathrm{r}}C]^{-1}e_l^{\mathrm{i}}$. Integration of Green's function is done over a disk, which leads to an analytical expression of [7, 8]. As a first step, the forward problem is solved to get the scattered electric field due to incident electric field. As a next step the inverse problem is solved to reconstruct the contrast profile by using Levenberg–Marquardt method.

10.1.2 Inverse problem solution by using Levenberg–Marquardt

The formulation of equations (10.5) and (10.6) is by using method of moment discretization. It is written as equation (10.11).

$$F(c) = E^{s} \tag{10.11}$$

In equation (10.11), E^s is a vector composed of different E_l^s and F is a nonlinear vector function. Now, equation (10.11) is solved by using least square approach of equation (10.12).

$$Q(c) = ||F(c) - E^{s}||^2 = \min \tag{10.12}$$

c_{sol} and c_{sol}^0 are the solutions of equation (10.12) corresponding to noisy data E^s and original data E^s0. The Gauss–Newton method approximates $F(c)$ in equation (10.12) with affine model around the current iterate c_c and choosing the minimizer of the obtained quadratic approximation to $Q(c)$ as the next iterate. The above statements can be expressed as equation (10.13).

$$D^{*}D\Delta c = D^{*}\Delta E^{s} \tag{10.13}$$

In equation (10.13), D^* indicates the conjugate transpose, where $\Delta E^s = E^s - F(c_n)$, $\Delta c = c_{n+1} - c_n$, D is derivate matrix of the form $[\partial F(c_n)/\partial c]$ with $[D]_{ij} = \partial F_i/\partial c_j$. An analytical expression of the Jacobian matrix is derived below. Consider the first-order variations of equations (10.5) and (10.6).

$$\delta e_l = G^{r}\delta[Ce_l] \tag{10.14}$$

$$\delta e_l^{s} = G_l^{s}\delta[E_l c] \tag{10.15}$$

where $E_l c = Ce_l$.

$$\delta[Ce_l] \approxeq [\delta C]e_l + C[\delta e_l] \tag{10.16}$$

Equation (10.17) is obtained by substituting equation (10.14) into equation (10.16).

$$\delta[Ce_l] = [I - CG^{r}]^{-1}[\delta C]e_l \tag{10.17}$$

Now, equation (10.18) is obtained after substituting equation (10.17) into (10.15).

$$D_l = G_l^{s}[I - CG^{r}]^{-1}E_l \tag{10.18}$$

Derivative matrix D_l of size $M \times N$ is relating electric field variations δe_l^s and contrast variations δc. The computation of $[I - CG^r]^{-1}$ is straightforward since its transpose is already calculated in the forward problem as $[I - G^rC]^{-1}$. Gathering L matrices D_l finally produces the Jacobian matrix D. Hessian matrix, second-order derivatives of $Q(c)$ are neglected in the Gauss–Newton method which is not the case with the Newton method. Correction Δc is never locally uphill because D^*D is a positive semi-definite matrix. If the problem is not too nonlinear and residuals are not too large then this approximation is valid. It may be possible to have worst reconstruction in next iterations if objects have high contrast or C_n as still far from c_{sol}. If the condition number of D^*D is large then Δc is very sensitive to the noise in the data and method can again diverge. Levenberg–Marquardt algorithm [1, 2, 9–12] is applied such that the correction factor Δc satisfies the condition of equation (10.19).

$$[D^*D + \alpha I_N]\Delta c + \alpha = D^*\Delta E^s \tag{10.19}$$

Equation (10.19), α is a real positive number, I_N is the $N \times N$ identity matrix. It is equivalent to write equation (10.20) from equation (10.19).

$$||D\Delta c_\alpha - \Delta e^s||^2 + \alpha||\Delta c_\alpha||^2 = min \tag{10.20}$$

There is a twofold effect of equation (10.19). If the solution is very far from actual or the problem is very nonlinear, then it increases chances of the convergence with large value of α. The effect of noise amplification on Δc is reduced by controlling the condition number of D^*D [13, 14]. Equation (10.19) is solved by using singular value decomposition (SVD) because it provides base for the application of generalized cross-validation (GCV) method to choose regularization parameter. The SVD of matrix D is calculated as $D = U\Sigma V^*$, where U and V are $LM \times LM$ and $N \times N$ unitary matrices, Σ is a $LM \times N$ diagonal matrix with $[\Sigma]_{kk} = \sigma_k$, $k = 1\ldots\min(LM, N)$, σ_k are the singular values $|\sigma_1| \geqslant |\sigma_2| \geqslant \ldots \geqslant |\sigma_k| \geqslant \ldots \geqslant 0$, with $[\Sigma]_{ij} = 0$ for $i \neq j$. Now consider K to be the rank of D, $\sigma_k = 0$ for $k > K$. The zero singular values and associated vectors do not intervene so U and V are denoted as $LM \times K$ and $K \times K$ matrices, respectively, and Σ as the diagonal matrix diag$[\sigma_k, k = 1\ldots K]$. The Levenberg–Marquardt correction is given by the equation (10.21).

$$\Delta c_\alpha = V\text{diag}\left[\frac{1}{|\sigma_k|^2 + \alpha}, k = 1\ldots K\right]V^*D^*\Delta e^s \tag{10.21}$$

Equation (10.21) reduces to Gauss–Newton correction for $\alpha = 0$. The same mesh grids are used for direct and inverse problems. *A priori* known upper and lower bounds are enforced on the complex permittivity values at the end of each iteration.

10.1.3 Choice of the regularization parameter

There are two approaches described here for choosing the regularization parameter. The first approach is based on the empirical formula of [15, 16] that controls the step length to avoid overcorrections because of nonlinearity. The similar approach is also used in the trust region methods [9, 11, 12]. The second approach is about reduction of ill-conditioning on the correction for noisy data. The basic idea is to regularize the correction such that it gets close to the exact Gauss–Newton correction corresponding to exact data. Regulation term is not included in this approach for avoiding overcorrections due to nonlinearity. Initial guess should not be too far from the solution. Practically value of α is computed by minimizing the error between the exact and predicted data through regularized correction. This computation is possible by using GCV method. White noise complex vector is defined with zero mean ($E[n] = 0$) and σ^2 as the variance of n, where $E[nn^*] = 2\sigma^2 I_{LM}$. The empirical method uses equation (10.22) to compute the value of α.

$$\alpha_{\text{emp}} = \beta\frac{\text{Trace}[D^*D]}{N}\frac{||F(c_n) - e^s||^p}{||e^s||^p} \tag{10.22}$$

The value of α is proportional to the normalized field error Err e^s raised to the power p. The normalization with respect to eigenvalue is included by the trace of D^*D and some regulation is included by parameter β. The initial value of β is chosen in a random fashion. and it is updated at each iteration depending on the variation of error in the e_c^s with respect to error in e^s as follows.

$$\beta_+ = \begin{matrix} \beta_c & \text{if Err } e_c^s - \text{Err } e^s < -0.1 \text{ Err } e_c^s \\ \frac{1}{2}\beta_c & \text{if } -0.1\text{Err } e_c^s \leqslant \text{Err } e_c^s - \text{Err } e^s \leqslant 0.1\text{Err } e_c^s \\ 2\beta_c & \text{if Err } e_c^s - \text{Err } e^s > 0.1\text{Err } e_c^s \end{matrix} \quad (10.23)$$

If the process converges too slowly or error increases slightly then the constraint over $||\Delta c||$ is weakened, this eventually allows escaping from a local minimum. The initial values of p and β affect the convergence speed but this is not too crucial. The second method is generalized cross-validation for choosing value of regularization parameter. A practical approach to find an optimal regularization parameter is proposed in [17] for an ill-conditioned linear system. The minimization of true prediction error (error between exact data and the data predicted by the regularized solution) is achieved by this approach. The value that minimizes equation (10.24) is denoted by α_T.

$$T(\alpha) = \frac{1}{LM}||D\Delta c_\alpha - \Delta e^{s0}||^2 \quad (10.24)$$

Let

$$A_\alpha = D[D^*D + \alpha I_{LM}]^{-1}D^* \quad (10.25)$$

The reconstructed data satisfies equation (10.26).

$$D\Delta c_\alpha = A_\alpha \Delta e^s \quad (10.26)$$

The true prediction error $T(\alpha)$ cannot be computed in a real experiment because it depends on exact data. However, there are methods proposed for estimating α_T in [17–21], which estimate α_T from the data without the knowledge of the noise variance σ^2. Equation (10.27) shows the minimizer α_{GCV} of the GCV function.

$$V(\alpha) = \frac{\frac{1}{LM}||[A_\alpha - I_{LM}]\Delta e^s||^2}{\left(\frac{1}{LM}\text{Trace}[A_\alpha - I_{LM}]\right)^2} \quad (10.27)$$

Equation (10.27), is an estimate of the α_T, if Δe^{s0} is very smooth, noise is white with fixed variance σ^2 and $LM \to \infty$. The above solution is not valid if $\sigma^2 \to 0$. The difference between $E[T(\alpha) + \sigma^2]$ and $E[V(\alpha)]$ is shown to be small with respect to $E[T(\alpha)]$ with $LM \to \infty$ and certain conditions on the traces of A_α and $[A_\alpha]^2$ are satisfied [3]. Equation (10.28) is used to give the unbiased estimate $\hat{T}$ for the $E[T]$ (expectation of T).

$$\hat{T}(\alpha) = \frac{1}{LM}||[A_\alpha - I_{LM}]\Delta e^s||^2 - \frac{2\sigma^2}{LM}\text{Trace}[A_\alpha - I_{LM}]^2 + \frac{2\sigma^2}{LM}\text{Trace}[A_\alpha]^2 \tag{10.28}$$

The α_{RR} of the above equation is known as the range risk estimate [18, 19]. The value of α which satisfies the discrepancy principle of equation (10.29) is known as $\alpha_{\text{discrepancy}}$.

$$||D\Delta c_\alpha - \Delta e^s||^2 = 2LM\sigma^2 \tag{10.29}$$

Now, major steps of numerical implementation are described which simplify the computations of equations (10.27) and (10.28) to accelerate the process of minimization [22]. The optimization problem of equation (10.20) is transformed into the equivalent problem of equation (10.30) by applying coordinate transformation through a well chosen orthogonal basis of dimension K in the range of D.

$$||\hat{D}\Delta c_\alpha - \Delta \hat{e}^s||^2 + \alpha||\Delta c_\alpha||^2 = \min \tag{10.30}$$

The orthogonal basis is chosen as the column vector of the unitary matrix U.

$$\hat{D} = U^* D = \Sigma V^* \tag{10.31}$$

$$\Delta \hat{e}^s = U^* \Delta e^s \tag{10.32}$$

The solution of the minimization problem of equation (10.30) also minimizes equation (10.20) because both the equations just differ at most by a constant which is independent of Δc_α. Problems of equations (10.20) and (10.30) have the same optimum value for α.

$$T(\alpha) = \frac{1}{K}||\hat{D}\Delta c_\alpha - \Delta \hat{e}^{s0}||^2 \tag{10.33}$$

Performing some linear algebra calculations and by using equation (10.32), equation (10.34) can be derived.

$$\hat{A}_\alpha = \hat{D}\hat{D}^*[\hat{D}\hat{D}^* + \alpha I_K]^{-1} = \text{diag}\left[\frac{|\sigma_k|^2}{|\sigma_k|^2 + \alpha}\right] \tag{10.34}$$

and

$$\Delta \hat{e}^s = \text{diag}\left[\frac{\sigma_k}{|\sigma|^2 + \alpha} - \frac{1}{\overline{\sigma_k}}\right] V^* D^* \Delta e^s \tag{10.35}$$

In the above equations $\hat{A}_\alpha$ is a $K \times K$ matrix and the hat stands for complex conjugate. The $V(\alpha)$ is given by equation (10.36).

$$V(\alpha) = K\frac{\Delta e^s D V \text{diag}\left[\frac{1}{(|\sigma|^2 + \alpha)^2 |\sigma_k|^2}\right] V^* D^* \Delta e^s}{\left(\sum_{k=1}^{K}\frac{1}{|\sigma_k|^2 + \alpha}\right)^2} \tag{10.36}$$

$T(\alpha)$ is shown by equation (10.37).

$$\hat{T}(\alpha) = \frac{1}{K}||[\hat{A}_\alpha - I_k]\Delta\hat{e}^s||^2 - \frac{2\sigma^2}{K}\text{Trace}[\hat{A}_\alpha - I_K]^2 + \frac{2\sigma^2}{K}\text{Trace}[\hat{A}_\alpha]^2 \quad (10.37)$$

The signal-to-noise ratio is defined by equation (10.38).

$$SNR = 10\log_{10}\frac{||e^{s0}||^2}{||n||^2} \quad (10.38)$$

The norm of the exact data is obtained through summation over views and receivers and where $||n||^2 = 2LM\sigma^2$, where σ^2 is the variance used for generating the Gaussian white noise. Noise level with respect to the difference between exact field data e^{s0} and the field e_c^s during each iteration for the current contrast c_c. The electric field error, the permittivity error and contrast error are given by equations (10.39), (10.40) and (10.41), respectively.

$$\text{Err } e^s = \frac{||e^s - e_c^s||}{||e^s||} \quad (10.39)$$

$$\text{Err}\epsilon = \frac{||\epsilon_{sol}^0 - \epsilon_c}{\epsilon_{sol}^0} \quad (10.40)$$

$$\text{Err}c = \frac{||c_{sol}^0 - c_c||}{c_{sol}^0} \quad (10.41)$$

In the above equations, e^s is the noisy electric field data, c_{sol}^0 is the exact solution. The regularization parameters α_{EMP} and α_{GCV} are computed with equations (10.22) and (10.36), respectively. The parameters α_T, α_{RR} and α_{DISC} are computed for comparison of different regularization parameter estimation methods. Equations (10.24) (10.28) and (10.37) are minimized by computing those functions in a range $[\alpha_{min}, \alpha_{max}]$ with a logarithmic increment $\log\alpha = 1/30$. The larger increment is chosen for the computation of α_{GCV} since a further refinement with a golden section search is performed. Now, the parameter α_{OPT} is given by equation (10.42).

$$||c_+(\alpha) - C_{sol}^0||^2 = \min \quad (10.42)$$

The correction Δc_α is obtained with α_{OPT} producing a next iterate c_+ which tends to the exact solution better than with any other choice of α.

10.2 Gauss–Newton method

The regularized Gauss–Newton method is described for three-dimensional microwave imaging [28]. A 3-D inhomogeneous lossy dielectric object with arbitrary shape and complex permittivity $\epsilon(r) = \epsilon'(r) - j\epsilon''(r)$, where $r = x\hat{x} + y\hat{y} + z\hat{z}$ denotes the location or position. All materials are non-magnetic and have permeability of free space μ_0. A boundary domain D is defined which completely includes the object, and $\epsilon(r)$ is to be reconstructed as the permittivity contrast within D.

$$X(r) = \epsilon(r) - \epsilon_b \tag{10.43}$$

The time harmonic incident electric fields E^{inc} for successive multiview illuminations are applied to the object. The corresponding scattered electric fields E^{scat} are measured at different receiver locations r in the observation domain D. The time dependence is assumed as $e^{j\omega t}$ with ω as the angular frequency. In microwave imaging, a contrast-source integral equation is used where scattered electric field E^{scat} is radiated by a contrast current density J^{scat} in the medium with background permittivity ϵ_b which is zero outside of source volume D.

$$J^{scat}(r) = j\omega x(r)E(r) \tag{10.44}$$

Total electric field is the sum of incident electric field and scattered electric field, $E = E^{inc} + E^{scat}$. At any arbitrary point r, the contrast-source integral equation for the total electric field can be written as equation (10.45) [23, 24].

$$E(r) = -j\omega\mu_0\left[I + \frac{1}{k_b^2}\nabla\nabla\right]\int_{R^3} G_b(r - r')[J^{inc}(r') + J^{scat}(r')]\mathrm{d}r' \tag{10.45}$$

In equation (10.45), I is 3×3 identity matrix, k_b is the background permittivity of the medium, J^{inc} is the source current density for E^{inc}, $G_b(r - r')$ is the scalar Green's function of homogeneous medium. The Green's function is given by equation (10.46).

$$G_b(r - r') = \frac{e^{-jk_b||r-r'||}}{4\pi||r - r'||} \tag{10.46}$$

The Green's function of equation (10.46) satisfies equation (10.47).

$$\nabla^2 G_b(r - r') + k_b^2 G_b(r - r') = -\delta(r - r') \tag{10.47}$$

The nonlinear inverse scattering problem is described by domain integral and observation equations.

$$E^{inc}(r) = E(r) + j\omega A^{scat}(r) + \nabla\phi^{scat}(r) \tag{10.48}$$

$$E^{scat}(r) = \frac{k_b^2}{\epsilon_b}\int_D G_b(r - r')\cdot x(r')E(r')\mathrm{d}r' \tag{10.49}$$

Equations (10.48) and (10.49) are useful to compute scattered electric field for the nonlinear inverse scattering problem. Equation (10.49) relates the scattered electric field at the observation points to the unknown contrast sources. Equation (10.49) is nonlinear as scattered electric field depends on E and E depends on the contrast in permittivity. In equation (10.49), scattered field is expressed in terms of vector and scalar potentials A^{scat} and ϕ^{scat} [25]. In equation (10.49), tensor G_b is the dyadic Green's function of homogeneous space such that the field is generated by an elementary dipole with current density.

$$J_\delta(r) = -\frac{1}{j\omega\mu_0}\delta(r - r')\hat{u} \tag{10.50}$$

It is necessary to express the unknown permittivity $\epsilon(r)$ in terms of parameters in domain D. The domain is expressed as a uniform grid D_ϵ with N_ϵ cubic cells with side Δ_ϵ. The shape of this parameter grid D_ϵ can be chosen so that the wave does not travel faster than the speed of light. The total number of cells $N_\epsilon = F \times G \times H$. The grid points are denoted as $r_{f,g,h} = f\Delta_\epsilon\hat{x} + g\Delta_\epsilon\hat{y} + h\Delta_\epsilon\hat{z}$. The approximate permittivity is computed by a piecewise cost function that has one value in each cell.

$$\epsilon(r) \approx \sum_{f=0}^{F-1}\sum_{g=0}^{G-1}\sum_{h=0}^{H-1}\epsilon_{f,g,h}\epsilon_b\phi_{f,g,h}(r) \tag{10.51}$$

In equation (10.51), $\phi_{f,g,h}$ is a 3-D pulse function which assumes the value 1 inside the cell (f, g, h) and is zero elsewhere, the unknown coefficients $\epsilon_{f,g,h}$ represent relative complex permittivity values. These values are collected in an N_ϵ dimensional complex permittivity vector.

$$\epsilon = [\epsilon_{0,0,0}\ldots\epsilon_{F-1,G-1,H-1}]^T = [\epsilon_v]^T \tag{10.52}$$

In equation (10.52), T stands for transpose of the matrix, the triplet (f, g, h) is replaced with a single index v. The measured scattered electric field is denoted by E^{meas}. The nonlinear equation (10.49) is solved for complex permittivity vector ϵ with the help of domain equation (10.48) and by using Newton type iterative optimization methods. The above iterative methods rely on the minimization of the cost function which is the distnce between the measured and predicted values of scattered electric field data. The full forward problem is solved for each iteration and derivative of scattered fields are computed for updating directions. In order to simplify the notations, operator G_b^v is introduced that acts on the vector function p with support V.

$$[G_b^v(p)](r) = -j\omega\mu_0\left[I + \frac{1}{k_b^2}\nabla\nabla\right]\cdot\int_V G_b(r - r')p(r')dr' \tag{10.53}$$

The total electric field of equation (10.45) at an arbitrary point r is equation (10.54).

$$E(r) = [G_b^S(J^{\text{inc}})](r) + [G_b^D(j\omega XE)](r) \tag{10.54}$$

The dyadic Green's function of the inhomogeneous medium G_{inh}, such that $G_{\text{inh}}(r, r')\cdot\hat{u}$ corresponds to the total field in r due to an elementary dipole at r' due to the object. The total electric field of equation (10.54) is given by equation (10.55).

$$E(r) = -j\omega\mu_0\int_S G_{\text{inh}}(r, r')\cdot J^{\text{inc}}(r')dr' \tag{10.55}$$

Now, the derivative of equation (10.49) or (10.54) with respect to the permittivity parameter ϵ_v gives

$$\frac{\partial E^{\text{scat}(r)}}{\partial \epsilon_v}(r) = k_{\text{b}}^2 \int_D \phi_v(r') G_{\text{inh}}(r, r') \cdot E(r') \text{d}r' \tag{10.56}$$

Equation (10.56) satisfies equation (10.54) with J^{inc} replaced with a current density $j\omega\epsilon_b\phi_v E$ in the cell v. Equation (10.56) can be rewritten by following equation (10.55).

$$\frac{\partial E^{\text{scat}}}{\partial \epsilon_v} = k_{\text{b}}^2 \int_D \phi_v(r') G_{\text{inh}}(r, r') \cdot E(r') \text{d}r' \tag{10.57}$$

It is shown in [26] that a unique solution exists for the scalar 3D inverse scattering problem if the scattered far electric field is known in all directions due to plane incident waves from all possible directions. The problem of non-uniqueness can be dealt with if there is sufficient data due to finite number of illuminations and measurements. There are a total of N_{A} antenna positions, denoted with r_a^{A}, $a = 1, \ldots, N_{\text{A}}$, for the transmitting and receiving antennas. The number of different polarizations $N_{\text{P}} \leqslant 3$ and is defined for each antenna position r_a^{A}. In a spherical geometry, the antenna positions typically lie on circles with proper polarization directions. An elementary dipole is chosen as the transmitter r_{t}^{A} oriented along $\hat{u}_{t,p}^{\text{A}}$, where t is a subset of a. Total number of illuminations is denoted by the number of transmitter positions N^{T} times the number of polarizations N^P. The electric field measured at N_t^{R} receiver positions r_r^{A} along the polarization directions $\hat{u}_{r,p}^{\text{A}}$, here the subset r and N_t^{R} is different for each illumination t. The total amount of measured scattered electric field data in a vector is e^{meas} with dimension $N^D = (N^P)^2 \sum_t N_t^{\text{R}} \leqslant (N^P)^2 (N^A)^2$. The vector contains the scattered electric field components $E_{t,p}^{\text{meas}}(r_r^{\text{A}}) \cdot \hat{u}_{r,p'}^{\text{A}}$ at points r_r^{A} and polarized along p' due to p-polarized dipole excitations at r_t^{A}. The scattered electric field components $Et,\ p^{\text{scat}}(r_r^{\text{A}}) \cdot \hat{u}_{r,p}^{\text{A}}$ collected in an N^{D} dimensional vector e^{scat} for a given permittivity vector ϵ, are collected in an N^{D} dimensional vector e^{scat}. The derivatives of these components with respect to to ϵ_v are derived by using (10.57).

$$\frac{\partial E_{t,p}^{\text{scat}}}{\partial \epsilon_v}(r_r^{\text{A}}) \cdot \hat{u}_{r,p'}^{\text{A}} = k_{\text{b}}^2 \int_D \phi_v(r') \hat{u}_{r,p'}^{\text{A}} \cdot G_{\text{inh}}(r_r^{\text{A}}, r') \cdot E_{t,p}(r') \text{d}r' \tag{10.58}$$

According to reciprocity $G_{\text{inh}}(r_r^{\text{A}}, r') = G_{\text{inh}}^T(r', r_r^{\text{A}})$ and since

$$E_{r,p'}(r') = G_{\text{inh}}(r', r_r^{\text{A}}) \cdot \hat{u}_{r,p'}^{\text{A}} \tag{10.59}$$

It follows equation (10.60).

$$\frac{\partial E_{t,p}^{\text{scat}}}{\partial \epsilon_v}(r_r^{\text{A}}) \cdot \hat{u}_{r,p'}^{\text{A}} = k_{\text{b}}^2 \int_D \phi_v(r') E_{t,p}(r') \cdot E_{r,p'}(r') \text{d}r' \tag{10.60}$$

The derivative of scattered field is computed by solution of the forward problem for excitations along all polarizations $\hat{u}_{a,p}^{\text{A}}$ at all antenna locations. On the other hand, computation of the cost function requires only the transmitting positions r_t^{A}. This computation results in $N^{\text{A}} N^{\text{P}}$ forward problems for a given permittivity vector ϵ.

The total number of forward problems is very large due to full 3D imaging technique. If the measurement domain configuration has a transmitter at all antenna positions then $E_{t,p'}(r')$ and $E_{r,p'}(r')$ in equation (10.60) are already computed for the cost function. This is the advantage of this method over modified gradient approach where workload is increased due to inrease in number of transmitters [27]. The dimension of single forward problem often results in thousands of unknowns. Efficient algorithms are needed for optimum use of memory and computation time.

10.2.1 Forward problem formulation

Galerkin method of moments is applied to solve a forward problem [27, 28]. N^{B} vectorial functions are used to expand the equation (10.47). Uniform cuboidal grid is used with $L \times M \times N$ cubic cells in this formulation. The N_{B} dimensional linear system of equations is solved iteratively with the stabilized bi-conjugate gradient method [29]. The convolutional property of integral equation, matrix multiplications and fast Fourier transform are used to solve forward problem [23, 30, 31]. The computational complexity of BICGSTAB-FFT method is $O(PN_{\mathrm{B}} \log N_{\mathrm{B}})$, with P number of iterations to reach the required accuracy, and memory complexity is $O(N_{\mathrm{B}})$. The forward problem is solved multiple times in the inversion scheme with varying contrast, source positions and polarizations. A proper choice of initial guess can accelerate the iterative solution of the linear systems. In a practical measurement system the transmitter is moved to successive positions r_t^{A} in small steps, the fields vary accordingly. The forward problem in matrix form is given by equation (10.61).

$$E_t^{\mathrm{inc}} = Zd_t \tag{10.61}$$

In equation (10.61), the N_{B} dimensional vector d_t has the coefficients of electric flux density. The initial guess d_t^0 is an extrapolation of solutions d_{t-1}, d_{t-2}, ... computed for different transmitter positions as shown by equation (10.62).

$$d_t^0 = \sum_{i=1}^{I} a_{t,i} d_{t-i} \tag{10.62}$$

In equation (10.62), the coefficients are chosen to minimize the error $||Zd_t^0 - e_t^{\mathrm{inc}}||^2$.

$$\sum_{i=1}^{I} [E_{t-j}^{\mathrm{inc}}]^H E_{t-i}^{\mathrm{inc}} a_{t,i} = [E_{t-j}^{\mathrm{inc}}]^H E_t^{\mathrm{inc}} \tag{10.63}$$

In equation (10.63), $j = 1, 2, \ldots, I$. The coefficients of equation (10.62) are the solution of equation (10.63).

10.2.2 The inverse problem formulation

The cost function with an additive multiplicative regularization is proposed in equation (10.64).

$$F(\epsilon) = F^{\mathrm{LS}}(\epsilon)[1 + \alpha F^{\mathrm{R}}(\epsilon)] \tag{10.64}$$

In equation (10.64), F^{LS} is the least square data error, F^{R} is a regularizing function, α is a regularization parameter and ϵ is the complex permittivity vector. The least square data error is given by equation (10.65).

$$F^{\mathrm{LS}}(\epsilon) = \frac{1}{N^{\mathrm{LS}}}||E^{\mathrm{scat}} - E^{\mathrm{meas}}||^2 \tag{10.65}$$

In equation (10.65), $N^{\mathrm{LS}} = ||e^{\mathrm{meas}}||^2$ a normalization constant and $||.||$ is the L^2 norm. The least square data error of equation (10.65) is used as a cost function in many research articles. The minimum is not well-defined due to the ill-posedness of the inverse problem. Consequently a coarse grid D_ϵ for the parameterization of $\epsilon(r)$ is often preferred to reduce unwanted fluctuations in the reconstruction for noisy data. In this work, regularization is applied by adding multiplicative terms to equation (10.65).

$$\begin{aligned} F^{\mathrm{R}}(\epsilon) = \frac{1}{N_R}\Bigg[&\sum_{f=0}^{F}\sum_{g=0}^{G-1}\sum_{h=0}^{H-1}|\epsilon_{f,g,h} - \epsilon_{f-1,g,h}|^2 + \\ &\sum_{f=0}^{F-1}\sum_{g=0}^{G}\sum_{h=0}^{H-1}|\epsilon_{f,g,h} - \epsilon_{f,g-1,h}|^2 + \sum_{f=0}^{F-1}\sum_{g=0}^{G-1}\sum_{h=0}^{H}|\epsilon_{f,g,h} - \epsilon_{f,g,h-1}|^2\Bigg] \end{aligned} \tag{10.66}$$

In equation (10.66), F^{R} is the positive function, N^R is a normalization constant, which relates to the object dimensions and cell discretization. The optimization in this work is going to start from a constant relative permittivity ϵ_{int} for all cells. The discrete version of $(1/D)\int_D|\nabla_\epsilon(r)|^2 dr$ is denoted by function F^{R}, it penalizes strong local fluctuations in the permittivity. The total variation regularization is included as a multiplicative regularization to a modified gradient cost function [32]. The cost function F is always greater than the data error F^{LS}, except for $F^{\mathrm{LS}} = 0$ at the solution in the absence of measurement noise. The regularized solution is automatically equal to the exact solution. In this case, regularization is not strictly needed, the multiplicative term appears to have a positive effect on the convergence of the optimization algorithm in terms of dealing with the nonlinearity. The minimization of cost function is stopped when the data error F^{LS} is equal to the noise level h for nosisy data. The regularization provides a smoothed solution which is dependent on the value of α. This regularization provides a solution between the desired smoothing and the capability to reconstruct strong inhomogeneous objects. The reconstruction is not very sensitive to the specific choice of α until data error F^{LS} can reach the noise level. This condition is known as the discrepancy principle [33]. The value of $\alpha F^{\mathrm{R}}0 \approxeq 10^{-3} to 10^{-2}$, with F^{R0} as the value of F^{R} at the true solution. Magnitude order of F^{R0} can be considered from *a priori* information about object size and upper limit for permittivity.

10.2.3 Gauss–Newton optimization in general

Newton's method can approximate a nonlinear cost function by using a quadratic model based on the first- and second-order derivatives of the cost function for the current iteration, and chooses the minimum of this model as the next iterate. There is an important basic property known as super linear convergence if the initial guess is close enough to the solution [34]. If the initial guess is far from the solution then Newton's correction step may lead to an increase in the cost function. If the model is not a good approximation to the function at the stationary point or the Hessian matrix is not positive definite then cost function may increase in the next iteration. If the number of cells is large then it results in the heavy computation of second-order derivatives or Hessian matrix. A modified Gauss–Newton method is proposed to deal with the above problems of Newton's method. The cost function $F(\epsilon)$ and $F^{\mathrm{LS}}(\epsilon)$ and $F^{\mathrm{R}}(\epsilon)$ are real functions of N_ϵ complex variables $\epsilon_v = \epsilon_v{}' - j\epsilon_v{}''$. The gradient is defined as shown in equation (10.67).

$$g = \begin{bmatrix} \dfrac{\partial F}{\partial \epsilon_v} \\ \dfrac{\partial F}{\partial \epsilon_v^*} \end{bmatrix} \tag{10.67}$$

The Hessian matrix is defined as shown in equation (10.68).

$$H = \begin{bmatrix} \dfrac{\partial^2 F}{\partial^2 \epsilon_v} & \dfrac{\partial^2 F}{\partial \epsilon_v \partial \epsilon_v^*} \\ \dfrac{\partial^2 F}{\partial \epsilon_v^* \partial \epsilon_v} & \dfrac{\partial^2 F}{\partial^2 \epsilon_v^*} \end{bmatrix} \tag{10.68}$$

The gradient equation (10.67) has partial derivatives with respect to permittivity ϵ_v and its complex conjugate ϵ_v^*, where $v = 1 \ldots N_\epsilon$. The gradient equation is denoted by (10.69) for least squares data error F^{LS}.

$$g^{\mathrm{LS}} = \frac{1}{N^{\mathrm{LS}}} \begin{bmatrix} J^T[E^{\mathrm{scat}} - E^{\mathrm{meas}}]^* \\ J^H[E^{\mathrm{scat}} - E^{\mathrm{meas}}] \end{bmatrix} \tag{10.69}$$

In equation (10.69), J is the Jacobian matrix ($N_D \times N_\epsilon$) with first-order derivatives of the scattered electric field components, $J_{dv} = \partial E_d^{\mathrm{scat}} / \partial \epsilon_v$. The Hessian matrix is given by equation (10.70).

$$H^{\mathrm{LS}} = \frac{1}{N^{\mathrm{LS}}} \begin{bmatrix} B & J^T J^* \\ J^H J & B^* \end{bmatrix} \tag{10.70}$$

In equation (10.70), B is $N_\epsilon \times N_\epsilon$ matrix having second-order derivatives of the scattered electric field with the residue, $B_{vv} = (\partial^2 E^{\mathrm{scat}} / \partial \epsilon_v \partial \epsilon_v)^T [E^{\mathrm{scat}} - E^{\mathrm{meas}}]^*$. g^{R} is denoted by equation (10.71) for the regularization function F^{R}.

$$g^{\mathrm{R}} = \begin{bmatrix} \Omega \\ \Omega^* \end{bmatrix} \tag{10.71}$$

with $\Omega_v = \partial F^{\mathrm{R}} / \partial \epsilon_v$

$$H^{\mathrm{R}} = \begin{bmatrix} 0 & \Sigma \\ \Sigma & 0 \end{bmatrix} \tag{10.72}$$

In equation (10.72), Σ is a real and constant matrix with $\Sigma_{vv} = \partial^2 F^{\mathrm{R}} / \partial\epsilon_v \partial\epsilon_v^*$. Now, the gradient and Hessian matrix of the regularized cost function F is written as equations (10.73) and (10.74), respectively.

$$g = g^{\mathrm{LS}}(1 + \alpha F^{\mathrm{R}}) + F^{\mathrm{LS}}\alpha g^{\mathrm{R}} \tag{10.73}$$

$$H = \frac{1}{N^{\mathrm{LS}}}\begin{bmatrix} B' & A^* \\ A & B'^* \end{bmatrix} \tag{10.74}$$

In equation (10.74), H is a complex symmetric matrix with

$$B' = B(1 + \alpha F^{\mathrm{R}}) + \alpha J^T[E^{\mathrm{scat}} - E^{\mathrm{meas}}]^*\Omega^T + \alpha\Omega[E^{\mathrm{scat}} - E^{\mathrm{meas}}]^H J \tag{10.75}$$

$$\begin{aligned} A = {} & J^H J(1 + \alpha F^{\mathrm{R}}) + \alpha J^H[E^{\mathrm{scat}} - E^{\mathrm{meas}}]\Omega^T + \alpha\Omega^*[E^{\mathrm{scat}} - E^{\mathrm{meas}}]^H J \\ & + \alpha N^{\mathrm{LS}} F^{\mathrm{LS}}\Sigma \end{aligned} \tag{10.76}$$

In an optimization scheme the complex permittivity vector is updated iteratively as equation (10.77).

$$\epsilon_{n+1} = \epsilon_n + \Delta\epsilon_n \tag{10.77}$$

In equation (10.77), $\Delta\epsilon_n$ is the permittivity correction at iterate n. The Newton correction of F is given by equation (10.78).

$$\begin{bmatrix} \Delta\epsilon_k \\ \Delta\epsilon_k^* = -H_k^{-1} g_k \end{bmatrix} \tag{10.78}$$

The search direction can be found by this correction factor with an approximate line search [34]. It is shown in [23] that an optimization method that searches successively along different descent paths converges to a minimizer by using approximate line search [34].

10.2.4 Gauss–Newton method for the least squares

Gauss–Newton method is used as an alternative to the Newton method in the case of squares of nonlinear functions with data error F^{LS}. The function e^{scat} of equation (10.64) is converted to linear for the current iterate.

$$\Delta E_k^{\mathrm{scat}} = E^{\mathrm{scat}}(\epsilon_k + \Delta\epsilon_k) - E_k^{\mathrm{scat}}(\epsilon_k) \approxeq J_k \Delta\epsilon_k \tag{10.79}$$

In equation (10.79), $E^{\mathrm{scat}}(\epsilon_k + \Delta\epsilon_k) = E^{meas}$ and by applying least square method to solve the resulting system, the Gauss–Newton correction factor for F^{LS} is given by equation (10.80).

$$\Delta\epsilon_k = -(J_k^H J_k)^{-1} J_k^H [E_k^{\mathrm{scat}} - E^{\mathrm{meas}}] \tag{10.80}$$

Second-order derivatives of the scattered fields are not needed in the above formulation. The Hermitian matrix $J^H J$ is at least positive semi-definite, so the direction of update is never uphill. The condition number of Hermitian matrix is large due to small singular values of J. This numerical rank deficiency can prevent the convergence because of an orthogonal relationship between steepest descent vector and update directions. Improvement in Gauss–Newton method was done with a Levenberg–Marquardt trust region approach which gives a positive definite and better conditioned Hessian matrix. The cost function with regularization is given by equation (10.81).

$$A\Delta\epsilon + B'^{*}\Delta\epsilon^{*} = -J^H[E^{\mathrm{scat}} - E^{\mathrm{meas}}](1 + \alpha F^{\mathrm{R}}) + \alpha N\mathrm{LS}F^{\mathrm{LS}}\Omega^{*} \tag{10.81}$$

By using equations (10.75) and (10.76) with equation (10.79),

$$\begin{aligned} A\Delta\epsilon + B'^{*}\Delta\epsilon^{*} = {} & J^H J(1 + \alpha F^{\mathrm{R}})\Delta\epsilon + \alpha J^H[E^{\mathrm{scat}} - E^{\mathrm{meas}}][\Omega^T\Delta\epsilon + \Omega^H\Delta\epsilon^{*}] \\ & + \alpha\Omega^{*}[[E^{\mathrm{scat}} - E^{\mathrm{meas}}]^H\Delta E^{\mathrm{scat}} + [E^{\mathrm{scat}} - E^{\mathrm{meas}}]^T\Delta E^{\mathrm{scat}*}] \\ & + \alpha N^{\mathrm{LS}}F^{\mathrm{LS}}\Sigma\Delta\epsilon \end{aligned} \tag{10.82}$$

The constant initial permittivity, $\epsilon_{f,g,h} = \epsilon^{\mathrm{init}}$ is taken at the starting of optimization process. This permittivity vector minimizes the cost function and produces zero for Ω. The data residue $\Delta E^{\mathrm{meas}} = [E^{\mathrm{meas}} - E^{\mathrm{scat}}]$ is very small due to minimization so all the terms except the first in the right-hand side of equation (10.82) are negligible. The modified Gauss–Newton correction is given by equation (10.83).

$$\Delta\epsilon = -(J^H J + \lambda^2\Sigma)^{-1}(J^H[E^{\mathrm{scat}} - E^{\mathrm{meas}}] + \lambda^2\Omega^{*}) \tag{10.83}$$

The value of λ^2 is computed as $\alpha N^{\mathrm{LS}}F^{\mathrm{LS}}/(1 + \alpha F^{\mathrm{R}})$. The matrix $(J^H J + \lambda^2\Sigma)$ is always positive definite for $\lambda^2 \neq 0$ because Σ is positive definite. The presence of $\lambda^2\Sigma$ ensures a descent direction and the optimization is stopped when F^{LS} is equal to the noise level h with $F^{\mathrm{R}}_{\mathrm{max}}$ as bound in the region of interest, a lower bound $\lambda^2_{\mathrm{min}} = \alpha N^{\mathrm{LS}}h/(1 + \alpha F^{\mathrm{R}}_{\mathrm{max}})$. The update directions will be uniformly bounded with the steepest descent vector along the optimization path. The convergence to the stopping criteria or to a local minimum above this threshold can be established as proposed in [34]. The equation (10.83) approximates the Newton correction and super linear convergence as the data error is reduced. The solution to the regularized linear least square problem is given by equation (10.84).

$$\min||J\Delta\epsilon - \Delta E^{\mathrm{meas}}||^2 + \lambda^2||L^T\Delta\epsilon + L^{-1}\Omega^{*}||^2 \tag{10.84}$$

In equation (10.84), L is the Cholesky factor of $\Sigma = LL^T$. The second term of the above equation is known as the Tikhonov regularization term [13]. The above equation is minimized when $\Sigma\Delta\epsilon = -\Omega^{*}(\epsilon)$ when $\Omega^{*}(\epsilon + \Delta\epsilon) = 0$, since $\Sigma\Delta\epsilon = \Omega^{*}(\epsilon + \Delta\epsilon) - \Omega^{*}(\epsilon)$. This term tries to reduce F^{R}, or fluctuations in the permittivity ϵ, it is more appropriate than smoothing the correction $\Delta\epsilon$ [3, 35, 36]. The regularization parameter λ^2 in (10.84) is proportional to the data error F^{LS} with Tikhonov regularization [36].

10.2.5 The BFGS quasi-Newton method

The quasi-Newton method approximates the Hessian matrix in the Newton correction of equation (10.78) with a matrix that does not involve the explicit computation of second-order derivatives. This approximated Hessian matrix is updated based on the change in the gradient with respect to the previous iteration. The BFGS update formula for the inverse Hessian matrix H_k^{-1}.

$$\hat{H}_{k+1} = \hat{H}_k + \left(1 + \frac{\gamma_k^T \hat{H}_k \gamma_k}{\delta_k^T \gamma_k}\right)\frac{\delta_k \delta_k^T}{\delta_k^T \gamma_k} - \left(\frac{\delta_k \gamma_k^T \hat{H}_k + H_k \hat{\gamma_k} \delta_k^T}{\delta_k^T \gamma_k}\right) \tag{10.85}$$

In equation (10.85), $\delta_k = \Delta\epsilon_k$, $\gamma_k = g_{k+1} - g_k$, where $\hat{H}_k$ is a symmetric matrix for which $g_k^T \hat{H}_k g_k > 0$, it means that the updates $\Delta\epsilon_k = -\hat{H}_k g_k$ are descent directions. Select the $\hat{H}$ equal to the identity matrix. $\hat{H}_k$ is a close approximation to H_k^{-1} after a sufficient number of iterations [34]. Equation (10.85) directly approximates the inverse Hessian matrix so only single matrix vector multiplication is required to compute the quasi-Newton correction $\Delta\epsilon_k = -\hat{H}_k g_k$. The rate of convergence is much slower with this BFGS quasi-Newton method as compared to modified Gauss–Newton method.

10.3 Born iterative method

The Born iterative method is used for microwave reconstruction of the weak scatterer objects. The object to be reconstructed in given by equation (10.86).

$$O(\rho') = \epsilon(\rho') - \epsilon_b \tag{10.86}$$

In equation (10.86), ϵ_b is the known background permittivity. Permittivity of the homogeneous background medium, such that $g(\rho, \rho', t - t') = g_0(\rho, \rho', t - t')$. The wave equation with TM incidence is given by (10.88).

$$\nabla^2 E(\rho, t) - \mu_0 \epsilon(\rho) \frac{\partial^2}{\partial t^2} E(\rho t) = \mu_0 \frac{\partial}{\partial t} J_z(\rho, t) \tag{10.87}$$

In equation (10.86), $J_z(\rho, t)$ is an electric line source with a time-dependent excitation. $E(\rho, t)$ is the z component of the electric field. The scattered electric field due to the object satisfies the volume integral of equation (10.88) [37–39].

$$E^{\text{scat}}(\rho, t) = -\mu_0 \int_{t'} \int\int_S G(\rho, \rho', t - t') \times \frac{\partial^2}{\partial t'^2} E(\rho', t') O(\rho') \partial\rho' \mathrm{d}t' \tag{10.88}$$

In equation (10.88), ρ' is the locations or points in the domain of the object, $E^{\text{scat}}(\rho, t)$ is the scattered electric field, $G(\rho, \rho', t - t')$ is the time domain Green's function and $E(\rho', t')$ is the total electric field inside the object or scatterer. The object function or profile is unknown and it is reconstructed when other quantities are known.

$$E^{\text{scat}}(\phi, t) = -\mu_0 \int_{t'} \int\int_S G_0(\rho, \rho', t - t') \frac{\partial^2}{\partial t'^2} E(\rho', t') \times [\epsilon(\rho') - \epsilon_b] \, \mathrm{d}\rho' \mathrm{d}t' \tag{10.89}$$

Equation (10.89) is converted into matrix form by applying dicretization to the object function.

$$E^{\text{scat}} = \bar{M} \cdot O \tag{10.90}$$

In equation (10.90), E^{scat} has scattered electric field at all the receiver locations due to each of the incident field waves. The unknown parameters are represented by using vector O. The elements of matrix $\bar{M}$ are given by equation (10.91).

$$M_{(i,j,k),\rho} = -\mu_0 \int_{t'} \int\int_{S_p} g_0(\rho_i^{\text{r}}, \rho', t_j - t') \times \frac{\partial^2}{\partial t'^2} \phi(\rho', \rho_k^{\text{t}}, t') \mathrm{d}\rho' \mathrm{d}t' \tag{10.91}$$

In equation (10.91), (ij, k) represent the data measured at receiver i and jth time sample due to the kth transmitter, the subscripts r and t refer to receiver and transmitter locations. In order to reduce computations, fast Fourier transform is applied to both sides of equation (10.90).

$$\tilde{E}^{\text{scat}} = \tilde{\bar{M}} \cdot O \tag{10.92}$$

Now equation (10.91) can be rewritten as equation (10.93).

$$\tilde{M}_{(i,j,k),\rho} = \frac{i}{4} \mu_0 \int\int_{S_p} H_0^{(1)}(k_j|\rho_i^{\text{r}} - \rho^{\text{t}}|) \omega_j^2 \tilde{\phi}(\rho^{\text{r}}, \rho_k^{\text{t}}, \omega_j) \mathrm{d}\rho' \tag{10.93}$$

In equation (10.93), $H_0^{(1)}(k_j|\rho_i^{\text{r}} - \rho^{\text{t}}|)$ is the Hankel function of the first kind. The unknown vector O is found by solving equation (10.94).

$$||\tilde{\bar{M}} \cdot O - \mathbb{E}_{\text{meas}}^{\text{scat}}||^2 + \gamma ||O||^2 = \text{minimum} \tag{10.94}$$

where, γ is the regularization parameter. The object function is found from equation (10.95).

$$\tilde{\bar{M}}^T \cdot \tilde{\bar{M}} \cdot O + \gamma O = \tilde{\bar{M}}^T \cdot \tilde{E}_{\text{meas}}^{\text{scat}} \tag{10.95}$$

Born iterative method is implemented by using following steps.

1. $\tilde{E}_n = \tilde{f}(\rho^{\text{r}}, \rho^{\text{t}}, t, \omega; \epsilon_n)$ $E_n^{\text{scat}} = f(\rho^{\text{r}}, \rho^{\text{t}}, t; \epsilon_n) - E^{\text{inc}} \Rightarrow$ Object field
2. $\Delta = ||\phi_n^{\text{scat}} - \phi_{\text{meas}}^{\text{scat}}||$
3. If $\Delta <$ tolerance then stop
4. $\tilde{\bar{M}}_n^T \cdot \tilde{\bar{M}}_n \cdot O_{n+1} + \gamma O_{n+1} = \tilde{\bar{M}}_n^T \cdot \tilde{E}_{\text{meas}}^{\text{scat}}$ conjugate gradient solution $\Rightarrow O_{n+1}$
5. $\epsilon_{n+1} = \epsilon_b + O_{n+1}$, Go to (i)

In the above steps, E^{inc} is the vector containing the time samples of the incident field values at the receivers due to each transmitter, f and $\tilde{f}$ are the solutions of the time domain forward problem and its Fourier transformed version, respectively. The forward solver is used once every iteration. The iterations are stopped, when error Δ is less than the tolerance value. Nonlinear inverse scattering problems are approximated through successive linear formulation in distorted Born iterative method (DBIM). Conjugate gradient least square method uses the gradient based iterative method to solve inverse scattering problems.

10.4 Stochastic optimization methods for microwave imaging

Stochastic optimization methods are also used to solve inverse scattering problems. Genetic, differential evolution, memetic, particle swarm, ant colony optimization algorithms are covered briefly in this section. The cost function of equation (10.96) is calculated by considering multiple illuminations and frequencies approach.

$$f_{\text{data}}(\tau, E_{\omega}^{\text{tot}}) = \sum_{\omega}\sum_{v=1}^{V}\sum_{m=1}^{M} |E_{\omega_{\text{meas}}}^{\text{tot},v}(x_m) - E_{\omega}^{\text{inc},v}(x_m) - \sum_{n}\tau_n E_{\omega,n}^{\text{tot},v} g_{n,m}|^2 \tag{10.96}$$

In equation (10.96),the first summation is over frequencies, V is the number of electromagnetic sources, M is the number of measurement points, $\tau_n = \tau(y_n)$ and $E_{\omega,n}^{\text{tot},v} = E_{\omega}^{\text{tot},v}(y_n)$, $n = 1, \ldots, N$, $g_{n,m}$ is a coefficient calculated by the integral of the Green's function over the area of the nth subdomain.

10.4.1 Genetic algorithm

Genetic algorithm (GA) optimizes a function known as chromosomes and it acts simultaneously on populations of trial solutions. Let $\zeta_k(i)$, $i = 1, \ldots, P$, P = population dimension be the ith element of the population at the kth iteration. The chromosomes are randomly constructed on the basis of the some *a priori* information about the specific problem about the problem in the intialization phase ($k = 0$). The population in the next iteration is generated by applying the genetic operators of selection, mutation and crossover. There are several ways (e.g. tournament and roulette wheel) to implement selection operator. The selection is done through reproduction of only the chromosomes that better perform on the objective function. The crossover operator creates new chromosomes by combining the selected chromosomes of the previous population. Mutation operator randomly perturbs some genes of the elements of the new elements of the population and it prevents a premature convergence to a local minimum. The GA operators are used with certain probabilities which control the iterative method depending upon the application. In the problem formulation, the problem unknowns are quantized and coded in bit strings and genetic operators applied on these strings. An integer between 1 and P is randomly chosen in a single point crossover. From the two selected chromosomes $\zeta_k(j)$ and $\zeta_k(l)$ of the kth population, two chromosomes $\zeta_{k+1}(j)$ $\zeta_{k+1}(l)$ are generated. The first n genes are kept unchanged and the last $P - n$ genes are swapped. The simplest way to extend the previously defined genetic operators is shown by equations (10.97) and (10.98).

$$\zeta_{k+1}(j) = r\zeta_k(j) + (r - 1)\zeta_k(l) \tag{10.97}$$

$$\zeta_{k+1}(l) = r\zeta_k(l) + (r - 1)\zeta_k(j) \tag{10.98}$$

In equations (10.97) and (10.98) r is a random number between 0 and 1. The mutation operator can be implemented by adding random numbers to certain genes. The steps of genetic algorithms to solve the microwave imaging problems are as follows.

- Population (collection or subset of all possible solutions) initialization.
- Fitness function (which takes possible solution as input and produces suitability of solution as output) is calculated.
- Selection of the two fittest chromosomes for creating the next generation. Roulette wheel selection, rank selection, steady state selection, tournament selection, elitism selection are some methods for selecting two fittest chromosomes.
- Crossover is the equivalent of two parents having a child. Each parent chromosome contributes a certain number of genes to the new one. Single point crossover, K-point crossover and uniform crossover are some methods to perform crossover.
- Mutation provides diversity and reduces duplication. It can be done by randomly changing the value.

Tha above steps are performed till the convergence where algorithm terminates with a set of solutions.

10.5 Summary

Traditional microwave image reconstruction methods are discussed in this chapter. Levenberg–Marquardt method is discussed with forward problem, inverse problem and choice of regularization parameter. Gauss–Newton method is discussed with forward problem and inverse problem formulations. Gauss–Newton method for least squares and BFGS quasi-Newton method are given with necessary mathematical details. Born iterative optimization and overview of different stochastic optimization methods are discussed for microwave imaging.

References

[1] Levenberg K 1944 A method for the solution of certain non linear problems in least squares *Quart. Appl. Math.* **2** 164–8

[2] Marquardt D W 1963 An algorithm for least-squares estimation of non linear parameters *J. Soc. Zndust. Appl. Math.* **11** 431–41

[3] Franchois A and Pichot C 1997 Microwave imaging-complex permittivity reconstruction with a Levenberg–Marquardt method *IEEE Trans. Antennas Propag.* **45** 203–15

[4] Jofre L, Hawley M S and Broquetas A 1990 Medical imaging with a microwave tomographic scanner *IEEE Trans. Biomed. Eng.* **37** 303–12

[5] Broauetas A, Romeu J, Rius J M, Elias-FustB A R, Cardama A and Iofre L 1991 Cylindrical geometry: a further step in active microwave imaging *IEEE Trans. Microw. Theory Tech.* **39** 836–44

[6] Harrington R F 1968 *Field Computation by Moment Methods* (New York: Macmillan)

[7] Richmond J H 1965 Scattering by a dielectric cylinder of arbitrary cross section shape *IEEE Trans. Antennas Propagat.* **AP-13** 334–41
[8] Franchois A 1993 Contributionila tomographie microonde: algorithmes de reconstruction quantitative et vkrifications expkrimentales *PhD Thesis* Université Paris-Sud, France
[9] Dennis J E and Schnabel R B 1983 *Numerical Methods for Unconstrained Optimization and Nonlinear Equations* (Englewood Cliffs, NJ: Prentice-Hall)
[10] McKeown J J 1980 Nonlinear least-squares problems *Nonlinear Optimization Theory and Algorithms* ed E Spedicato and G P Szego (Boston, MA: Birkhanser Dixon) pp 91–105
[11] Gill P E and Murray W 1974 *Numerical Methods for Constrained Optimization* (London: Academic)
[12] Vogel C R 1990 A constrained least squares regularization method for nonlinear ill-posed problems *SIAM J. Control Optim.* **28** 34–49
[13] Tikhonov A N and Arsenine V Y 1977 *Solutions of Ill-Posed Problems* (Washington, DC: Winston)
[14] De Mol C 1992 A critical survey of regularized inversion methods *Inverse Problems in Scattering and Imaging* ed M Imaging, Bertero and E R Pike (Bristol: Hilger)) pp 345–70
[15] Hugonin J P, Joachimowicz N and Pichot C 1990 Quantitative reconstruction of complex permittivity distributions by means of microwave tomography *Inverse Methods in Action* ed P C Sabatier vol 11 (Berlin: Springer) pp 302–3
[16] Chew W C and Wang Y M 1990 Reconstruction of two-dimensional permittivity distribution using the distorted born iterative method *IEEE Trans. Med. Imaging* **9** 218–25
[17] Wahba G 1977 Practical approximate solutions to linear operator equations when the data are noisy *SIAM J. Numer. Anal.* **14** 651–67
[18] Craven P and Wahba G 1979 Smoothing noisy data with spline functions *Numer. Math.* **31** 377–403
[19] Golub G H, Heath M and Wahba G 1979 Generalized cross validation as a method for choosing a good ridge parameter *Technometrics* **21** 215–23
[20] Stone M 1974 Cross-validation, choice and assessment of statistical prediction (with discussion) *J. Roy. Stat. Soc. Ser.* B **36** 117–47
[21] Reinsch C M 1967 Smoothing by spline functions *Numer. Math.* **10** 177–83
[22] Girard D 1986 Practical optimal regularization of large linear systems *Math. Mod. Num. Anal.* **20** 75–87
[23] Zwamborn P and van den Berg P M 1992 The three-dimensional weak form of the conjugate gradient FFT method for solving scattering problems *IEEE Trans. Microw. Theory Tech.* **40** 1757–66
[24] Van Bladel J 1985 *Electromagnetic Fields* (New York: Springer)
[25] De Zaeytijd J, Bogaert I and Franchois A 2008 An efficient hybrid MLFMA–FFT solver for the volume integral equation in case of sparse 3D inhomogeneous dielectric scatterers *J. Comput. Phys.* **227** 7052–68
[26] Kirsch A 1996 *An Introduction to the Mathematical Theory of Inverse Problems* (New York: Springer)
[27] Abubakar A, van den Berg P M and Mallorqui J J 2002 Imaging of biomedical data using a multiplicative regularized contrast source inversion method *IEEE Trans. Microw. Theory Tech.* **50** 1761–70

[28] De Zaeytijd J, Franchois A, Eyraud C and Geffrin J-M 2007 Full-wave three-dimensional microwave imaging with a regularized Gauss–Newton method: theory and experiment *IEEE Trans. Antennas Propag.* **55** 3279–92
[29] da Cunha R D and Hopkins T 1995 The parallel iterative methods (PIM) package for the solution of systems of linear equations on parallel computers *Appl. Num. Math.* **19** 33–50
[30] Gan H and Chew W C 1995 A discrete BCG-FFT algorithm for solving 3-D inhomogeneous scatterer problems *IEEE Trans. Antennas Propag.* **9** 1339–57
[31] Sarkar T K, Sarvas E and Rao S M 1986 Application of FFT and the conjugate gradient method for the solution of electromagnetic radiation from electrically large and small conducting bodies *IEEE Trans. Antennas Propag.* **34** 635–40
[32] Abubakar A and van den Berg P M 2001 Total variation as a multiplicative constraint for solving inverse problems *IEEE Trans. Image Process* **10** 1384–92
[33] Morozov V A On the solution of functional equations by the method of regularization *Soviet Math. Dokl.* **7** 414–7
[34] Fletcher R 1990 *Practical Methods of Optimization* 2nd edn (New York: Wiley)
[35] Chew W C and Wang Y M 1990 Reconstruction of two-dimensional permittivity distribution using the distorted Born iterative method *IEEE Trans. Med. Imaging* **9** 218–25
[36] Joachimowicz N, Pichot C and Hugonin J 1991 Inverse scattering: An iterative numerical method for electromagnetic imaging *IEEE Trans. Antennas Propag.* **39** 1742–52
[37] Moghaddam M, Chew W C and Oristaglio M 1991 Comparison of the born iterative method and Tarantola's method for an electromagnetic time-domain inverse problem *Int. J. Imaging Syst. Technol.* **3** 318–33
[38] Chew W C 1990 *Waves and Fields in Inhomogeneous Media* (New York: Van Nostrand Reinhold)
[39] Tarantola A 1984 The seismic reflection inverse problem *Inverse Problems of Acoustic and Elastic Waves* ed F Santosa, Y H Pao, W Symes and C Holland (Philadelphia, PA: SIAM)

Chapter 11

The role of AI in diagnosis, treatment and monitoring of breast cancer during COVID-19 and ahead

COVID-19 has affected almost 213 countries throughout the globe, infecting 33 million people and causing a loss of one million lives. Scientists, researchers, and doctors are still investigating the behaviour of this novel corona virus (SARS-CoV-2) that has led to the pandemic of COVID-19. Some investigations have suggested the reasons of mortality due to this novel and mysterious disease. This includes co-morbid conditions like blood pressure, heart disease, diabetes, and asthma create higher risk due to this novel corona virus. Cancer patients are also at higher risk of having COVID-19 due to their compromised immunity. Breast and lung cancers are most important among all types of cancers due to their vicinity to chest area. Breast cancer diagnosis, treatment and monitoring are affected severely by this pandemic. Technology like artificial intelligence (AI) is needed to automate the process of breast cancer diagnosis, treatment, and monitoring. This chapter reviews the role of AI in breast cancer diagnosis, treatment, and monitoring during the COVID-19 pandemic and further proposes a state-of-the-art AI based breast cancer diagnosis, treatment, and monitoring system. The system is adaptive, robust, and modular, allowing the addition of new AI models in tandem without altering the current work of current AI models. Policy and guideline changes in breast cancer diagnosis, treatment, and monitoring can easily be incorporated due to unforeseen events like a pandemic or any other emergencies by using reinforcement learning. We conclude that the role of AI will ultimately be beneficial in diagnosis, treatment and monitoring of breast cancer during COVID-19 and beyond.

doi:10.1088/978-0-7503-2592-9ch11

11.1 Introduction

The corona virus (SARS-CoV-2) is spreading very fast in the world and causing CVOID19 disease. This virus has infected more than 30 million people and almost one million people have died due to this deadly disease. The disease was declared a pandemic on 11 March, 2020 by the World Health Organization (WHO). Breast cancer incidence and mortality rates are high in USA as compared to Asia and the whole world [1]. Thus, there is an alarming situation of breast cancer in USA which results in a significant economic burden on patients and their families [2, 3]. Breast cancer patients are at the highest risk due to their low immunity and comorbidity [4–13]. There are different imaging modalities for breast cancer screening, namely, mammography, ultrasound, magnetic resonance imaging (MRI), computed tomography (CT). Mammography, MRI and ultrasound are used for breast cancer diagnosis and all other medical imaging modalities are in the research phase. Medical imaging modalities have their advantages and disadvantages [14]. This pandemic has challenged the above imaging techniques due to disinfection requirements for the instruments. Diagnosis, treatment and monitoring of breast cancer have been changed due to this pandemic situation. Immunity of the breast cancer patient has been compromised due to different breast cancer treatments. AI is making machines intelligent enough to reduce human intervention. The world has been heavily dominated by technologies in the last two decades. AI is still in the research phase in most of the sectors but some of the sectors have implemented AI as an enabler. We are still very far from singularity in AI because none of the AI machines or robots have dominated over this pandemic. AI has assisted us during this pandemic but it has not dominated over this pandemic which shows the need of AI systems in healthcare [15–19]. The COVID-19 situation has forcing us to deploy AI in health and other sectors which have fallen victim of this pandemic [20]. Breast cancer management is very challenging even without the current pandemic. AI can play a crucial role as an enabler initially and it can even reduce human intervention slowly as it becomes smart with time [21–24]. Human intuition cannot be right all the time and the human brain cannot process or handle lots of features to make decisions. The above human limitations are forcing us to look for smarter solutions to reduce errors, as well as efforts in policy and decision-making processes [25–28]. An AI system can easily adapt changes due to COVID-19 pandemic situation or even other crises [19, 29]. COVID-19 has resulted in a lack of healthcare resources, higher risk for breast cancer patients, significant changes in decision making processes of breast cancer diagnosis, treatment and monitoring [6, 9, 11, 12, 30–34]. Now, different AI systems have been applied in the diagnosis of breast cancer [22, 35–47]. There are plenty of research articles about breast cancer diagnosis using AI. Now, AI techniques are also used to frame breast cancer treatment and monitoring policies or decisions [16, 25, 48–50]. All the AI techniques used for breast cancer management (diagnosis, treatment and monitoring) are in the research phase so there is no standard adopted by the breast cancer community. There are lots of AI techniques for COVID-19 management which can be used to manage breast cancer during this pandemic [5–8, 9–11, 13, 15–19, 30, 32–34, 51–61]. Researchers have proposed many ideas on breast cancer management during COVID-19, AI based breast cancer management and AI based COVID-19 management, but there are only few proposed research ideas on AI based breast cancer management during COVID-19 [14, 21, 24, 36, 45, 62–72]. We have proposed a general AI system to manage breast cancer under all circumstances including the current COVID-19 pandemic. There is a clear need for an adaptive, robust and modular AI system for the management of breast cancer which can deal with the COVID-19 pandemic as well as other emergencies that largely impact breast cancer patients. The following sections are pathophysiology of breast cancer and AI architecture, the role of AI in diagnosis of breast cancer, the role of AI in monitoring of breast cancer and the role of AI in treatment of breast cancer, AI based integrated system for breast cancer management and a conclusion.

11.2 AI architectures

AI is going to play the role of game changer in almost all areas of science, technology, engineering and management. AI is about creating intelligent machines which can improve performance on tasks with experience and time. Machine learning is a subset or part of AI and deep learning is a subset or part of machine learning. The relationship of AI, machine learning (ML) and deep learning (DL) is shown in figure 11.1. ML is about making machines learn without explicitly

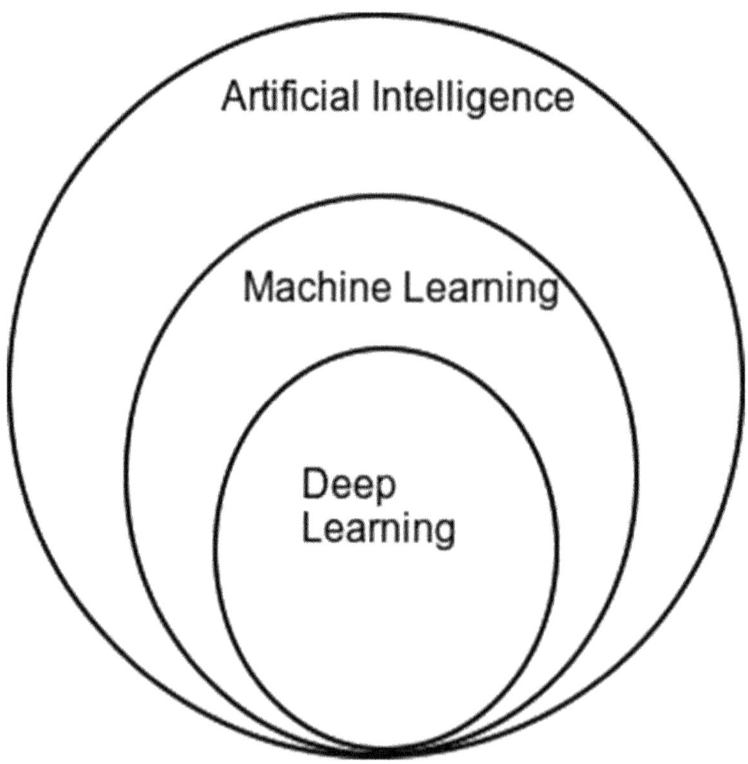

Figure 11.1. Relationship between AI, ML and DL.

programming them. Supervised learning, unsupervised learning, semi-supervised learning and reinforcement learning are different types of ML. In supervised learning, a training data set is required with the corresponding labels. In unsupervised learning, labelled training data is not required; it generally performs clustering of a data set. Semi-supervised learning is a combination of supervised and unsupervised learning. Neural networks are also part of ML. Neural networks have input layer, hidden layer and output layer in their architecture. If neural networks have more than two hidden layers (depth is greater than two) then solutions implemented by using such neural networks are known as DL. ML and DL are used widely in the diagnosis of breast cancer [22, 23, 35–37, 40–42, 44, 45, 47, 62, 63, 93–101, 104, 105]. ML and DL are used for detection, classification and risk classification of breast cancer (figure 11.2).

The above steps are performed to train, validate and implement an ML model irrespective of its type. DL models are neural networks with depth more than two and they include feature extraction as part of the model. Convolutional neural networks (CNNs), recurrent neural networks (RNNs), generative adversarial network (GAN), gated recurrent unit (GRU), long short term memory (LSTM) are different types of deep neural networks. Large data sets are required to train different types of deep neural networks which result in good performance. If AI models are implemented properly then they can learn with time and perform better in the future, which is not the case with non-AI models. CNNs and RNNs are used in medical image analysis for image classification and recognition. RNN is generally preferred for time series data and it is used for text and image classification. GRU and LSTM are different types of RNN which are used to learn a long-term recurring relationship or trend. A simple CNN architecture is shown in figure 11.3 to understand a deep neural network.

There are seven layers in the CNN of figure 11.3. The first layer is known as convolution layer which extracts the high level features from images. The second layer is max-pool which is used to reduce spatial size and number of parameters, which in turn reduce computations. Similarly, the third layer is a convolution layer which learns low level details of images. The fourth layer is max-pooling to reduce computations. The fifth and sixth layers are fully connected layers. The seventh layer is the output layer. Fully connected layers are useful in the classification and recognition tasks. The output layer is finally used to classify the images and it has neurons equal to the number of classes used in the problem. RNNs are also formed

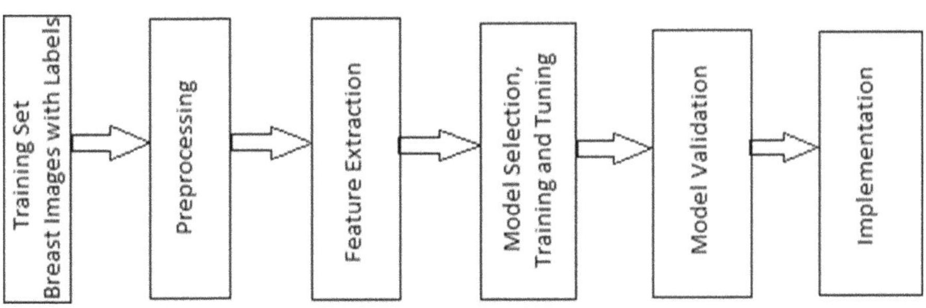

Figure 11.2. ML steps for breast cancer diagnosis.

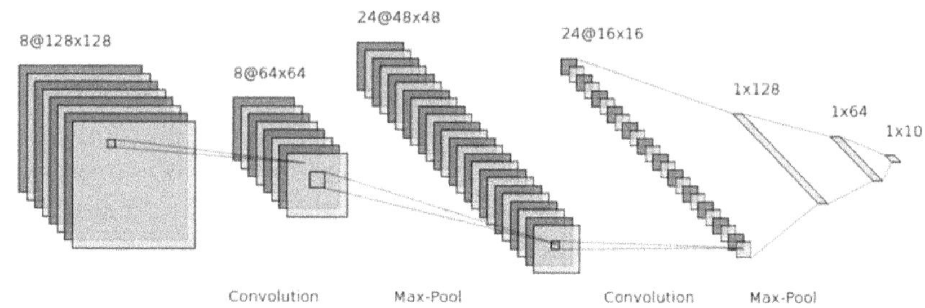

Figure 11.3. CNN example.

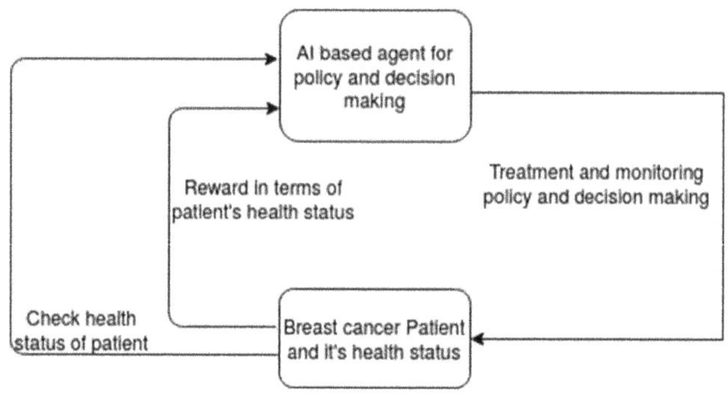

Figure 11.4. Reinforcement learning architecture for policy making.

like the CNN but the output is given in the input. GRU and LSTM are variants of RNN which are used to learn the long-term recurring trends in the data. RL is basically an environment and agent based approach [102, 103]. Here each patient and their health conditions can be treated as an environment and, based on an environmental AI based agent, takes an action to maximize the reward. Here reward is the patient's health condition, so the patient's condition improvement results in a positive reward and its condition degradation results in a negative reward. The architecture of figure 11.4 is useful in breast cancer monitoring and treatment policy formation and decision making.

Transfer learning is used to reduce the training time of the neural network. In transfer learning, exception, VGG-16, VGG-19, RestNet50, InceptionV3, InceptionRestNetV2, MobileNet, DenseNet121, DenseNet169, DenseNet201, LeNet-5, AlexNet and ResNet are the deep neural network architectures. These neural networks have been trained by using large dat asets for image classification for a long time. Researchers can directly use these network architectures by freezing the particular layers and changing only fully connected and output layers of these deep neural networks. Time series data is also used in breast cancer detection. Time series analysis is useful in breast cancer progression, monitoring and treatment predictions [106–108]. Different AI architectures have different applications in diagnosis, monitoring and treatment of breast cancer. There is no end-to-end AI based system architecture for breast cancer detection, so we have proposed a state-of-the-art AI system for breast cancer diagnosis, treatment and monitoring.

11.3 The role of artificial intelligence in diagnosis of breast cancer

Breast cancer diagnosis is extremely important to save lives. There are many traditional algorithms in literature for breast cancer diagnosis [14, 41, 109–117]. Breast cancer diagnosis process before the COVID-19 pandemic is shown in figure 11.5.

As shown in figure 11.5, the decision process marked by yellow colour can be replaced by AI. The yellow coloured decision processes can be replaced by AI models. Most of the research articles in AI based breast cancer diagnosis are focused on replacing this decision making processes by different AI models. Analysis of AI applications in breast cancer is given with the performance details in table 11.1 [118]. Most of the articles mentioned above deal with the diagnosis of breast cancer using AI. Analysis of AI based methods for breast cancer diagnosis using image processing is given, which covers research papers from different sources [43, 66, 116, 118].

Rapid spreading capability of corona virus has changed the breast cancer diagnosis process. The role of AI in diagnosis of breast cancer during COVID-19 is shown in figure 11.6. COVID-19 testing is essential to prevent the spread of this disease among breast cancer patients. The risk analysis based on COVID-19 and immunity can also be included with the testing of this disease.

It is necessary to detect COVID-19 before breast cancer. Machine and medical staff are involved in the breast screening, so it is better to avoid COVID-19 infection risk by testing the patient for COVID-19 before breast imaging.

According to table 11.2, The percentage usage of support vector machine (SVM), neural network and discriminant analysis is about 42%, 31% and 8%, respectively. Overall usage of the above three models is about 81%. Other AI models are used only 19% in the imaging research. Diagnosis of breast cancer includes segmentation of images produced by the imaging modality used in the screening. Classification, detection and recognition are applied after segmentation of the breast images provided by imaging modality. There are four decision making processes involved in breast cancer diagnosis where AI can play a crucial role as an enabler. The role of AI in the treatment of breast cancer is described in the next section.

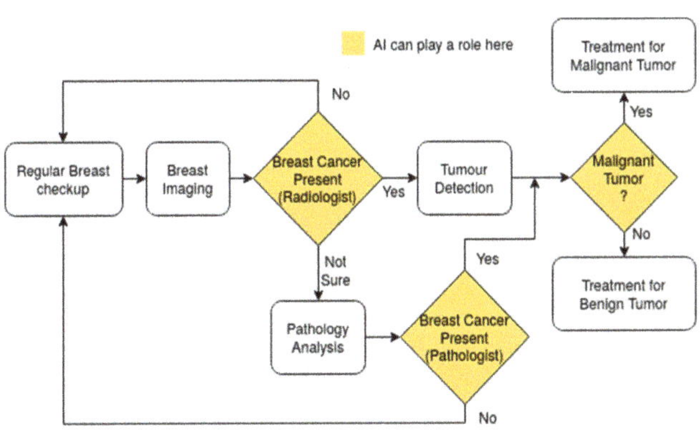

Figure 11.5. Role of AI in diagnosis of breast cancer before COVID-19.

Table 11.1. Analysis of AI applications in breast cancer.

Ref.	Applications, No. of cases	Imaging modality	ML Algorithm	Results
[119]	Microcalcification, 34	Mammography	CNN	AUC, 0.91
[120]	Mass lesions, 500	Mammography	Classification	Same as radiologists
[121]	Mass lesions, 21	Tomosynthesis	Classification	Sn, 90%
[122]	Microcalcification, 72	Tomosynthesis	Classification	Sn, 90%
[123]	Mass lesions, 27	DCE-MRI	Classification	AUC, 0.96
[39]	Microcalcifications, 104	Mammography	Classification	AUC, 0.75
[124]	Mass lesions, 121	DCE-MRI	Engineered	Better than 2D
[125]	Differentiate bening, 353	DCE-MRI	Bayesian NN	AUC, 0.79–0.85
[126]	Mass lesions, 1126	multimodal	t-SNE and NN	AUC, 0.88
[127]	Breast cancer risk, 495	Mammography	Classification	AUC, 0.57–0.66
[100]	Mass lesions, 219	Mammography	Deep learning	AUC,0.81
[37]	Mass lesions, 1125	Multimodal	Deep learning	AUC, 0.89
[128]	Mutation status, 237	Mammography	Bayesian ANN	AUC, 0.68–0.72
[129]	Molecular subtype classification, 91	DCE-MRI	LDA	AUC, 0.65–0.89
[46]	Mutation status, 456	Mammography	CNN, SVM	AUC 0.73–0.86
[65]	Survival prediction, 284	DCE-MRI	–	HR, 2.28–4.81
[35]	Classification	Mammography	Deep belief network	Acc = 92.86
[96]	Detection, classification	Mammography	YOLO	Detection acc = 99.7

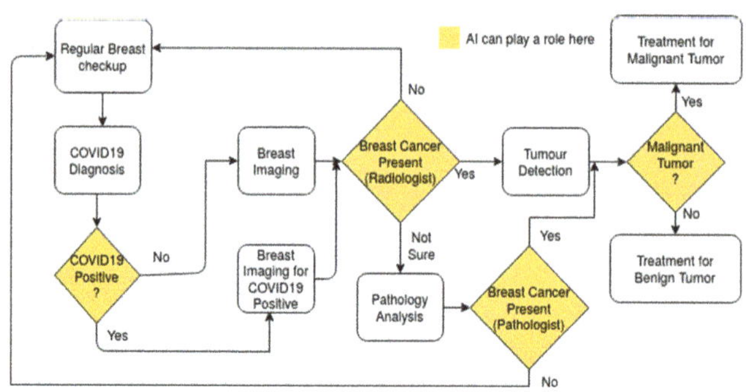

Figure 11.6. Role of AI in diagnosis of breast cancer during COVID-19.

11.4 The role of AI in treatment of breast cancer

Chemotherapy, radiotherapy, immunotherapy and bone marrow transplant result in reduction of immunity and increase the risk of COVID-19 disease. It is important to consider breast cancer management during this pandemic because existing patients who have gone through the above treatments are more vulnerable to COVID-19. Classification of patients for treatment based on risk, comorbidity, health resources and hormone status of breast cancer are included in breast cancer management

Table 11.2. Analysis of AI applications in breast cancer.

Sr. No.	AI Models	Usage (%)
1	Support vector machine (SVM)	42
2	Neural network	31
3	Discriminant analysis	8
4	Nearest neighbour	3
5	Linear regression	3
6	Logistic regression	2
7	Naive Bayes	2
8	Random forest	1
9	Others	8

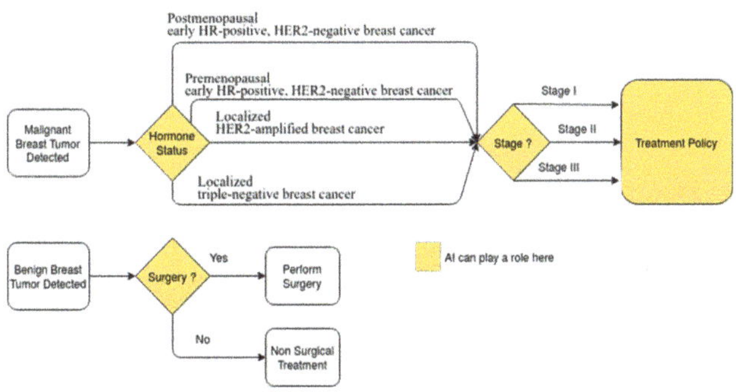

Figure 11.7. Role of AI in treatment of breast cancer before COVID-19.

policies during COVID-19 [6, 94, 130]. The role of AI in treatment of breast cancer before COVID-19 is shown in figure 11.7. All benign and secondary reconstruction surgeries should be delayed to avoid long surgeries and hospitalization [131]. Impact of COVID-19 on diagnosis of breast cancer and think about doubling time of tumor before taking post diagnosis decisions [132]. Detailed diagnosis, treatment and monitoring strategies for triple-negative, HER2-positive, hormone receptor positive cases are described in [11]. Cancer management challenges and strategies are proposed for low- and middle-income countries (LMICs) in [51]. The negative effects of COVID-19 pandemic will be worst for cancer management in LMICs due to the following reasons [51].

One should delay lengthy, complex surgeries and prefer telephonic or teleconferencing for meetings to reduce risk of COVID-19 in breast cancer patients [131]. The MRI machine should be avoided due to complexity in its disinfection process [131].

Newly diagnosed post-menopausal early HR-positive, HER2-negative breast cancer typical management before pandemic and modified management, during the pandemic are represented by figure 11.8 [12]. Newly diagnosed pre-menopausal early HR-positive, HER2-negative breast cancer typical management before the

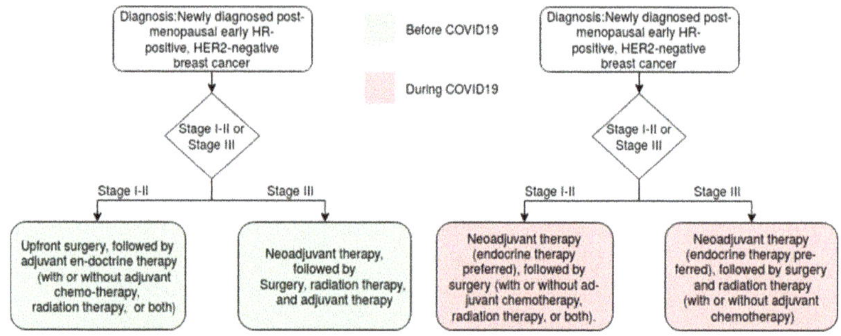

Figure 11.8. Newly diagnosed post-menopausal early HR-positive, HER2-negative breast cancer: (left) typical management before the pandemic; (right) modified management during the pandemic.

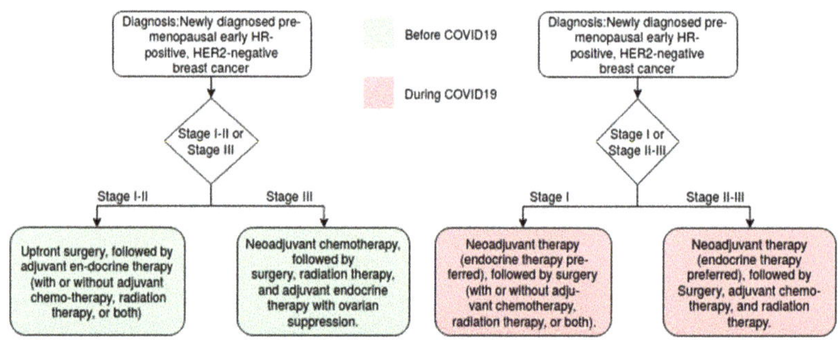

Figure 11.9. Newly diagnosed pre-menopausal early HR-positive, HER2-negative breast cancer: (left) typical management, before the pandemic; (right) modified management, during the pandemic.

pandemic, and modified management during the pandemic are represented by figure 11.9 [12]. Newly diagnosed localized HER2-amplified breast cancer typical management before the pandemic and modified management during the pandemic using an AI system can easily adapt to changes due to the pandemic situation or even other crises [17, 56].

(i) Cancer is diagnosed at an advanced stage in LMIC countries; (ii) there is delay in cancer diagnosis and treatment due to limited healthcare resources; (iii) COVID-19 patient management affects cancer management; (iv) the economic impact of the COVID-19 pandemic affects investment in cancer management. Breast cancer management and treatment guidelines based on breast cancer subtypes are proposed by considering the COVID-19 pandemic in Spain [9]. Authors from different countries with different stages of the COVID-19 pandemic have suggested to keep breast cancer surgical treatment simple and reconstruction, autologous, complex oncoplastic should be delayed [133]. High efficiency of breast cancer management and treatment guidelines based on breast cancer subtypes are proposed by considering the COVID-19 pandemic in Spain [9].

High efficiency same day breast reconstruction approach is proposed with less healthcare resources and 5.02 ± 1.29 h discharge time after completion of surgery [34]. This same day approach is useful to reduce the breast cancer patient's exposure to corona virus during this pandemic. 151 women with breast cancer have filled in a cross-sectional online survey with questionnaires on perceived health status, perceived susceptibility to anxiety, coping resources, health services utilization (contact with healthcare professionals and cancellation of an appointment by the oncology/haematology clinic), and socio-demographics [32]. Breast cancer patients, especially with comorbidity, have reduced their physical contacts with healthcare professionals during this pandemic period [32]. An interesting case study of a 62 year-old Italian early breast cancer patient is published with detailed subtype based breast cancer management during the pandemic in [11]. This pandemic has resulted in a lack of healthcare resources, higher risk for breast cancer patients, significant changes in decision making processes of breast cancer diagnosis, treatment and monitoring.

All the AI techniques used for breast cancer management (diagnosis, treatment and monitoring) are in the research phase so there is no standard adopted by the breast cancer community. We have a proposed general AI system to manage breast cancer under all circumstances including the current pandemic. Newly diagnosed localized HER2-amplified breast cancer typical management before the pandemic and modified management during the pandemic are represented by figure 11.10 [12]. Newly diagnosed localized triple-negative breast cancer typical management before the pandemic and modified management during the pandemic are represented by figure 11.11 [12]. The impact of AI is proposed on patients and breast cancer care including lack of healthcare resources and dilemma of patients due to this unforeseen pandemic [8]. Primary ER+ HER2− breast cancer management is proposed by using evidence-based guidelines in [7]. Detailed guidelines are proposed for diagnosis and treatment by considering breast cancer subtypes [7]. The surgery selection criteria are proposed which prioritize the treatment of malignant breast lesions at immediate risk of life [5]. Detailed guidelines for breast cancer patients are described by considering the possibility of next outbreak and load at the end of the pandemic [5]. Lung, colorectal and breast cancers are more susceptible to SARS-COV-2 virus according to the study of [134]. The role of AI in treatment of breast cancer during COVID-19 is shown in figure 11.12. Treatment and monitoring policy has two inputs based on COVID-19. Now, the treatment and monitoring policy is decided by considering the impact of COVID-19.

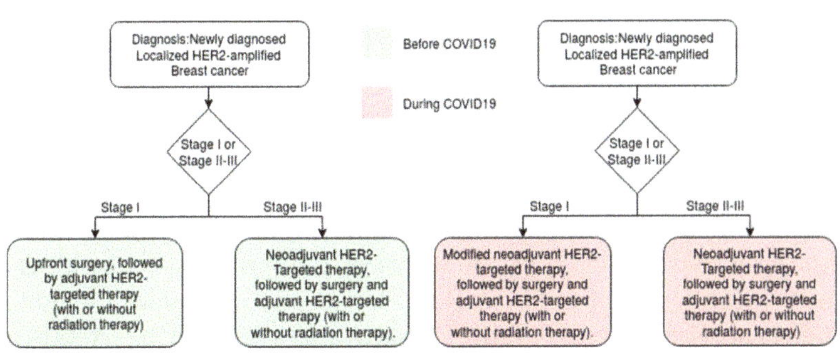

Figure 11.10. Newly diagnosed localized HER2-amplified breast cancer: (left) typical management, before the pandemic; (right) modified management, during the pandemic.

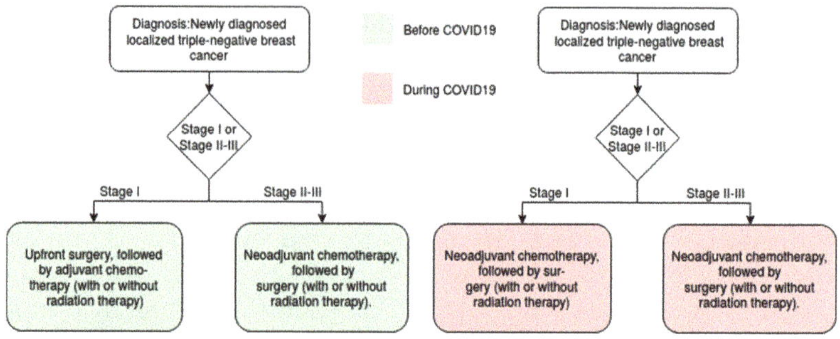

Figure 11.11. Newly diagnosed localized triple-negative breast cancer: (left) typical management, before pandemic; (right) modified management, during pandemic.

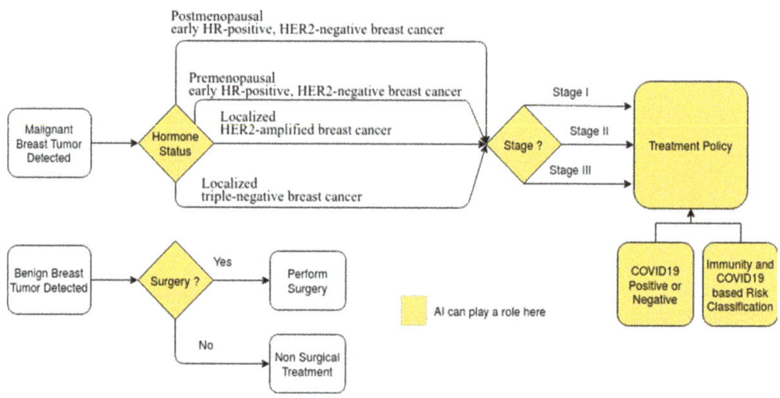

Figure 11.12. Role of artificial intelligence in treatment of breast cancer during COVID-19.

11.5 The role of AI in monitoring of breast cancer

Continuous monitoring of an existing breast cancer patient is also challenging during the emergency created by this pandemic. At the same time, diagnosis and treatment of new breast cancer patients are crucial during this pandemic. This pandemic has created an unforeseen crisis in breast cancer management including diagnosis, treatment and monitoring [6]. Breast cancer monitoring was mostly done through offline consultation before this COVID-19 pandemic. There are two main changes in the breast cancer monitoring process during this COVID-19 pandemic. Most patients have preferred online consultation and immunity monitoring is now part of breast cancer monitoring due to COVID-19 risk [32]. Monitoring is done to check the health status of the patient during different stages of treatment. Patient monitoring is still manual and often done through online or offline consultation.

Monitoring is required to check the response and progress of treatment and it is helpful in the decision and policy making based on the patient's condition. The monitoring process before COVID-19 is shown in figure 11.13. A breast cancer monitoring system during COVID-19 is shown in figure 11.14. Online consultation and immunity observation are two important aspects of monitoring during this

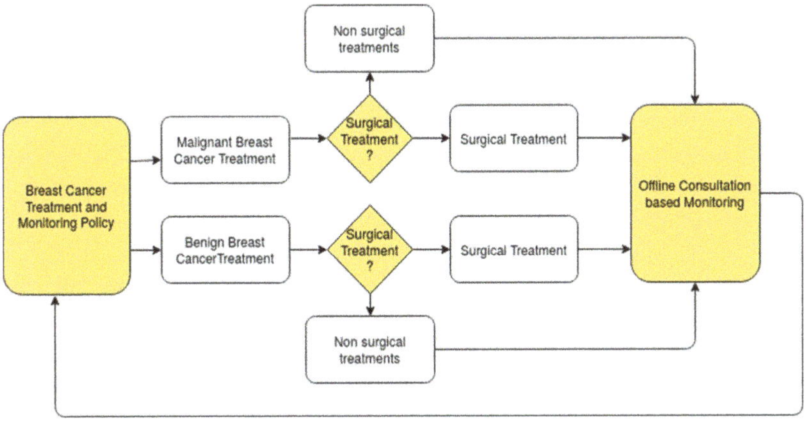

Figure 11.13. Role of AI in monitoring of breast cancer before COVID-19.

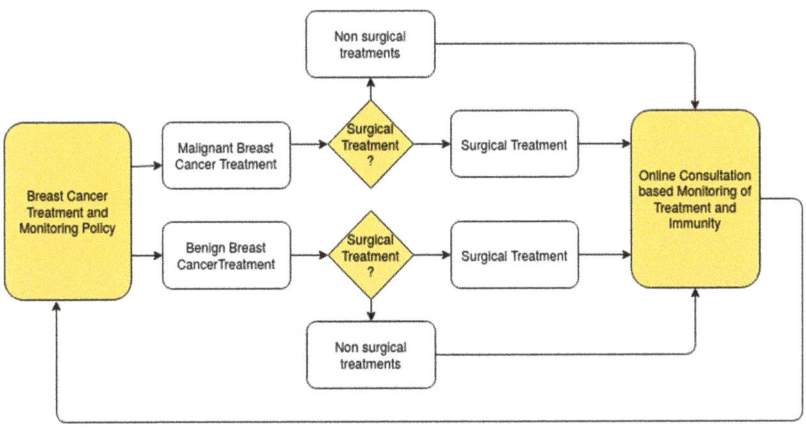

Figure 11.14. Role of AI in monitoring of breast cancer during COVID-19.

pandemic. Telemedicine can play a role in the monitoring of breast cancer by providing data through wearable devices and special mobile applications [135, 136]. Data collected by telemedicine can be used to train an AI model for monitoring of breast cancer patients.

11.6 AI based integrated system for breast cancer management

There are lots of research articles available on AI based diagnosis of breast cancer. At the same time, there are only few articles available on AI based treatment and monitoring of breast cancer. There are very few articles which integrate AI based diagnosis, treatment and monitoring for breast cancer management. Breast cancer patients are in dilemma about their visits to hospitals during this pandemic. Breast cancer management can be done in a better way by using AI as an enabler. Most of the literature has focused on applications of AI in diagnosis, treatment and monitoring. Only few articles have focused on using AI to develop a breast cancer management system which integrates diagnosis, treatment and monitoring. Bi *et al* have proposed AI in cancer imaging with clinical challenges and applications which covers lung, brain, breast, and prostate cancers [118]. A breast screening system is used to generate images of breasts by using different imaging modalities. Then the AI classifier detects the presence of the tumor in breast images. If a tumor is not detected then the patient may have to go through breast screening in future. If a tumor is detected then the AI classifier characterizes the tumor as either benign or malignant. If the tumor is found to be benign then treatment and monitoring AI models take the decision of surgery or another diagnostic procedure. The important characteristic of this system is its adaptive nature to include a benign tumour as well as the impact of the treatment even in this pandemic. Surgeries can be delayed in the case of a benign tumor during a pandemic. An AI model can be added to the treatment part of a benign tumor and this model can be trained with existing data to take surgery related decisions during this pandemic. A monitoring AI model can assist doctors to track the growth of a malignant tumor that has been detected by the AI model then monitoring and treatment decisions are taken by the AI model, which is trained specifically for malignant tumor cases.

Subtype based classification is described above with different treatment options before as well as during this pandemic. There are four subtypes: (I) newly diagnosed post-menopausal early HR-positive, HER2-negative breast cancer; (II) Newly diagnosed pre-menopausal early HR-positive, HER2-negative breast cancer; (III) newly diagnosed localized HER2-amplified breast cancer; (IV) newly diagnosed localized triple-negative breast cancer. As per figure 11.15, an AI model of detailed characterization can classify patients in different categories and treatment decisions

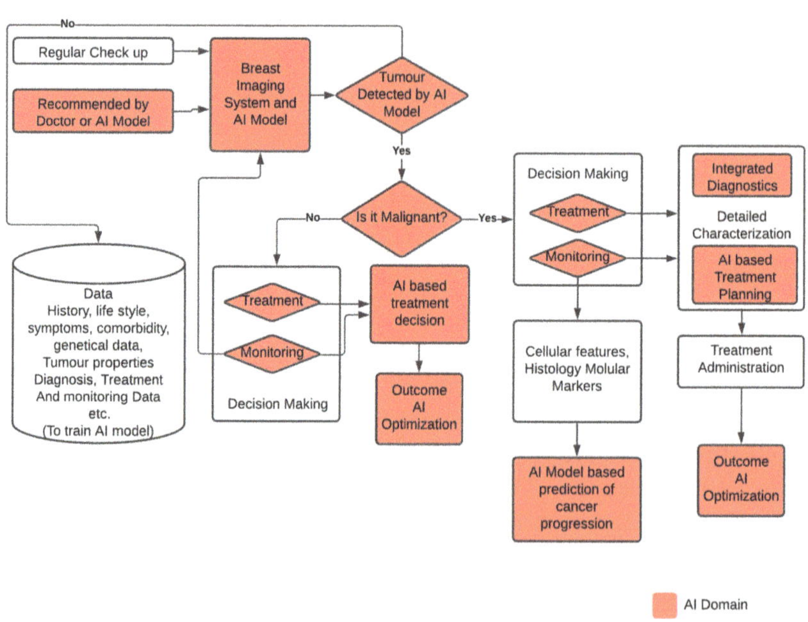

Figure 11.15. AI based diagnosis, treatment and monitoring system for breast cancer.

are taken based on suggestions of an AI model of treatment planning before as well as during the pandemic. Figures 11.6, 11.12 and 11.14 are included as a part of the architecture of figure 11.15. If hospitals or certain care centres decide to use their own data to train AI models for this breast cancer management system then this can be done with this proposed system. The monitoring part of the AI model uses cellular, histology and molecular markers as features and predicts progression of malignant breast cancer. These treatment and monitoring AI models assist doctors to take breast cancer decisions even during the pandemic with some overheads of adding a new trained model. Our proposed AI based diagnosis, treatment and monitoring system is robust, adaptive and modular. New AI models can be added without any effect on the working of current AI models. Our state-of-the-art AI system can improve breast cancer management and it becomes better with time. All the AI techniques used for breast cancer management (diagnosis, treatment and monitoring) are in the research phase so there is no standard adopted by the breast cancer community. We have proposed a general AI system to manage breast cancer under all circumstances including the current pandemic. There is a clear need for an adaptive, robust and modular AI system for the management of breast cancer which can deal with this pandemic as well as other emergencies that greatly impact breast cancer patients.

11.7 Summary

The pandemic has forced the healthcare industry to set new healthcare policies and guidelines for breast cancer patients. It is impossible for humans to make decisions by considering comorbidity, genetic history, lifestyle, other medical problems etc. This pandemic has impacted diagnosis, treatment and monitoring of breast cancer patients such that the new guidelines and policies are designed to deal with breast cancer patients. Breast cancer patients are also at high risk of infection due to ongoing treatment and comorbidity. Our proposed state-of-the-art AI system has the ability to manage breast cancer in all circumstances including this pandemic or any other emergencies. Our proposed AI system has the ability to apply new guidelines and policies without changing or affecting current working of the system. As a future work, we would like to do research on individual AI components of this whole breast cancer management system.

References

[1] Ferlay J *et al* 2019 Estimating the global cancer incidence and mortality in 2018: GLOBOCAN sources and methods *Int. J. Cancer* **144** 1941–53

[2] Zheng Z *et al* 2016 Annual medical expenditure and productivity loss among colorectal, female breast, and prostate cancer survivors in the United States *J. Natl. Cancer Inst.* **108** djv382

[3] Ginsburg O *et al* 2017 The global burden of women's cancers: a grand challenge in global health *Lancet* **389** 847–60

[4] Dai M *et al* 2020 Patients with cancer appear more vulnerable to SARS-CoV-2: a multicenter study during the COVID-19 outbreak *Cancer Discov.* **10** 783–91

[5] Casella D *et al* 2020 The patient's pathway for breast cancer in the COVID-19 era: an Italian single-center experience *Breast J.* **26** 1589–92
[6] Citgez B *et al* 2020 Management of breast cancer during the COVID-19 pandemic *Med. Bull. Sisli Etfal Hospital* **54** 132
[7] Dowsett M *et al* 2020 Evidence-based guidelines for managing patients with primary ER+ HER2− breast cancer deferred from surgery due to the COVID-19 pandemic *Breast Cancer* **6** 1–10
[8] Ghidinelli F and Bianchi A 2020 COVID-19 and breast cancer: impact on patients and breast care centers *Eur. J. Surg. Oncol.* **46** P2158–9
[9] Martin M *et al* 2020 GEICAM Guidelines for the management of patients with breast cancer during the COVID-19 pandemic in Spain *Oncologist* **25** e1339–45
[10] Poggio F *et al* 2020 Assessing the impact of the COVID-19 outbreak on the attitudes and practice of Italian oncologists toward breast cancer care and related research activities *JCO Oncol. Pract.* **16** e1304–14
[11] Sheng J Y *et al* 2020 Management of breast cancer during the COVID-19 pandemic: a stage-and subtype-specific approach *JCO Oncol. Pract.* **16** 665–74
[12] Spring L M *et al* 2020 Case 22-2020: A 62-year-old woman with early breast cancer during the Covid-19 pandemic *N. Engl. J. Med.* **383** 262–72
[13] Vanni G *et al* 2020 Breast cancer diagnosis in coronavirus-era: alert from Italy *Front. Oncol.* **10** 938
[14] Patel H N 2019 Microwave imaging for breast cancer detection using 3D level set based optimization, FDTD method and method of moments *PhD Thesis* Dhirubhai Ambani Institute of Information and Communication Technology
[15] Alimadadi A *et al* 2020 *Artificial Intelligence and Machine Learning to Fight COVID-19* (Bethesda, MD: American Physiological Society)
[16] Jamshidi M *et al* 2020 Artificial intelligence and COVID-19: deep learning approaches for diagnosis and treatment *IEEE Access* **8** 109581–95
[17] Lalmuanawma S, Hussain J and Chhakchhuak L 2020 Applications of machine learning and artificial intelligence for Covid-19 (SARS-CoV-2) pandemic: a review *Chaos Solit. Fractals* **139** 110059
[18] Obeid J S *et al* 2020 An artificial intelligence approach to COVID-19 infection risk assessment in virtual visits: a case report *J. Am. Med.J. Am. Med. Inform. Assoc*
[19] Zhu J *et al* 2020 Deep transfer learning artificial intelligence accurately stages COVID-19 lung disease severity on portable chest radiographs *PLoS One* **15** e0236621
[20] Guillermin Y *et al* 2018 What does this mutation mean? The tools and pitfalls of variant interpretation in lymphoid malignancies *Int. J. Mol. Sci.* **19** 1251
[21] Rodriguez-Ruiz A *et al* 2019 Stand-alone artificial intelligence for breast cancer detection in mammography: comparison with 101 radiologists *J. Natl. Cancer Inst.* **111** 916–22
[22] Houssami N *et al* 2019 Artificial Intelligence (AI) for the early detection of breast cancer: a scoping review to assess AI's potential in breast screening practice *Expert Rev. Med. Devices* **16** 351–62
[23] Jiang Y *et al* 1999 Improving breast cancer diagnosis with computer-aided diagnosis *Acad. Radiol.* **6** 22–33
[24] McKinney S M *et al* 2020 International evaluation of an AI system for breast cancer screening *Nature* **577** 89–94

[25] Ahmed Z *et al* 2020 Artificial intelligence with multi-functional machine learning platform development for better healthcare and precision medicine *Database (Oxford)* **2020** baaa010
[26] Cruz-Roa A *et al* 2017 Accurate and reproducible invasive breast cancer detection in whole-slide images: a deep learning approach for quantifying tumor extent *Sci. Rep.* **7** 46450
[27] Lamy J B *et al* 2019 Explainable artificial intelligence for breast cancer: a visual case-based reasoning approach *Artif. Intell. Med.* **94** 42–53
[28] Rodriguez-Ruiz A *et al* 2019 Detection of breast cancer with mammography: effect of an artificial intelligence support system *Radiology* **290** 305–14
[29] Obeid J S *et al* 2020 An artificial intelligence approach to COVID-19 infection risk assessment in virtual visits: a case report *J. Am. Med. Inform. Assoc.* **27** 1321–5
[30] Al-Shamsi H O *et al* 2020 A practical approach to the management of cancer patients during the novel coronavirus disease 2019 (COVID-19) pandemic: an International Collaborative Group *Oncologist* **25** e936–45
[31] Belkacemi Y *et al* 2020 A review of the international early recommendations for departments organization and cancer management priorities during the global COVID-19 pandemic: applicability in low- and middle-income countries *Eur. J. Cancer.* **135** 130–46
[32] Shinan-Altman S, Levkovich I and Tavori G 2020 Healthcare utilization among breast cancer patients during the COVID-19 outbreak *Palliat. Support. Care* **18** 385–91
[33] Soran A, Gimbel M and Diego E 2020 Breast cancer diagnosis, treatment and follow-up during COVID-19 pandemic *Eur. J. Breast Health* **16** 86
[34] Specht M *et al* 2020 High-efficiency same-day approach to breast reconstruction during the COVID-19 crisis *Breast Cancer Res. Treat.* **182** 679–88
[35] Al-antari M A *et al* 2018 An automatic computer-aided diagnosis system for breast cancer in digital mammograms via deep belief network *J. Med. Biol. Eng* **38** 443–56
[36] Al-Masni M A *et al* 2018 Simultaneous detection and classification of breast masses in digital mammograms via a deep learning YOLO-based CAD system *Comput. Methods Programs Biomed.* **157** 85–94
[37] Antropova N, Huynh B Q and Giger M L 2017 A deep feature fusion methodology for breast cancer diagnosis demonstrated on three imaging modality datasets *Med. Phys.* **44** 5162–71
[38] Drukker K, Sennett C A and Giger M L 2014 Computerized detection of breast cancer on automated breast ultrasound imaging of women with dense breasts *Med. Phys.* **41** 012901
[39] Jiang Y *et al* 1999 Improving breast cancer diagnosis with computer-aided diagnosis *Acad. Radiol.* **6** 22–33
[40] Ng E Y *et al* 2002 Computerized detection of breast cancer with artificial intelligence and thermograms *J. Med. Eng. Technol.* **26** 152–7
[41] Rangayyan R M and Suri J S 2006 *Recent Advances in Breast Imaging, Mammography, and Computer-aided Diagnosis of Breast Cancer* (Bellingham, WA: SPIE Publications)
[42] Robertson S *et al* 2018 Digital image analysis in breast pathology: from image processing techniques to artificial intelligence *Transl. Res.* **194** 19–35
[43] Sadoughi F *et al* 2018 Artificial intelligence methods for the diagnosis of breast cancer by image processing: a review *Breast Cancer: Targets Ther.* **10** 219
[44] Sharma A, Kulshrestha S and Daniel S 2017 Machine learning approaches for breast cancer diagnosis and prognosis *2017 International Conference on Soft Computing and its Engineering Applications (icSoftComp)* (Piscataway, NJ: IEEE)

[45] Sheth D and Giger M L 2020 Artificial intelligence in the interpretation of breast cancer on MRI *J. Magn. Reson. Imaging.* **51** 1310–24
[46] Wu Y *et al* 1993 Artificial neural networks in mammography: application to decision making in the diagnosis of breast cancer *Radiology* **187** 81–7
[47] Xie J *et al* 2019 Deep learning based analysis of histopathological images of breast cancer *Front. Genet.* **10** 80
[48] Bi W L *et al* 2019 Artificial intelligence in cancer imaging: clinical challenges and applications *CA Cancer J. Clin.* **69** 127–57
[49] Jiang F *et al* 2017 Artificial intelligence in healthcare: past, present and future *Stroke Vasc. Neurol.* **2** 230–43
[50] Xu F *et al* 2019 Artificial intelligence treatment decision support for complex breast cancer among oncologists with varying expertise *JCO Clin. Cancer Inform.* **3** 1–15
[51] Belkacemi Y *et al* 2020 A review of the international early recommendations for departments organization and cancer management priorities during the global COVID-19 pandemic applicability in low- and middle-income countries *Eur. J. Cancer* **135** P130–46
[52] Chavez S *et al* 2020 Coronavirus Disease (COVID-19): a primer for emergency physicians *Am. J. Emerg. Med.* **44** 220–9
[53] Dai M *et al* 2020 Patients with cancer appear more vulnerable to SARS-COV-2: a multicenter study during the COVID-19 outbreak *Cancer Discov.* **10** 783–91
[54] Diao B *et al* 2020 Reduction and functional exhaustion of T cells in patients with coronavirus disease 2019 (COVID-19) *Front. Immunol.* **11** 827
[55] Omranipour R *et al* 2020 Recommendations for breast surgical care during COVID-19 outbreak in Iran: setting priorities of management *World Cancer Res. J.* **7** e158
[56] World Health Organization 2020 *Coronavirus disease 2019 (COVID-19): situation report 82* https://apps.who.int/iris/handle/10665/331780
[57] Salman F M and Abu-Naser S S 2020 Expert system for COVID-19 diagnosis *Int. J. Acad. Inform. Syst. Res. (IJAISR)* **4** 1–13
[58] Toraman S, Alakus T B and Turkoglu I 2020 Convolutional capsnet: a novel artificial neural network approach to detect COVID-19 disease from x-ray images using capsule networks *Chaos Solit. Fractals* **140** 110122
[59] Vuagnat P *et al* 2020 COVID-19 in breast cancer patients: a cohort at the Institut Curie hospitals in the Paris area *Breast Cancer Res.* **22** 1–10
[60] Wu Z and McGoogan J M 2020 Characteristics of and important lessons from the coronavirus disease 2019 (COVID-19) outbreak in China: summary of a report of 72 314 cases from the Chinese Center for Disease Control and Prevention *JAMA* **323** 1239–42
[61] Zheng M *et al* 2020 Functional exhaustion of antiviral lymphocytes in COVID-19 patients *Cell. Mol. Immunol.* **17** 533–5
[62] Albarqouni S *et al* 2016 Aggnet: deep learning from crowds for mitosis detection in breast cancer histology images *IEEE Trans. Med. Imaging* **35** 1313–21
[63] Bejnordi B E *et al* 2017 Diagnostic assessment of deep learning algorithms for detection of lymph node metastases in women with breast cancer *JAMA* **318** 2199–210
[64] Cruz-Roa A *et al* 2017 Accurate and reproducible invasive breast cancer detection in whole-slide images: a deep learning approach for quantifying tumor extent *Sci. Rep.* **7** 46450
[65] Drukker K, Sennett C A and Giger M L 2014 Computerized detection of breast cancer on automated breast ultrasound imaging of women with dense breasts *Med. Phys.* **41** 012901
[66] Gardezi S J S *et al* 2019 Breast cancer detection and diagnosis using mammographic data: systematic review *J. Med. Internet Res.* **21** e14464

[67] Houssami N *et al* 2019 Artificial Intelligence (AI) for the early detection of breast cancer: a scoping review to assess AI's potential in breast screening practice *Expert Rev. Med. Devices* **16** 351–62
[68] Kharya S, Dubey D and Soni S 2013 Predictive machine learning techniques for breast cancer detection *Int. J. Comput. Sci. Inform. Technol.* **4** 1023–8
[69] Ng E-K *et al* 2002 Computerized detection of breast cancer with artificial intelligence and thermograms *J. Med. Eng. Technol.* **26** 152–7
[70] Rodríguez-Ruiz A *et al* 2019 Detection of breast cancer with mammography: effect of an artificial intelligence support system *Radiology* **290** 305–14
[71] Sahiner B *et al* 2012 Computer-aided detection of clustered microcalcifications in digital breast tomosynthesis: a 3D approach *Med. Phys.* **39** 28–39
[72] Shen L *et al* 2019 Deep learning to improve breast cancer detection on screening mammography *Sci. Rep.* **9** 1–12
[73] Chen W *et al* 2016 Cancer statistics in China *CA: Cancer J. Clin.* **66** 115–32
[74] Kamboj M and Sepkowitz K A 2009 Nosocomial infections in patients with cancer *Lancet Oncol.* **10** 589–97
[75] Paules C I, Marston H D and Fauci A S 2020 Coronavirus infections—more than just the common cold *JAMA* **323** 707–8
[76] Centers for Disease Control and Prevention 2016 People at high risk of developing flu-related complications http://www. cdc. gov/h1n1flu/highrisk.htm
[77] Centers for Disease Control and Prevention *et al* 2020 Coronavirus disease 2019 in children —United States *Morbidity and Mortality Weekly Report (MMWR)* **69** 422–6
[78] Liang W *et al* 2020 Cancer patients in SARS-CoV-2 infection: a nationwide analysis in China *Lancet Oncol.* **21** 335–7
[79] Raab M S, Breitkreutz P K, Richardson I and Anderson P G 2009 Multiple myeloma *Lancet* **374** 324–39
[80] Lainey E *et al* 2013 EGFR inhibitors exacerbate differentiation and cell cycle arrest induced by retinoic acid and vitamin D3 in acute myeloid leukemia cells *Cell Cycle* **12** 2978–91
[81] Zheng R *et al* 2019 Report of cancer epidemiology in China *Zhonghua zhong liu za zhi [Chin. J. Oncol.]* **41** 19–28
[82] Travlos G S 2006 Normal structure, function, and histology of the bone marrow *Toxicol. Pathol.* **34** 548–65
[83] Hijano D R, Maron G and Hayden R T 2018 Respiratory viral infections in patients with cancer or undergoing hematopoietic cell transplant *Front. Microbiol.* **9** 3097
[84] Kim Y-J *et al* 2014 Respiratory syncytial virus in hematopoietic cell transplant recipients: factors determining progression to lower respiratory tract disease *J. Infect. Dis.* **209** 1195–204
[85] Ménétrier-Caux C *et al* 2019 Lymphopenia in cancer patients and its effects on response to immunotherapy: an opportunity for combination with cytokines? *J. Immunother. Cancer* **7** 1–15
[86] Ellsworth S G 2018 Field size effects on the risk and severity of treatment-induced lymphopenia in patients undergoing radiation therapy for solid tumors *Adv. Radiat. Oncol.* **3** 512–9
[87] Lewis A L *et al* 2020 Immune checkpoint inhibitors: a narrative review of considerations for the anaesthesiologist *Br. J. Anaesth.* **124** 251–60

[88] Weber J S *et al* 2015 Toxicities of immunotherapy for the practitioner *J. Clin. Oncol.* **33** 2092
[89] Echeverry G, Fischer G W and Mead E 2019 Next generation of cancer treatments: chimeric antigen receptor t-cell therapy and its related toxicities: a review for perioperative physicians *Anesth. Analg.* **129** 434–41
[90] Hakim H *et al* 2016 Acute respiratory infections in children and adolescents with acute lymphoblastic leukemia *Cancer* **122** 798–805
[91] Fisher B T *et al* 2018 A multicenter consortium to define the epidemiology and outcomes of inpatient respiratory viral infections in pediatric hematopoietic stem cell transplant recipients *J. Pediatric Infect. Dis. Soc.* **7** 275–82
[92] Ogonek J *et al* 2016 Immune reconstitution after allogeneic hematopoietic stem cell transplantation *Front. Immunol.* **7** 507
[93] Sadoughi F *et al* 2018 Artificial intelligence methods for the diagnosis of breast cancer by image processing: a review *Breast Cancer* **10** 219–30
[94] Sherbet G V, Woo W L and Dlay S 2018 Application of artificial intelligence-based technology in cancer management: a commentary on the deployment of artificial neural networks *Anticancer Res.* **38** 6607–13
[95] Wu Y *et al* 1993 Artificial neural networks in mammography: application to decision making in the diagnosis of breast cancer *Radiology* **187** 81–7
[96] Al-Masni M A *et al* 2018 Simultaneous detection and classification of breast masses in digital mammograms via a deep learning YOLO-based CAD system *Comput. Methods Programs Biomed.* **157** 85–94
[97] Coccia M 2020 Deep learning technology for improving cancer care in society: New directions in cancer imaging driven by artificial intelligence *Technol. Soc.* **60** 101198
[98] Danaee P, Ghaeini R and Hendrix D A 2017 A deep learning approach for cancer detection and relevant gene identification *Pacific Sympos. on Biocomputing 2017* (Singapore: World Scientific)
[99] Fakoor R *et al* 2013 Using deep learning to enhance cancer diagnosis and classification *Proceedings of the Int. Conf. on Machine Learning* (New York: ACM)
[100] Huynh B Q, Li H and Giger M L 2016 Digital mammographic tumor classification using transfer learning from deep convolutional neural networks *J. Med. Imaging* **3** 034501
[101] Li H *et al* 2017 Deep learning in breast cancer risk assessment: evaluation of convolutional neural networks on a clinical dataset of full-field digital mammograms *J. Med. Imaging* **4** 041304
[102] Mahmud M *et al* 2018 Applications of deep learning and reinforcement learning to biological data *IEEE Trans. Neural Netw. Learn. Syst.* **29** 2063–79
[103] Maicas G *et al* 2017 Deep reinforcement learning for active breast lesion detection from DCE-MRI *Int. Conf. on Medical Image Computing and Computer-assisted Intervention* (Berlin: Springer)
[104] Shen L *et al* 2019 Deep learning to improve breast cancer detection on screening mammography *Sci. Rep.* **9** 12495
[105] Wei B *et al* 2017 Deep learning model based breast cancer histopathological image classification *IEEE 2017 2nd Int. Conf. on Cloud Computing and Big Data Analysis (ICCCBDA)* (Piscataway, NJ: IEEE)
[106] Biswas A, Al Nazi Z and Abir T A 2019 Invasive ductal carcinoma detection by a gated recurrent unit network with self attention *2019 4th Int. Conf. on Electrical Information and Communication Technology (EICT)*

[107] Yang Y, Fasching P A and Tresp V 2017 Predictive modeling of therapy decisions in metastatic breast cancer with recurrent neural network encoder and multinomial hierarchical regression decoder *IEEE 2017 Int. Conf. on Healthcare Informatics (ICHI)* (Piscataway, NJ: IEEE)
[108] Yang Y, Fasching P A and Tresp V 2017 Modeling progression free survival in breast cancer with tensorized recurrent neural networks and accelerated failure time models *Machine Learning for Healthcare Conf.*
[109] Guo Y *et al* 2006 Breast image registration techniques: a survey *Med. Biol. Eng. Comput.* **44** 15–26
[110] Huang S-F *et al* 2008 Analysis of tumor vascularity using three-dimensional power Doppler ultrasound images *IEEE Trans. Med. Imaging* **27** 320–30
[111] Ng Y *et al* 2013 *Multimodality Breast Imaging* (Bellingham, WA: SPIE Press)
[112] Singh B K *et al* 2017 Risk stratification of 2D ultrasound-based breast lesions using hybrid feature selection in machine learning paradigm *Measurement* **105** 146–57
[113] Sun Y *et al* 2006 A new approach for breast skin-line estimation in mammograms *Pattern Anal. Appl.* **9** 34
[114] Chen W *et al* 2007 Volumetric texture analysis of breast lesions on contrast-enhanced magnetic resonance images *Magn. Reson. Med.* **58** 562–71
[115] Guo Y *et al* 2006 Breast image registration techniques: a survey *Med. Biol. Eng. Comput.* **44** 15–26
[116] Robertson S *et al* 2018 Digital image analysis in breast pathology—from image processing techniques to artificial intelligence *Transl. Res.* **194** 19–35
[117] Patel H N and Ghodgaonkar D K 2017 3D level set based optimization of inverse scattering problem for microwave breast imaging *IEEE 2017 First MTT-S Int. Microwave Bio Conf. (IMBIOC)* (Piscataway, N J: IEEE)
[118] Bi W L *et al* 2019 Artificial intelligence in cancer imaging: clinical challenges and applications *CA: Cancer J. Clin.* **69** 127–57
[119] Zhang W *et al* 1994 Computerized detection of clustered microcalcifications in digital mammograms using a shift-invariant artificial neural network *Med. Phys.* **21** 517–24
[120] Karssemeijer N *et al* 2006 Computer aided detection of masses in mammograms as decision support *Br. J. Radiol.* **79** S123–6
[121] Reiser I *et al* 2006 Computerized mass detection for digital breast tomosynthesis directly from the projection images *Med. Phys.* **33** 482–91
[122] Sahiner B *et al* 2012 Computer-aided detection of clustered microcalcifications in digital breast tomosynthesis: a 3D approach *Med. Phys.* **39** 28–39
[123] Gilhuijs K G, Giger M L and Bick U 1998 Computerized analysis of breast lesions in three dimensions using dynamic magnetic-resonance imaging *Med. Phys.* **25** 1647–54
[124] Chen W *et al* 2007 Volumetric texture analysis of breast lesions on contrast-enhanced magnetic resonance images *Magn. Reson. Medi.* **58** 562–71
[125] Bhooshan N *et al* 2010 Cancerous breast lesions on dynamic contrast-enhanced MR images: computerized characterization for image-based prognostic markers *Radiology* **254** 680–90
[126] Jamieson A R *et al* 2010 Exploring nonlinear feature space dimension reduction and data representation in breast CADx with Laplacian eigenmaps and t-SNE *Med. Phys.* **37** 339–51
[127] Nielsen M *et al* 2011 A novel and automatic mammographic texture resemblance marker is an independent risk factor for breast cancer *Cancer Epidemiol.* **35** 381–7

[128] Gierach G L *et al* 2014 Relationships between computer-extracted mammographic texture pattern features and BRCA1/2mutation status: a cross-sectional study *Breast Cancer Res.* **16** 424

[129] Li H *et al* 2016 Quantitative MRI radiomics in the prediction of molecular classifications of breast cancer subtypes in the TCGA/TCIA data set *NPJ Breast Cancer* **2** 1–10

[130] Fisher B T *et al* 2018 A multicenter consortium to define the epidemiology and outcomes of inpatient respiratory viral infections in pediatric hematopoietic stem cell transplant recipients *J. Pediatric Infect. Dis. Soc.* **7** 275–82

[131] Daraï E, Mathelin C and Gligorov J *et al* 2020 Breast cancer diagnosis in coronavirus-era: alert from Italy *Eur. J. Breast Health* **16** 160

[132] Vanni G *et al* 2020 Breast cancer diagnosis in coronavirus-era: alert from Italy *Front. Oncol.* **10** 938

[133] Vidya R *et al* 2020 Should breast reconstruction and breast oncoplastic procedures be performed during the coronavirus pandemic? *Ecancermedicalscience* **11** 1041

[134] Wang B and Huang Y 2020 Which type of cancer patients are more susceptible to the SARS-COX-2: evidence from a meta-analysis and bioinformatics analysis *Crit. Rev. Oncol./ Hematol.* **153** 103032

[135] Chung I Y *et al* 2019 An assessment of physical activity data collected via a smartphone app and a smart band in breast cancer survivors: observational study *J. Med. Internet Res.* **21** e13463

[136] Dorri S *et al* 2020 A Systematic Review of Electronic Health (eHealth) interventions to improve physical activity in patients with breast cancer *Breast Cancer* **27** 25–46

IOP Publishing

Breast Image Reconstruction and Cancer Detection Using Microwave Imaging

Hardik N Patel, Deepak K Ghodgaonkar and Jasjit S Suri

Appendix A

Numerical breast phantom, antenna placement and immersion (surrounding) medium

A.1 Numerical breast phantom

Anatomically realistic numerical breast phantoms are required to make a reliable microwave breast imaging system. A 3D view of class III numerical breast phantom is shown in figure A.1 [1]. Breast density classification is discussed in the introduction. Class III or class IV numerical breast phantoms are an obvious choice for testing a microwave breast imaging system. *Y–Z*, *X–Z*, and *X–Y* views of class III numerical breast phantom are shown in figure A.2. Fibro-glandular tissues are represented by white (bright) colour and adipose tissues are represented by black or gray (dark) colour. An MRI derived numerical breast phantom makes an imaging system more realistic because it captures heterogeneity well. In a numerical breast phantom, dielectric properties of fibro-glandular and adipose breast tissues are assigned to regions with one and zero, respectively.

A.2 Antenna placement surrounding a numerical breast phantom

Antenna placement surrounding a numerical breast phantom for an inverse scattering problem formulation is discussed in this appendix. Antenna placement is shown in figure A.3. The middle point of a numerical breast phantom is the origin of the coordinate system. There are five rings of antennas around a numerical breast phantom [2]. Each circular ring has eight short dipoles of length 1 cm, which lead to 40 antennas in the system. The distance between two consecutive rings is 3 cm. The radius of each ring is 6 cm.

A.3 Immersion (surrounding) medium

A surrounding medium is required in a microwave breast imaging system for better matching with a human breast model. An oil based surrounding medium is

doi:10.1088/978-0-7503-2592-9ch12

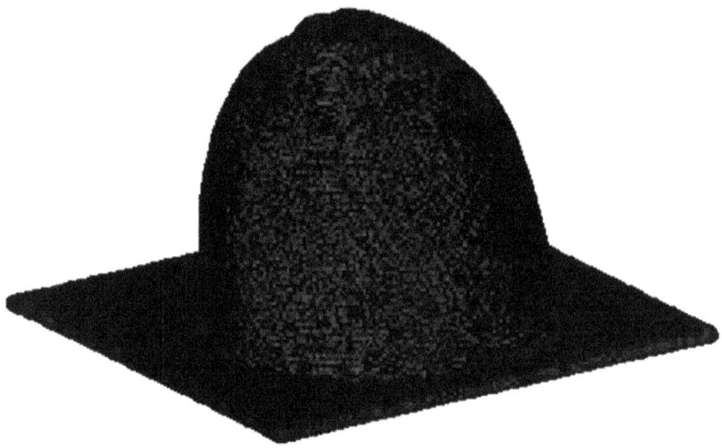

Figure A.1. 3D view of numerical breast phantom.

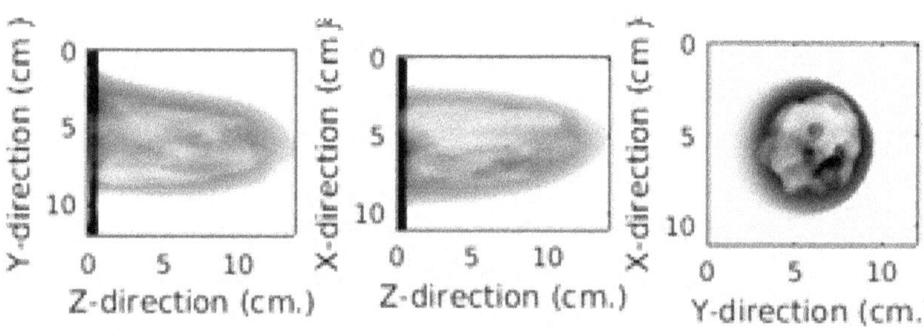

Figure A.2. *Y–Z*, *X–Z* and *X–Y* view of class 3 MRI derived numerical breast phantom.

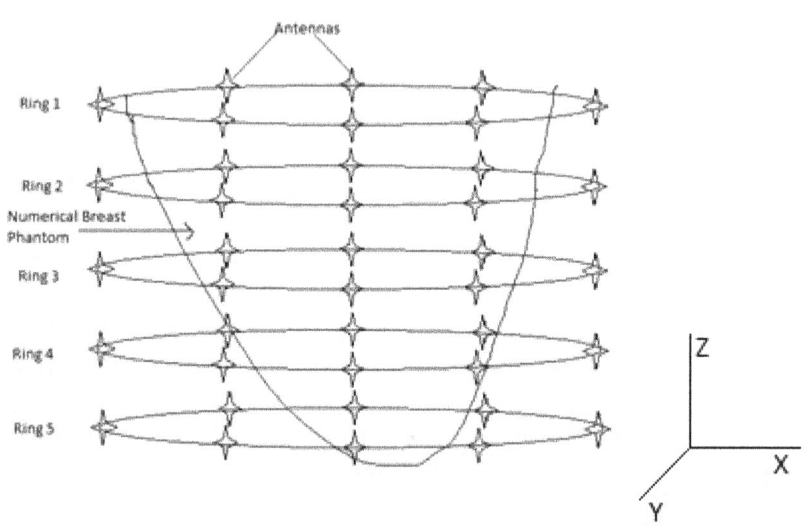

Figure A.3. Antenna placement surrounding the numerical breast phantom.

considered in this microwave breast imaging system [2, 3]. The infinite frequency permittivity (ϵ_{∞}) of this surrounding medium is 2.6 because it matches the average dielectric properties of the human breast tissues. Difference permittivity ($\Delta\epsilon$) and static conductivity (σ_s) are zero for this surrounding medium.

Method of moment is a frequency domain method. Saline is used as the surrounding medium in method of moments [4]. Performance of saline is better than air as surrounding medium because it provides better matching than air. Error in complex permittivity reconstruction is less for saline as the surrounding medium.

References

[1] Zastrow E, Davis S K, Lazebnik M, Kelcz F, Van Veen B D and Hagness S C 2008 Development of anatomically realistic numerical breast phantoms with accurate dielectric properties for modelling microwave interactions with the human breast *IEEE Trans. Biomed. Eng.* **55** 2792–800

[2] Shea J D, Kosmas P, Hagness S C and Van Veen B D 2010 Three-dimensional microwave imaging of realistic numerical breast phantoms via a multiple-frequency inverse scattering technique *Med. Phys.* **37** 4210–26

[3] Patel H N and Ghodgaonkar D K 2017 3D level set based optimization of inverse scattering problem for microwave breast imaging *IEEE MTT-S Int. Microwave Bio Conf., (15–17 May 2017, Gothenburg, Sweden)* 1–4

[4] Ghodgaonkar D K, Gandhi O P and Hagmann M J 1983 Estimation of complex permittivities of 3D inhomogeneous biological bodies *IEEE Trans. Microw. Theory Tech.* **31** 442–6

IOP Publishing

Hardik N Patel, Deepak K Ghodgaonkar and Jasjit S Suri

Appendix B

Important derivations

B.1 Debye model

The biological molecules are polar molecules with relaxation frequencies in the range of high frequency (HF) to microwave frequencies. Complex permittivity of human breast tissues is a function of temperature and frequency. Temperature is assumed to be constant. Dispersion and polarization effect of human breast tissues are incorporated by using a single-pole Debye model given by equation (B.4).

Transient response of dielectric medium is shown in figure B.1 [1]. D is electric displacement, τ is relaxation time constant. D_∞ is initial value of electric displacement. D_0 is final value of electric displacement. The situation of figure B.1 is expressed in terms of equation (B.1).

$$D = D_\infty + (D_0 - D_\infty)(1 - e^{-\frac{t}{\tau}}) \tag{B.1}$$

Now, equation (B.2) is obtained by substituting $D = \epsilon_0\epsilon_r E$, $D_\infty = \epsilon_0\epsilon_\infty E$ and $D_0 = \epsilon_0\epsilon_s E$ in equation (B.1).

$$\epsilon_r = \epsilon_\infty + (\epsilon_s - \epsilon_\infty)(1 - e^{-\frac{t}{\tau}}) \tag{B.2}$$

In equation (B.2), ϵ_r is relative permittivity, ϵ_∞ is infinite (high) frequency permittivity, ϵ_s is static (low) frequency permittivity. Now, equation (B.3) is obtained by applying Laplace transform to equation (B.2).

$$\frac{\epsilon_r}{s} = \frac{\epsilon_\infty}{s} + \frac{(\epsilon_s - \epsilon_\infty)}{s} - \frac{(\epsilon_s - \epsilon_\infty)}{s + \dfrac{1}{\tau}} \tag{B.3}$$

In order to obtain equation (B.4), equation (B.3) is simplified after multiplying both sides by s and substituting $s = j\omega$.

doi:10.1088/978-0-7503-2592-9ch13

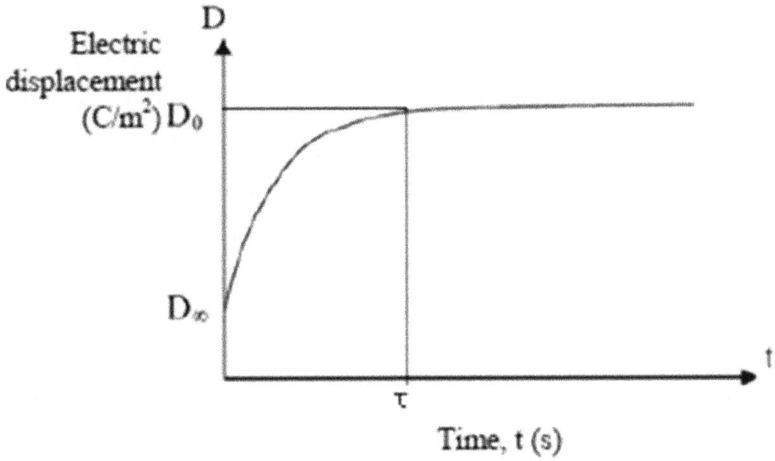

Figure B.1. Transient response of dielectric medium.

$$\epsilon_r = \epsilon_\infty + \frac{(\epsilon_s - \epsilon_\infty)}{1 + j\omega\tau} \tag{B.4}$$

B.2 Derivation of electric field update equations for numerical breast phantom region

The finite-difference time-domain (FDTD) electric field update equation is derived by using the polarization density equation. The polarization property of human breast tissues is included by substituting the Debye model into the Ampere's law equation. All derivations are done by assuming air as surrounding medium. In the case of a specific surrounding medium replace impedance and velocity of light values according to the surrounding medium.

$$\nabla \times \vec{H} = \epsilon_0 \epsilon_\infty j\omega \vec{E} + j\omega\epsilon_0 \frac{\Delta\epsilon}{1 + j\omega\tau}\vec{E} + \sigma_s \vec{E} \tag{B.5}$$

σ_s is static conductivity. $\Delta\epsilon$ is the difference between static permittivity and infinite permittivity. Equation (B.6) is obtained by rearranging equation (B.5).

$$\nabla \times \vec{H} = \epsilon_0 \epsilon_\infty j\omega \vec{E} ++ \sigma_s \vec{E} + j\omega\epsilon_0 \frac{\Delta\epsilon}{1 + j\omega\tau}\vec{E} \tag{B.6}$$

The polarization current density equation is important for derivation of the FDTD electric field update equations. The equation of polarization current density is given below.

$$\vec{J}_p = j\omega\epsilon_0 \frac{\Delta\epsilon}{1 + j\omega\tau}\vec{E} \tag{B.7}$$

$\vec{J}_{\mathrm{p}}$ is polarization current density vector and $\vec{E}$ is electric field intensity vector. Equation (B.8) is obtained by rearranging equation (B.7).

$$\vec{J}_{\mathrm{p}}(1 + j\omega\tau) = j\omega\epsilon_0\Delta\epsilon\vec{E} \tag{B.8}$$

By applying inverse Fourier transform.

$$\vec{J}_{\mathrm{p}} + \tau\frac{\partial\vec{J}_{\mathrm{p}}}{\partial t} = \epsilon_0\Delta\epsilon\frac{\partial\vec{E}}{\partial t} \tag{B.9}$$

Now, by applying FDTD [2] and rearranging the terms

$$\frac{\tau}{\Delta t}\vec{J}_P^{t+\Delta t}\left(1 + \frac{\Delta t}{2\tau}\right) = \frac{\tau}{\Delta t}\vec{J}_P^{t}\left(1 - \frac{\Delta t}{2\tau}\right) + \epsilon_0\Delta\epsilon\frac{\vec{E}_{t+\Delta t} - \vec{E}_t}{\Delta t} \tag{B.10}$$

Whatever the time-constant τ is, it can be expressed as a multiple of the time-step, $\tau = N_t\Delta t$ where N_t does not need to be an integer. Put $\tau = N_t\Delta t$ and multiplying both sides by $\Delta x = \delta$

$$\delta\vec{J}_P^{t+\Delta t} = \left(\frac{1 - \dfrac{1}{2N_t}}{1 + \dfrac{1}{2N_t}}\right)\delta\vec{J}_P^{t} + \left(\frac{\epsilon_0\Delta\epsilon\delta}{N_t\Delta t\cdot\left(1 + \dfrac{1}{2N_t}\right)}\right)(\vec{E}_{t+\Delta t} - \vec{E}_t) \tag{B.11}$$

$$\delta\vec{J}_P^{t+\Delta t} = (mj1)\delta\vec{J}_P^{t} + (mj2)(\vec{E}_{t+\Delta t} - \vec{E}_t) \tag{B.12}$$

Divide both sides by $\Delta x = \delta$ to get the polarization current density equation.

$$\delta\vec{J}_P^{t+\frac{\Delta t}{2}} = \frac{\delta\vec{J}_P^{t+\Delta t} + \delta\vec{J}_P^{t}}{2} \tag{B.13}$$

By applying inverse Fourier transform to equation (B.6)

$$\nabla\times\vec{H}_{t+\frac{\Delta t}{2}} = \epsilon_0\epsilon_\infty\frac{\partial\vec{E}}{\partial t} + \sigma_{\mathrm{s}}\vec{E} + \vec{J}_P^{t+\frac{\Delta t}{2}} \tag{B.14}$$

By applying FDTD and multiplying both sides by $\Delta x = \delta$.

$$\delta\nabla\times\vec{H}_{t+\frac{\Delta t}{2}} = \delta\epsilon_0\epsilon_\infty\frac{\vec{E}_{t+\Delta t} - \vec{E}_t}{\Delta t} + \delta\sigma_{\mathrm{s}}\frac{\vec{E}_{t+\Delta t} + \vec{E}_t}{2} + \delta\vec{J}_P^{t+\frac{\Delta t}{2}} \tag{B.15}$$

By substituting $\delta J_P^{t+\frac{\Delta t}{2}}$ in the above equation

$$\begin{aligned}\delta\nabla\times\vec{H}_{t+\frac{\Delta t}{2}} = \delta\epsilon_0\epsilon_\infty\frac{\vec{E}_{t+\Delta t} - \vec{E}_t}{\Delta t} + \delta\sigma_{\mathrm{s}}\frac{\vec{E}_{t+\Delta t} + \vec{E}_t}{2}\\ + 1/2[(1 + mj1)\delta\vec{J}_P^{t} + mj2(\vec{E}_{t+\Delta t} - \vec{E}_t)]\end{aligned} \tag{B.16}$$

By rearranging the above equation after normalizing electric field vector.

$$\frac{\delta\epsilon_0\epsilon_\infty}{\Delta t}\left(1+\frac{\sigma_s\Delta t}{2\epsilon_0\epsilon_\infty}+\frac{\Delta t\cdot mj2}{2\delta\epsilon_0\epsilon_\infty}\right)\vec{E}_{t+\Delta t}=\frac{\delta\epsilon_0\epsilon_\infty}{\Delta t}\left(1-\frac{\sigma_s\Delta t}{2\epsilon_0\epsilon_\infty}+\frac{\Delta t\cdot mj2}{2\delta\epsilon_0\epsilon_\infty}\right)\vec{E}_t + \frac{\delta}{\eta_0}\nabla\times\vec{H}_{t+\frac{\Delta t}{2}}-\frac{1}{2}(1+mj1)\delta\vec{J}_P^{\,t} \tag{B.17}$$

The electric field update equation is given by equation (B.18)

$$\vec{E}_{t+\Delta t}=\frac{\left(1-\frac{\sigma_s\Delta t}{2\epsilon_0\epsilon_\infty}+\frac{\Delta t\cdot mj2}{2\delta\epsilon_0\epsilon_\infty}\right)}{\left(1+\frac{\sigma_s\Delta t}{2\epsilon_0\epsilon_\infty}+\frac{\Delta t\cdot mj2}{2\delta\epsilon_0\epsilon_\infty}\right)}\vec{E}_t+\frac{c_0\Delta t}{2\delta\epsilon_\infty\left(1+\frac{\sigma_s\Delta t}{2\epsilon_0\epsilon_\infty}+\frac{\Delta t\cdot mj2}{2\delta\epsilon_0\epsilon_\infty}\right)}\cdot\left(2\delta\nabla\times\vec{H}_{t+\frac{\Delta t}{2}}-\eta_0(1+mj1)\delta\vec{J}_P^{\,t}\right) \tag{B.18}$$

By substituting $\frac{\left(1-\frac{\sigma_S\Delta t}{2\epsilon_0\epsilon_\infty}+\frac{\Delta t\cdot mj2}{2\delta\epsilon_0\epsilon_\infty}\right)}{\left(1+\frac{\sigma_S\Delta t}{2\epsilon_0\epsilon_\infty}+\frac{\Delta t\cdot mj2}{2\delta\epsilon_0\epsilon_\infty}\right)}=me1$ and $\frac{c_0\Delta t}{2\delta\epsilon_\infty\left(1+\frac{\sigma_S\Delta t}{2\epsilon_0\epsilon_\infty}+\frac{\Delta t\cdot mj2}{2\delta\epsilon_0\epsilon_\infty}\right)}=me2$

$$\vec{E}_{t+\Delta t}=me1\cdot\vec{E}_t+me2\cdot\left[\left(2\Delta x\cdot\nabla\times\vec{H}_{t+\frac{\Delta t}{2}}\right)-\left(\eta_0\cdot(1+mj1)\cdot\Delta x\cdot\vec{J}_P^{\,t}\right)\right] \tag{B.19}$$

B.3 Derivation of electric field update equations for PML region

A perfectly match layer (PML) is required at grid boundaries to avoid reflection of microwave signals in FDTD. Artificial losses in x-direction are given below [3, 4].

$$S_x=\begin{bmatrix}\left(1+\frac{\sigma_x}{j\omega\epsilon_0}\right)^{-1} & 0 & 0\\ 0 & \left(1+\frac{\sigma_x}{j\omega\epsilon_0}\right) & 0\\ 0 & 0 & \left(1+\frac{\sigma_x}{j\omega\epsilon_0}\right)\end{bmatrix} \tag{B.20}$$

σ_x in the above matrix is defined as below.

$$\sigma_x=\frac{0.5\epsilon_0}{\Delta t}\left(\frac{x}{L_x}\right)^3 \tag{B.21}$$

In the above equation, L_x is length of PML in x-direction. x is particular cell number of PML. Artificial losses in Y-direction are given below.

$$S_y = \begin{bmatrix} \left(1 + \frac{\sigma_y}{j\omega\epsilon_0}\right) & 0 & 0 \\ 0 & \left(1 + \frac{\sigma_y}{j\omega\epsilon_0}\right)^{-1} & 0 \\ 0 & 0 & \left(1 + \frac{\sigma_y}{j\omega\epsilon_0}\right) \end{bmatrix} \tag{B.22}$$

In the above equation, L_y is length of PML in z-direction. z is particular cell number of PML. Artificial losses in Z-direction are given below.

$$S_z = \begin{bmatrix} \left(1 + \frac{\sigma_z}{j\omega\epsilon_0}\right) & 0 & 0 \\ 0 & \left(1 + \frac{\sigma_z}{j\omega\epsilon_0}\right) & 0 \\ 0 & 0 & \left(1 + \frac{\sigma_z}{j\omega\epsilon_0}\right)^{-1} \end{bmatrix} \tag{B.23}$$

Artificial losses in all three directions can be combined as

$$[S] = [S_x][S_y][S_z] \tag{B.24}$$

The Ampere's law equation can be written to incorporate artificial losses in all directions.

$$\nabla \times \vec{H} = j\omega[S]\vec{D} \tag{B.25}$$

Writing the x component of the above equation after substituting $[S]$ in it.

$$j\omega\left(1 + \frac{\sigma_x}{j\omega\epsilon_0}\right)^{-1}\left(1 + \frac{\sigma_y}{j\omega\epsilon_0}\right)\left(1 + \frac{\sigma_z}{j\omega\epsilon_0}\right)D_x = \left[\frac{\partial H_z}{\partial y} - \frac{\partial H_y}{\partial z}\right] \tag{B.26}$$

By substituting $\left[\frac{\partial H_z}{\partial y} - \frac{\partial H_y}{\partial z}\right] = (CH)_x$ and rearranging the terms

$$j\omega\left(1 + \frac{\sigma_y}{j\omega\epsilon_0}\right)\left(1 + \frac{\sigma_z}{j\omega\epsilon_0}\right)D_x = \left(1 + \frac{\sigma_x}{j\omega\epsilon_0}\right)(CH)_x \tag{B.27}$$

equation (B.28) by simplifying equation (B.27).

$$j\omega D_x + \frac{\sigma_y + \sigma_z}{\epsilon_0}D_x + \frac{\sigma_y\sigma z}{j\omega\epsilon_0^2}D_x = (CH)_x + \frac{\sigma_x}{j\omega\epsilon_0}(CH)_x \tag{B.28}$$

By applying inverse Fourier transform

$$\frac{\partial}{\partial t}D_x + \frac{\sigma_y + \sigma_z}{\epsilon_0}D_x + \frac{\sigma_y \sigma z}{\epsilon_0^2}\int_{-\infty}^{t} D_x d\tau = (CH)_x + \frac{\sigma_x}{\epsilon_0}\int_{-\infty}^{t}(CH)_x d\tau \quad \text{(B.29)}$$

By applying FDTD and normalizing the electric field density component.

$$\frac{D_x^{t+\Delta t} - D_x^t}{\Delta t} + \frac{\sigma_y + \sigma_z}{\epsilon_0}\frac{D_x^{t+\Delta t} + D_x^t}{2} + \frac{\sigma_y \sigma_z \Delta t}{\epsilon_0^2}\left[\frac{D_x^{t+\Delta t} + D_x^t}{4} + \sum_{T=0}^{t} D_x\right] = c_0 CH_x + \frac{c_0 \sigma_x}{\epsilon_0}\sum_{T=0}^{t+\frac{\Delta t}{2}} CH_x \quad \text{(B.30)}$$

By rearranging the above equation.

$$D_x^{t+\Delta t} = \frac{\left(\frac{1}{\Delta t} - \frac{\sigma_y + \sigma_z}{2\epsilon_0} - \frac{\sigma_y \cdot \sigma_z \cdot \Delta t}{4\epsilon_0^2}\right)}{\left(\frac{1}{\Delta t} + \frac{\sigma_y + \sigma_z}{2\epsilon_0} + \frac{\sigma_y \cdot \sigma_z \cdot \Delta t}{4\epsilon_0^2}\right)} D_x^t + \frac{c_0 \cdot CH_x}{\left(\frac{1}{\Delta t} + \frac{\sigma_y + \sigma_z}{2\epsilon_0} + \frac{\sigma_y \cdot \sigma_z \cdot \Delta t}{4\epsilon_0^2}\right)} + \frac{c_0 \cdot \Delta t \cdot \sigma_x}{\left(\frac{1}{\Delta t} + \frac{\sigma_y + \sigma_z}{2\epsilon_0} + \frac{\sigma_y \cdot \sigma_z \cdot \Delta t}{4\epsilon_0^2}\right) \cdot \epsilon_0}(Ich)_x - \frac{\Delta t \cdot \sigma_y \cdot \sigma_z \cdot ID_x}{\left(\frac{1}{\Delta t} + \frac{\sigma_y + \sigma_z}{2\epsilon_0} + \frac{\sigma_y \cdot \sigma_z \cdot \Delta t}{4\epsilon_0^2}\right) \cdot \epsilon_0^2} \quad \text{(B.31)}$$

The electric field can be updated as given below.

$$E_x = \frac{D_x}{\epsilon_{xx}} \quad \text{(B.32)}$$

The electric field update equations in y- and z-directions are obtained by repeating the above procedure.

B.4 Power calculations

Power calculations are extremely important to validate the implementation. Steps are given below to calculate power [2].

- Transverse wave vector expansion

$$\vec{k}_{xy}(m, n) = k_x(m)\hat{x} + k_y(n)\hat{y} \quad \text{(B.33)}$$

$k_x(m)\hat{x}$ and $k_y(n)\hat{y}$ are wave vectors in the above equation.

$$k_x(m) = \frac{2\pi m}{S_x} \quad \text{(B.34)}$$

S_x is total number of cells in the x-direction. m is varying from $-S_x/2$ to $+S_x/2$.

$$k_y(n) = \frac{2\pi n}{S_y} \quad \text{(B.35)}$$

S_y is total number of cells in the y-direction. n is varying from $-S_y/2$ to $+S_y/2$.

- Longitudinal wave vector expansion for reflection and transmission.

$$k_{zr}(m, n) = \sqrt{(k_0 n_{\text{ref}})^2 - k_x^2(m) - k_y^2(n)} \tag{B.36}$$

$$k_{zt}(m, n) = \sqrt{(k_0 n_{\text{tm}})^2 - k_x^2(m) - k_y^2(n)} \tag{B.37}$$

k_0 is the wave number for free space. n_{ref} and n_{tm} are refractive indices of reflection and transmission, respectively, on the grid.
- Normalize reflected and transmitted fields using the source field
- Calculate spatial harmonics Sp_{x_r}, Sp_{y_r}, Sp_{x_t}, Sp_{y_t} by using fast Fourier transform.
- Now find Sp_z.

$$Sp_{z_r} = -(k_x. *Sp_{x_r} + k_y. *Sp_{y_r})./k_{zr} \tag{B.38}$$

$$Sp_{z_t} = -(k_x. *Sp_{x_t} + k_y. *Sp_{y_t})./k_{zt} \tag{B.39}$$

- Calculate diffraction efficiencies

$$Spref = abs(Sp_{x_r}).^2 + abs(Sp_{y_r}).^2 + abs(Sp_{z_r}).^2 \tag{B.40}$$

$$Sptrn = abs(Sp_{x_t}).^2 + abs(Sp_{y_t}).^2 + abs(Sp_{z_t}).^2 \tag{B.41}$$

$$ref = real(k_{zr}/kzinc). *Spref \tag{B.42}$$

$$trn = real(k_{zt}/kzinc). *Sptrn \tag{B.43}$$

$$REF(nfreq) = sum(ref(:)) \tag{B.44}$$

$$TRN(nfreq) = sum(trn(:)) \tag{B.45}$$

REF and *TRN* are reflected and transmitted powers due to numerical breast phantom.

References

[1] Ikram-e-Khuda, Khatun S, Reza K J and Fakir Rahman Md M 2013 Improved Debye model for experimental approximation of human breast tissue properties at 6 GHz ultra-wideband centre frequency *Int. J. Eng. Technol.* **5** 4708–17

[2] Schneider J B 2010 *Understanding the Finite-Difference Time-Domain Method* 33–08 www.eecs.wsu.edu/schneidj/ufdtd

[3] Gedney S D 1996 An anisotropic perfectly matched layer-absorbing medium for the truncation of FDTD lattices *IEEE Trans. Antennas Propag.* **44** 1630–9

[4] Computational Electromagnetic Lecture 9, available at http://emlab.utep.edu/ee5390cem/Lecture9–PerfectlyMatchedLayer.pdf, accessed January 2015

www.ingramcontent.com/pod-product-compliance
Ingram Content Group UK Ltd.
Pitfield, Milton Keynes, MK11 3LW, UK
UKHW051857100926
8556IPUK00005B/674

9 780750 325905